AN APPLIED VISUAL SOCIOLOGY: PICTURING HARM REDUCTION

For Isabella, David and Amolwan 'Jaa' Parkin.

... social science research with an activist agenda can produce more than books alone.

An Applied Visual Sociology: Picturing Harm Reduction

STEPHEN PARKIN
University of Huddersfield, UK

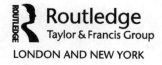

Routledge
Taylor & Francis Group

LONDON AND NEW YORK

First published 2014 by Ashgate Publishing

2 Park Square, Milton Park, Abingdon, Oxon OX14 4RN
711 Third Avenue, New York, NY 10017, USA

Routledge is an imprint of the Taylor & Francis Group, an informa business

First issued in paperback 2016

Copyright © 2014 Stephen Parkin

Stephen Parkin has asserted his right under the Copyright, Designs and Patents Act, 1988, to be identified as the author of this work.

All rights reserved. No part of this book may be reprinted or reproduced or utilised in any form or by any electronic, mechanical, or other means, now known or hereafter invented, including photocopying and recording, or in any information storage or retrieval system, without permission in writing from the publishers.

Notice:
Product or corporate names may be trademarks or registered trademarks, and are used only for identification and explanation without intent to infringe.

British Library Cataloguing in Publication Data
A catalogue record for this book is available from the British Library

The Library of Congress has cataloged the printed edition as follows:
Parkin, Stephen George.
 An applied visual sociology : picturing harm reduction / by Stephen Parkin.
    pages cm
 Includes bibliographical references and index.
 ISBN 978-1-4094-6839-4 (hardback)
1. Visual sociology. 2. Visual perception. 3. Drug abuse--Social aspects. 4. Sociology--Research. I. Title.
 HM500.P37 2014
 301.072--dc23

2013032331

ISBN 978-1-4094-6839-4 (hbk)
ISBN 978-1-138-25060-4 (pbk)

Contents

List of Boxes, Tables and Figures   *vii*
Acknowledgements   *xi*

PART I   REVIEW

Introduction   3

1   Considering an Applied Visual Sociology?   7

2   Harm Reduction and Injecting Drug Use   35

PART II   EMPIRICISM

3   Methodology and Methods   61

4   Analysis   93

5   Drug Using Environments as a 'Continuum of Descending Safety'   105

6   Drug Related Litter as Visual Data   135

7   The Management of Drug Related Litter in UK Settings   175

PART III   AN APPLIED VISUAL SOCIOLOGY

8   The Value of Applied Visual Data in 'Real World' Settings   219

9   Towards an Applied Visual Sociology   239

10   Practical Exercises in Applied Visual Sociology   263

References 277
Appendix I: A Harm Reduction Response to Media
    Reports of Needlestick Injury/Drug Related Litter 293
Appendix II: Frontline: A Photo-Ethnography of Drug-Using Environments 297
Index 299

List of Boxes, Tables and Figures

Boxes

2.1	References Relevant to 'Safer' Injecting Drug Use	50
6.1	A Harm Reduction Response to Negative Media Accounts of Drug Related Litter in Community Settings	140
7.1	A 13-step Guide to Managing Drug Related Litter	178
7.2	Key Recommendations Relating to Public Conveniences and Drug Related Litter Bins	192

Tables

3.1	Methods of Research within a Methodological Framework	75
3.2	The Collapsed Dataset	76
5.1	Frequency and Type of Injecting Environment	107
8.1	Evaluation Respondents' Occupation/Profession	227
9.1	Visual Methods as 'the Bridge' between Applied and Academic Sociology	241

Figures

2.1	Paraphernalia Associated with Injecting Drug Use	51
2.2	Needles and Syringes Used for Injecting Drug Use	52
2.3	Drug-related Litter Associated with Injecting Drug Use	53
4.1	Inside the Medically Supervised Injecting Centre, Sydney (Australia)	94
5.1	Bin Chute Room	109
5.2	Category A (Controlled) Injecting Environment (1)	121
5.3	Category A (Controlled) Injecting Environment (2)	122
5.4	Category A (Controlled) Injecting Environment (3)	123

5.5	Category A (Controlled) Injecting Environment (4)	124
5.6	Category A (Controlled) Injecting Environment (5)	125
5.7	Category B (Semi-Controlled) Injecting Environments (1)	126
5.8	Category B (Semi-Controlled) Injecting Environments (2)	126
5.9	Category B (Semi-Controlled) Injecting Environments (3)	127
5.10	Category B (Semi-Controlled) Injecting Environments (4)	128
5.11	Category B (Semi-Controlled) Injecting Environments (5)	129
5.12	Category C (Uncontrolled) Injecting Environments (1)	130
5.13	Category C (Uncontrolled) Injecting Environments (2)	130
5.14	Category C (Uncontrolled) Injecting Environments (3)	131
5.15	Category C (Uncontrolled) Injecting Environments (4)	132
5.16	Category C (Uncontrolled) Injecting Environments (5)	133
6.1	Harmless Drug Related Litter (1)	146
6.2	Harmless Drug Related Litter (2)	146
6.3	Harmful Drug Related Litter (3)	148
6.4	Harmful Drug Related Litter (4)	149
6.5	Harmful Drug Related Litter (5)	149
6.6	Harmful Drug Related Litter (6)	150
6.7	Harmful Drug Related Litter (7)	150
6.8	Harmful Drug Related Litter (8)	151
6.9	Massed Harm (1)	153
6.10	Massed Harm (2)	154
6.11	Hidden Harm (1)	156
6.12	Hidden Harm (2)	156
6.13	Hidden Harm (3)	157
6.14	'Snapping and Dropping' (1)	160
6.15	'Snapping and Dropping' (2)	161
6.16	Facilitative Space (1)	163
6.17	Facilitative Space (2)	164
6.18	Facilitative Space (3)	165
6.19	Facilitative Space (4)	166
6.20	Facilitative Space (5)	167
6.21	Facilitative Space (6)	168
6.22	Shaping Space (7)	169
6.23	Shaping Space (8)	170
7.1	Protective Equipment (1)	181
7.2	Protective Equipment (1)	181
7.3	Semi-Formal Drug Related Litter Collection	184
7.4	Drug Related Litter Bins in Public Place (1)	193
7.5	Drug Related Litter Bins in Public Place (2)	194
7.6	Drug Related Litter Bins in Public Place (3)	195
7.7	Drug Related Litter Bins in Public Place (4)	196

7.8	Drug Related Litter Bins in Public Place (5)	197
7.9	'Gold Standard' Public Toilet/Drug Related Litter Bin Design (1)	198
7.10	'Gold Standard' Public Toilet/Drug Related Litter Bin Design (2)	200
7.11	'Gold Standard' Public Toilet/Drug Related Litter Bin Design (3)	200
7.12	'Gold Standard' Public Toilet/Drug Related Litter Bin Design (4)	201
7.13	'Gold Standard' Public Toilet/Drug Related Litter Bin Design (5)	202
7.14	'Gold Standard' Public Toilet/Drug Related Litter Bin Design (6)	203
7.15	'Gold Standard' Public Toilet/Drug Related Litter Bin Design (7)	204
7.16	'Gold Standard' Public Toilet/Drug Related Litter Bin Design (8)	204
7.17	'Gold Standard' Public Toilet/Drug Related Litter Bin Design (9)	205
7.18	Ambiguous Signage	212
7.19	'Hiding Places' (1)	213
7.20	'Hiding Places' (2)	213
7.21	'Hiding Places' (3)	214
10.1	Gum and Butt Bin	270
10.2	Colliding Interventions	272

Acknowledgements

The views, opinions and academic interpretations expressed in this book are those of the author. These views, opinions and interpretations should not necessarily be associated with any previous body associated with the research described in this text. This includes the relevant research funders, commissioners and the relevant academic institutions (and colleagues) to which the author has been attached during all research and the writing of this book. This disclaimer also extends to all statutory, non-statutory and third sector bodies (and all associated employees, clients, service users) that contributed to the research during 2006–2011. Any technical or factual error made in this text is therefore the responsibility of the author and fault lies with none of the above.

The author acknowledges the Economic and Social Research Council (of Great Britain) and Plymouth Drug and Alcohol Action Team (Devon) for providing funding and financial support as part of a Collaborative Award in Science Engineering (CASE) studentship towards doctoral research (2006–2009). Similarly, the author acknowledges the support of Barking and Dagenham Drug and Alcohol Action Team and Southend-on-Sea Drug and Alcohol Action Team for the commission of research during the period 2010–2011. These latter studies were commissioned as part of the Public Injecting Rapid Appraisal Service (PIRAS) initiative under the direction of Professor Ross Comber at the Drug and Alcohol Research Unit (Plymouth University).

The author acknowledges the permission granted by all Drug and Alcohol Action Teams involved in this study to reuse the data collected for this academic text. The author is particularly thankful to Messrs Gary Wallace, Jaye Foster and Glyn Halksworth for their support and enthusiasm for this combined project as well as for the technical/local advice and assistance each individual provided during the relevant periods of fieldwork.

The author acknowledges the contributions of all individuals and organisations that agreed to participate in this study. This includes that of the 169 frontline service personnel (often employed in challenging working conditions) and the 71 injecting drug users (often reporting challenging living experiences) who agreed to be interviewed during the period 2006–2011. This acknowledgement extends to all the relevant harm reduction services (and associated personnel) that accommodated the author in various roles and settings throughout the same period. It is a cliché, but without this collective assistance, this book simply would not have happened.

The author would also like to acknowledge the support and enthusiasm expressed by all relevant individuals employed at Ashgate Publishing for this project – and its companion text, *Habitus and Drug Using Environments* (2013). In particular, the author remains indebted to the assistance provided by Neil Jordan and Philip Stirups throughout the production and publication of both texts.

Finally, on a more personal level, I thank Isabella, David and Jaa Parkin for their unwavering patience, support and understanding throughout the writing of both books.

PART I
Review

Introduction

Location: A British University
Event: Inter-departmental Research Seminar
Year: 2012

The researcher concluded their presentation, stood back and surveyed the audience with a smile that emanated self-satisfaction and confident self-assurance. The presentation on men's experience of degenerative disease had been made verbally and visually explicit and subsequently considered for academic discussion. The researcher stood in silence for a few moments before speaking, further emphasising the funereal hush that had permeated the seminar room. (The power of video; the shock and awe of suffering made portable and brought into the lives of the unaffected via digital technology). As the researcher closed down the online video-recorded interviews, featuring desperately unhappy and mentally scarred individuals, voices audibly shaken and stirred began to ripple around the room, breaking the silent reverie and dark contemplation that had descended.

Discussion followed. An audience (united in grief) voiced sympathy and support for those 'unfortunate' research participants in the videos; men who were 'clearly suffering' from illness, so obviously 'despairing' in their need and 'visibly affected' by the negative health experiences, 'social exclusion' and 'loneliness' they had endured. More theorisation followed. 'Can these experiences be compared to those of women and a feminist perspective? More debate. The re-contextualisation of masculinity, femininity and transgendered individuals in a society morphed by changing gender roles. Descartes' construct of dualism and the never ending battle between mind and body ... and then ...

A single voice: Can you explain what you think your use of video images – of these men's physical and mental suffering – adds to your study?

The researcher's reply: Using video adds extra context to the research interview, you can see the distress in the men's faces. You can also learn a little more about class. About social class. You see this in the clothes they are wearing, the furniture in their house and the type of accent they have. Americans like to hear the different British accents ...

A single voice: Excuse me?! *Class*? Why is *any of what you just said relevant*? Could you not have used soundfiles instead of video to avoid identifying the men with video? I don't understand why you need to include their image on video. I don't understand what these visual data add to the research findings.

A researcher supporter: But don't you see? If I was sick with this illness and I wanted to go online and find out more, I could possibly relate to these men's experiences.

A single voice: Seriously? But what about the Hawthorne Effect? How did you address this – or did you think it was something that you even had to address? (A blank expression falls on the researcher's face). You know, when you place a camera in front of someone, their behaviour, their performance can change ...

The researcher: The interview was not a performance and the responses would be the same if we had only used audio-recorders ...

A single voice: (*Sighs*) ... (*And lost for words*)

The above vignette, based on actual events, *is why this book had to be written*. Indeed, the above event also explains why this book *has been* written. Visual methods in the social sciences are undoubtedly *à la mode* in the early 21st century and the above event perhaps underscores the way in which visual data and associated images *should not* be used for research purposes.

As a visual sociologist involved in the field of public health, this author found the justifications for video presentations of physical suffering in the above seminar offensive and grossly insensitive. In short, the relevant researcher's use and public projection of visual images of men describing harrowing and stressful health-related experiences was completely unnecessary and used almost entirely for *illustrative* purposes. To *illustrate* the distress on the men's faces. To *illustrate* the clothes they wore during interview. To *illustrate* the furniture in the house. To '*illustrate*' their accents to an American audience! And ultimately to *illustrate* their social class. These blasé explanations of visual data, concerning sensitive topics and individual health events that have severely affected *people's lives*, are absurd, crass and pitiful validations. In this author's view, visual data used in this manner is devoid of respect for the individuals involved in the research; the methods fail to represent research participants in a dignified manner and, as discussed in the above seminar, such video material may emphasise individual guilt, shame and stigma associated with a particular health issue. Indeed, the flagrant *misuse* of visual methods and associated material in such circumstances represents the actual manifestation of 'a specialised form of pornography, a voyeuristic interest in the intimate details of other people's lives and the fetishistic cathexis of the Other' (Henley 1998, 52).

Visual methods in social science may be *en vogue*, may be relatively easy to apply and consider in almost any qualitative research project. But they should not be applied and conducted simply 'because we can'. The mass production of digital equipment should not penalise research integrity, should not forfeit the right to research anonymity and the internet does not give licence to ignore esteem, dignity and courtesy when working with *people* in research endeavours. Accordingly, in recognition of these fallacies, there is perhaps an enhanced need to conduct/ present visual research within a *humanistic* framework (relating to compassion, consideration, respect and dignity) as much as there is a need to apply ethical, methodological and theoretical principles to visual methods. Failure to observe these fundamental issues, especially within inquiries located in the field of health, may only generate a 'salacious social science illustrated' that serves to shock, titillate and/or glamourise.

... So this is why there is a need for *another* book in the ever-expanding literature on visual research within the social sciences. The purpose of this book, its *actual raison d'être*, is to advocate a reclamation of visual research from individuals promoting 'illustration' as academic inquiry. Whilst the author does not claim to have produced the quintessential text regarding the design, methods and application of visual-based inquiry, it is envisaged that this book will generate interest in a more methodologically-focused consideration of photography and video in academic and applied research, in which the implications of presenting visual data are fully understood – by researchers and research participants.

This text concerns visual-based, sociologically-driven, inquiries of injecting drug use as part of applied research that prioritises the practice and principles of harm reduction. For the reasons described above, the reader *should not* expect to find images of people injecting drugs in order to *illustrate* particular concerns. Instead, the reader will find photographs of drug-related issues that have been used as data in their own right, as data to formulate outcome and as data that complements and consolidates other qualitative information generated during fieldwork. In 'picturing harm reduction' in this way it is envisaged that the relevant photographic images within this text will emphasise Pierre Bourdieu's challenge that 'nothing *may* be photographed apart from that which *must* be photographed' (Bourdieu 1965, 23). Indeed, this is a book that aims to foster a disciplinary push towards an *applied visual sociology*.

Chapter 1
Considering an Applied Visual Sociology?

After penning such a provocative Introduction, the remainder of this book seeks to better situate the use of visual methods (photography and video) within the context of applied and academic research. In the following chapter the author aims to provide a more persuasive argument alongside a more measured account of how and why visual research may be appropriately considered within the various disciplines of the social sciences, humanities and, especially, within *applied sociological* inquiries of contemporary issues.

As noted earlier, the topics central to this book are injecting drug use, drug-using environments and harm reduction as observed in various street-based settings located throughout the south of England during 2006–2011. In addition, the associated research findings presented throughout this text were obtained from *applied* studies of street-based injecting drug use and were commissioned by various statutory bodies with a vested interest in solution-focused research (see Chapter 3). These empirical studies were, in the main, undertaken to inform local service intervention concerning public health development. As such, this book has been informed by previously conducted *visual* research that has already demonstrated *applied* impact in the settings concerned (see Chapter 9). Accordingly, this book essentialises the various ways in which field-based visual methods, (and the analyses of visual data), assisted in generating applied outcome to the issues of injecting drug use and harm reduction intervention (and by association drug-related harm) in local settings throughout the south of England.

Clarifying Intent

The aim of this book is to provide a text that suggests (not dictates) how visual research may provide both academic and applied value to social studies *per se*. The text also aims to demonstrate how visual data may assist wider qualitative methods in approaching questions regarding health concerns (in which injecting drug use may here be regarded as a suitable 'case study'). Similarly, the rationale regarding why visual methods was adopted as a means to 'visualise harm reduction' is implied (implicitly and explicitly) throughout Chapters 3–9. When considered holistically, it is envisaged that a reading of this text will subsequently clarify how visual methods (*when used in conjunction with other qualitative research techniques*) may inform wider issues (including public health, community safety and associated development) as part of an applied research agenda. Indeed, although using injecting drug use and harm reduction as the empirical platform, it is envisaged that the work described throughout this book will present a foundational template for conducting applied visual sociology in fields other than illicit substance use and that this framework may be used to influence/inform other researchers with a professional and applied interest in visual methods.

It should also be noted that this book represents the final section of the author's academic-applied triptych of projects concerning street-based injecting and harm reduction. The other components of this tripartite production are the 'companion' text to this book, (namely *Habitus and Drug Using Environments*) and a photographic exposition (titled *Frontline: A Photo-Ethnography of Drug Using Environments*). With *Habitus and Drug Using Environments* (Parkin 2013), the issues of street-based injecting and harm reduction are considered from various theoretical perspectives that totalise Pierre Bourdieu's (1977, 1984) habitus construct. For these reasons, *Habitus and Drug Using Environments* may be regarded as the 'academic-wing' of this collected work due to an emphasis upon sociological theory as a vehicle to inform and critique social policy in contemporary British society. In contrast, *this* text (*An Applied Visual Sociology: Picturing Harm Reduction*) may be regarded as the 'applied-wing' of the three projects due to an emphasis placed upon the drive to inform practitioner-based intervention in real world settings (with a specific focus upon harm reduction). *An Applied Visual Sociology: Picturing Harm Reduction* also aims to inform the academy on the way in which visually-focused research methods may be reclaimed and reinvigorated to provide a more applied focus rather than be a process for merely *illustrating* research output (Ball and Swan 1992, Silverman 2006). The academic and applied aspects of the two books are metaphorically bridged by the author's *Frontline* photography exhibition (Parkin 2012) that consists of over 100 mounted images of drug using environments that were visited in public locations throughout the south of England during 2006–2011. This latter project is completely visual in its design and delivery, due to the underlying intent to engage with audiences other than those with academic or applied interests in substance use, harm reduction and social policy. Instead, the visualisation of drug using environments (and not people) in the *Frontline* exhibition is a method of extending the impact of the research (and the harm reduction advocacy of the related research) in a way that is accessible to 'lay audiences' and commensurate with the academy's contemporary drive towards 'public engagement'.

Visual Research Methods in the Social Sciences:
An Unorthodox Literature Review

Whilst Chapter 3 provides a comprehensive account of the specific methodological design (and assorted research methods) that generated the aforementioned academic-applied triptych, the remainder of this chapter provides a more general overview of visual research *per se*. More accurately, this chapter provides a selective and succinct overview of what *should* be considered as the key themes and issues that underlie decisions to employ visual research whilst conducting sociological inquiries of people's lives. In recognising, acknowledging and applying the issues in the following outline, other researchers may subsequently avoid generating superfluous, illustrative and flippant data such as those noted in the introduction.

The following review focuses upon the suggested use of visual research as an aspect of an applied visual sociology, especially when concerning sensitive topics such as injecting drug use. Of course, this suggested application is only a tentative (albeit recommended) strategy that defines how an applied visual sociology may proceed. Similarly, such guidance may be fluid and subject to adaptation as required. However, consideration of the following issues is perhaps necessary in how researchers subsequently define their work, explain their actions and account for their findings. Furthermore, due to the applied nature of this positioning, adherence to following academic principles will more likely generate benefits to the intended target audience within real world settings than if they are ignored.

This chapter should therefore be regarded as a discerning review of the literature considered pertinent to an *applied* visual research project. It should not be regarded as a chapter that provides a comprehensive literature review of the historical development of visual research within the social sciences. This issue has been briefly addressed elsewhere by the author (Parkin 2008, Parkin and Coomber 2009b) and much more comprehensively by several distinguished and eminent visual researchers (Banks 2001, Collier and Collier 1986, Harper 1988, Pink 2007b, Prosser 1998). Nor should this chapter be regarded as an authoritative account of various issues that characterise the discourse of visual research (such as subjectivity, objectivity, image composition, photographic technique, colour/monochrome images, presentation and re-presentation). Again, these issues have been covered in detail in other works (Becker 1974, 1978, Collier and Collier 1986, Hockings 1995, Pink 2004a, b, Rose 2001). Slavishly reviewing and reproducing such material here in order to comply with academic convention would actually be surplus to requirements for this particular text.

Instead, the following chapter generalises the role of qualitative inquiry and visual research in the social sciences; underscores key methodological principles that underlie visual data collection and the interpretation of image, demonstrates the concept of 'disciplinary visuality' (Rose 2003) and introduces key ethical considerations pertaining specifically to visual sociology. Collectively these generalisations provide a suitable 'positioning' for conducting real world research for applied purposes.

Qualitative Research

Qualitative research is characterised and defined by the interpretation of naturally-occurring phenomenon (situated within specific settings) as part of an attempt to establish representations of the social meaning others hold within particular milieux (Ritchie and Lewis 2003). With qualitative sociology, such representations are typically obtained from observations, interrogations and interpretations of behaviour, beliefs, values and/or the lived-experience associated with particular social environments, in which the relationship between 'structure' and 'agency' is typically made explicit. The overall aim of qualitative research within this discipline (sociology) is therefore to unpack the way in which societies/individuals construct (and deconstruct) the social, physical and material world around them and to define what is significant and meaningful within these social realities in (Flick 2007) particularly in terms of *functionality*.

Qualitative research typically draws upon a wide range of overt techniques for generating data. These methods may include participant observation, direct observation, in-depth/focus group interviews and the use of assorted visual methods (including photography and video). Similarly, each of these methods may be serendipitously deployed as structured, semi-structured or unstructured techniques (in which decisions to adopt a particular format may best reflect the social/physical situation at a particular point in time during fieldwork). As noted by Bazeley (2007) qualitative research invariably generates voluminous amounts of data (due to the methods outlined above) and it is from these materials that on going and final analyses can occur. Analysis of qualitative data essentially aims to identify generalisations, consistencies, constants and patterns in behaviours and/or practice – and typically does not serve to accentuate specific anomalies. Although the latter may be of analytical value (in terms of 'Case Studies'), they do not necessarily reflect wider societal/social trends or shared experiences within a particular research cohort, sample or of shared values and representations within a specific setting, society, or culture (Flick 2007, Pearson, Parkin et al. 2011).

The defining and operative terms of qualitative research (of which visual research is clearly a component-part) each pertains to various methods of data manipulation: namely, 'generation of', 'gathering of', 'collection of', 'observation of' and 'analysis of'. Accordingly, the way in which data are obtained is of significance for the way in which they are interpreted and subsequently re-presented (as 'findings'). This is particularly relevant when attempting to make statements regarding *generalisations* (rather than comment upon *specific* individuals or 'Case Studies'). However, as previously noted by Guba and Lincoln (2004), *methods* of research are actually *secondary* to the more *methodological* concerns that underlie all research; namely epistemological and ontological orientations.

Guiding Paradigms

In research terms, a paradigm refers to the methodological structure used to guide and direct a particular form of academic inquiry, whether it is qualitative or quantitative in design. A research paradigm is essentially a theoretical framework from which questions and scholarship emerge, especially in relation to how constructions of reality are perceived and received. Within qualitative social science the three most dominant paradigms are termed 'positivism', 'interpretivism' (or 'constructivism') and those located under the umbrella-term of 'critical theory' (such as Marxism, neo-Marxism, feminism, post-structuralism and postmodernism). Each of these paradigms propose differing worldviews of how reality is constructed and understood; how reality may be understood and similarly inform different research methods for acquiring and extracting 'knowledge' about these perceived realities.[1]

A research paradigm therefore commences with a theoretical concept that encapsulates a particular worldview of the researcher. This paradigm is further informed by particular aspects of ontology and epistemology (as they are understood by the researcher). Simply stated, ontology is concerned with the nature of reality, the state of being and how relationships function from the perspective of, and within, a particular paradigm (whether 'positivist' etc.). Similarly, epistemology is concerned with the study of knowledge; how this is generated, acquired and applied. Epistemology therefore accounts for how people know what they claim to know and also reflects the paradigmatic worldviews attached to ontological affiliations.

In order to illustrate the construction of a methodological framework, one may consider the paradigm utilised by the author in the research described later in this book (and presented in full throughout Chapter 3). In selecting critical theory as the most appropriate paradigm for the study of street-based injecting, various ontological and epistemological traditions immediately become attached to the study. From an *ontological* perspective, critical theory prioritises the philosophical tradition of 'realism' that posits reality is a multiple, relative and independent structure that can be observed and experienced from a variety of oppositional perspectives. However, these multiple realities have also been historically constructed, influenced and shaped by society, politics, economics, ethnicity and gender that have subsequently permeated and filtered through all society in a historical and linear process (Guba and Lincoln 2004). Similarly, the concomitant *epistemology* (of critical theory) attached to this study is one that suggests knowledge is produced and shaped by the above ontological interactions (realism). For these reasons, researchers are often 'linked' to the social worlds they study in which their own values, knowledge and experiences of a given issue often influence a subjective mode of inquiry (ibid.). To illustrate, the influence of 'harm reduction' knowledge upon the author's experiences prior to this study influenced and guided the research described in this book. In this way, this study perhaps confirms that social scientists are *a part* of the societies they study – and not *apart* from the people they study (Mills 2000, Pink 2007b).

Social science researchers typically develop a methodological framework that reflects how they perceive reality and the construction of knowledge prior to commencing any fieldwork (Wagner 2001). This is because these details inform

---

1 Guber and Lincoln (2004) provide a detailed and tabular overview of the complex philosophical orientations attached to various paradigms, including those listed above. Their work is highly recommended reading for any individual who may wish to further pursue these fundamental qualities of social science research.

and direct how the topic at hand may be best studied with the most appropriate methods and types of question asked (Prosser and Schwartz 2004). In a critical theory paradigm, this methodology would primarily involve transactional, communicative research methods that incorporate researcher subjectivity and reflexivity (as part of the *critical* component) in which exposure to (and experience of) other realities is accepted as a valid means of inquiry. In following this tradition, one would anticipate that a research located within this paradigm would produce 'value-mediated' findings (Guber and Lincoln 2004, 26) that aim to reconstruct other realties from a critical-interpretative position.

At the risk of labouring this important and fundamental issue in social science research, further clarification of the above may be noted in a second (equally simplistic) illustration relating to the paradigm of positivism. For the positivist researcher, ontologically speaking, reality and human behaviour are shaped by natural laws and may be measured and tested in a manner similar to observations within the natural sciences. In this framework, reality is further regarded as a single, external and objective construct that can be rationalised and made apprehensible by controlled and equally objective research (Guber and Lincoln 2004). Similarly, positivist epistemology is one that maintains researcher and reality are mutually exclusive and exist as objective entities in their own right, in which the former can function in the latter without influence or distraction. Within this paradigm, a research methodology would almost certainly prioritise detached, quantitative methods (surveys, questionnaires, statistical measurements) and aims to provide conclusions that may be tested elsewhere on the basis of natural-science empiricism (Banks 2007).

Visual Methodologies: Function, Purpose and Rationale

A research project that incorporates a specifically *visual* methodology would therefore appear to sit more comfortably within the more constructivist-interpretivist spectrum of assorted paradigms, rather than those that emphasise objectivity and positivist detachment (Banks 2007). This relates to the naturally occurring qualitative content contained within visual data (including images, video and cultural artefacts) that is open to interpretation from various (often conflicting) viewpoints (Pink 2007b). In methodological terms, this ambiguity has been termed the multivocality of image (Rodman 2003) – or more frequently, as the polysemic content of visual data (for example, Banks 2007, Pink 2007b, Wagner 2001). As such, photographs and videos may be viewed from a number of perspectives that reflect ontological and epistemological orientation of the person viewing the visual image (or similar). This has implications for how an image is viewed and whether or not the person viewing it constructs reality as part of an objective/positivist or interpretivist/subjective paradigm (Pink 2007b, 2009).

Wagner (2001) perhaps simplifies this 'positivist-interpretivist continuum' (Prosser and Loxley 2008) in providing the following account of the overall ambiguity attached to visual data:

> The first (ambiguity) refers to how an image or artefact can and should be read – as an explicit, precise, and matter-of-fact communication or as a polysemic and ambiguous social and cultural artefact. The second ambiguity refers to how images in general can and should be used in social inquiry – as information–rich data for extending scientific investigations or as evocative artefacts for challenging ... a science too narrowly conceived. (Wagner 2001, 7)

As an illustration of the ambiguity noted above, one may consider the ways in which the visual dataset contained throughout this book may be viewed within alternative paradigms. For example, would the (positivist-oriented) 'matter-of-fact communication' of images containing blood-stained injecting equipment found in street-based settings (see Chapter 6) confirm reckless, anti-social behaviour, chaotic drug use and a need for increased policing or punitive action? Or would they provide bases for 'challenging' (via critical theory and interpretation) existing structural intervention and emphasise a drive for increased harm reduction services and amenities in settings affected by drug-related litter? Contradictory interpretations such as these have been previously explained by Bourdieu (1965, 77) who suggests that images will typically 'be judged with reference to the purpose that they fulfil for the person who looks at them'.

Accordingly, due to the challenges associated with the polysemic nature of visual images in applied settings (Parkin and Coomber 2009b) there is a need for researchers to be critically aware of the limitations of visual data (Becker 2004) whilst also be able to validate how such data reflect a particular *methodological* stance (Pink 2007b, 2009, Prosser and Schwartz 2004, Wagner 2001). In short, when working with visual data (or any data for that matter), the challenge for the social scientist when conducting applied research is to 'make sense of the interface between people and the image taken' (Pole 2004, 4) in any attempt to explain a particular reality, experience or knowledge-base – especially in terms of intervention.

As noted by several researchers (Banks 2007, Pink 2009, Prosser and Loxley 2008) the above challenge is typically addressed by the design and application of approaches that aim to reflect a methodological position. These approaches generally involve visual data collection that is researcher-generated, respondent-generated or involves the visual analysis of primary/secondary sources for contemporary comment.

Researcher Generated Visual Data

Primary qualitative research in the social sciences unavoidably involves an individual (or collective) accessing a particular field to generate data for analysis.

In visual studies of given phenomena this may involve the researcher spending time within a specific setting with particular people photographing and/or video-recording the immediate social, physical and material world as part of a wider qualitative inquiry. Therefore, the use of visual data in any subsequent research publication may be regarded as 'visual quotes' (Prosser and Schwartz 2004, 336) that visually articulate a particular issue or concern within the relevant text. In this way, visual data may be compared to the 'verbatim quotes' (extracted from interview transcripts) generated by qualitative social scientists as well as to 'numerical quotes' obtained from the quantitative analysis of statistical data.

The gathering of visual data from a field of enquiry may be regarded as a component of 'ethnographic' research (whether or not this involves limited stays of a few hours or extended periods covering several weeks, months and/or years) in which the influence of anthropological research may also be evident within this chosen terminology. Indeed, as noted by social anthropologist Sarah Pink (2007b), ethnography is not only a method of research but is also a term she uses to define a particular methodology. Accordingly, within Pink's (2007b) definition of ethnography, the overall rationale and justification for including researcher generated visual data from a particular field is made logical and coherent. Namely:

> (ethnography is) an approach to experiencing, interpreting and representing culture and society that informs and is informed by sets of different disciplinary agendas and theoretical principles. .... . *ethnography is a process of creating and representing knowledge (about society, culture and individuals) that is based on ethnographers' own experiences.* (Pink 2007b, 22 emphasis (of methodology) added)

When considering Pink's methodological definition of ethnography, it is perhaps a simple task to translate the use of cameras and video-recorders as devices that facilitate the visual and verbal recording of the above representations of other realties. Indeed, as demonstrated by Pink's own varied and multiple (anthropological) studies of disparate issues (such as housework, bullfighting and gardening), visual ethnography offers methodological innovation and thicker description of other experiences in a manner that significantly magnifies and enriches traditional observational studies of cultural/societal practices (Pink 2004a, 2007a, 2007b, 2008). Furthermore, Pink (2009) demonstrates how the process of conducting visual ethnography (and the practice of data generation) involves a physical, sensory, and spatial appreciation of materiality, sensoriality, sociality and physicality within the places, and of the people, that the visual researcher encounters during fieldwork. Elsewhere, Pink (2007b, 2008, 2011) also discusses 'doing' visual research methods as the embodiment of methodology. More specifically, when conducting visual methods in the field, associated actions become embodied practice (whether relating to walking, gardening and/or household chores) and – when coupled with reflexive analysis of those methods – provide physical and visual representations of place-making and knowledge construction within those particular settings. As such, the *physical* process of visually recording *social* experiences may assist in apprehending in the construction of 'place' especially in regard to the more mundane settings/events of everyday life.

For others, visual ethnography is a methodology and a method for conducting more critical inquiry of more problematic experiences. Schostak and Schostak (2008, 63) for example, regard ethnography as a process for unpacking the 'fault lines, the broken tracks, the derailments' of individual despair, dissatisfaction and social injustice associated with structural change and shifting communities. An exemplary visual ethnography of this variety may be noted in Bourgouis and Schonberg's (2009) *Righteous Dopefiend* that documents the lives and experiences of a cohort of homeless/roofless street injectors resident in 'encampments' located throughout San Francisco (USA). However, this work does not aim to merely provide a visiting snapshot of these lived-experiences, as it chronicles over a decade of sustained ethnographic inquiry by the authors (and various associates; described as the 'ethnographic team'). Furthermore, this ethnographic record is both textual and visual, in which words and pictures are used to articulate a theory of 'lumpen abuse' in regard to the way in which 'structurally imposed everyday suffering generates violent and destructive subjectivities' (ibid., 19). The inclusion of over 70 monochrome images throughout *Righteous Dopefiend* not only contribute to more nuanced depictions of the physicality of injecting drug use, but purposely aim to reflect constructions of power and powerlessness in advanced economies as well as (perhaps more fundamentally) portray the 'agony and the ecstasy of surviving on the street as a heroin injector' (ibid., 5).

In this study, all visual data were generated by the author. However as will be made apparent in Chapter 3, some aspects of this generation involved a collaborative process with research respondents (injecting drug users and frontline service personnel). Although all visual data were physically collected by the author, the process of how environmental setting influenced injecting episodes and affected employment procedures involved directional input and field-based teamwork with research participants. This process is explained in detail at a later point. However, in methodological terms, this researcher-led collaborative process provided opportunities for the author to experience drug using environments in a manner similar to those that directly informed the study (frontline service personnel and injecting drug users). As such, the application of visual methods provided opportunities for the author to conduct ethnographic 'observant-participation' (Wacquant 2004, 2005) as a means to fully appreciate and understand the various environments affected by injecting drug use from a variety of countering-perspectives. Observant-participation (as opposed to participant-observation) is an embodied learning process that has previously been utilised in studies of combat sports (Wacquant 2004, Crossley 2007). These techniques permitted the relevant researchers to gain first-hand experience and appreciation of practice associated with particular social worlds via their embodied physical and actual engagement with the people and places concerned. Observant-participation was included in this study as a method to understand the physical and social construction of street-based injecting environments.

Respondent Generated Visual Data (Photo-elicitation)

A second methodological approach towards constructing the meaning and significance of other realties involves visual data generated by respondents (or participants) within a given research project. In such studies, individuals are typically issued with disposable cameras and invited to record images of meaningful events, important environments and/or significant others associated with a given topic of inquiry. The images generated are then typically used as the bases of discussion in a research interview in which the photographs are explained in connection to the wider inquiry. This process is thus a method of extracting other realities in a communicative manner in which visually-informed experience is shared, clarified and verbalised to the researcher. For these reasons, this process is often termed 'photo-elicitation' (Collier and Collier 1986, Pink 2007b), as visual images of personal and intimate events become a mechanism for apprehending how other social worlds (and experiences) may be constructed and/or negotiated.

Photo-elicitation is a participatory process that has gained wide acceptance throughout the social sciences (Prosser and Loxley 2008). The aim of this approach, as noted by Banks (2007), is essentially to document personal connections to a particular social phenomenon from the privileged position of 'insider' (as a member of the community/setting involved). Similarly, Pink (2009) defines photo-elicitation techniques as involving the intersecting of (researcher-respondent) subjectivities towards renewed *understanding* of the 'other'. Pink further contends that photo-elicitation techniques can evoke memories and meaning that may otherwise have been omitted from the conventional research interview and can therefore assist in the *accessibility* to other social worlds. Collier and Collier (1986) however state that such strategies may also be a useful strategy for improving verbalisations in the unnatural situation established by the atypical (somewhat artificial) interaction that typifies the 'research interview'. Cumulatively, these benefits of photo-elicitation are consistent with the bridging of 'critical distance' (Prosser and Schwartz 2004, 339) that may exist between researcher and respondent. More specifically, photo-elicitation may reduce the gulf that often exists between the 'emic' (insider/member) world of the respondent and the 'etic' (outsider/non-member) world of the academic researcher. Banks (2007) stresses that this process of interaction also bridges different social statuses that may similarly exist between the researcher and the respondent (for example, such as that which may exist between adults and children).

For each of the aforementioned reasons, this visual technique has been widely used in studies that attempt to understand and access the socio-physical experiences of children and young people in a multitude of international settings. For example, Young and Barrett (2001) provide an account of how photo-elicitation was employed amongst street-involved youth located in Kampala (Uganda) and how the method constructed knowledge of the ways in which young people developed a particular survival strategy within hostile urban environments. Young and Barrett conclude that the visual component of their study greatly reduced an 'authoritarian' (ibid., 151) influence on data collection and facilitated a process in which children took control of data generation. In addition, the visual data subsequently permitted access to socio-spatial settings and behaviours that are normally hidden from the gaze of academics – especially those based in Western settings that may be geographically (and culturally) removed from 'ground-zero'.

Similarly, Walker et al. (2011) adopted this particular approach amongst pre-adolescent children involved in the criminal justice system in a variety of UK settings. This project focused upon the efficacy of 'family group conferences' as a means of empowering families and seeking appropriate restitution for children's participation in law-breaking activity and/or anti-social behaviour within community settings. As part of this particular participatory research process, children from 38 families were given disposable cameras and encouraged to photograph those aspects of their daily lives that were considered important and significant (post-intervention). Of the 19 cameras that were returned, Walker et al. comment that the images provided 'additional insight' (2011, 238) into the children's lives that assisted with a wider evaluation of family group conferences in the field of 'youth justice'. Furthermore, and perhaps most significantly, Walker et al. (ibid.) state that the images generated by young people also provided a useful strategy for informing and directing rapport (between child and adult) and the types of questions asked by (adults) during various stages of interviewing. That is, the photographs were believed to diminish the critical distance between the emic and etic worlds of young people and adult researchers respectively.

In these two examples of photo-elicitation – each located in two disparate geographical and economic locations – the shared methodological imperative seeks to unpack the assorted lived-experiences and social realities of children and young people involved in challenging circumstances. In utilising visual images generated by participatory research as a means of making rationalised abstractions of other worlds, researchers are able to provide a 'voice' to those that are not normally articulated in the 'adult' world. For these reasons this form of data generation is often termed 'photovoice'.[2] Photovoice is a popular communicative process used to support advocacy in action research projects concerning marginalised, vulnerable and disadvantaged individuals/communities. Furthermore, this form of visual research is often associated with addressing health inequalities and improving access to health-care for those most affected by exclusion and marginalisation (for example, see Bukowski and Buetow 2011, Pain 2012, Wang 1999).

In this study, photo-elicitation was *not* a chosen technique adopted by the author to reflect the social realities of street-based injecting. However, as will be noted in Chapter 3, elements of the method were adopted and appropriated as a

---

2   See http://www.photovoice.org (accessed: 11 July 2013)

means of informing interview schedules and recreating lived-experiences of drug-injecting episodes in street-based settings. Nevertheless, in this study, no cameras were issued to any research respondent for the purposes of generating data and no visual data generated by the author were shown to, or shared with, respondents/participants during fieldwork.

Visual Analysis of Secondary Sources

Whereas the two preceding accounts of visual data generation may be best regarded as exemplars of interpretivist paradigms, the following section may be better understood as constituent of a more positivist methodology. More specifically, in regard to some aspects of the gathering and analysis of primary and/or secondary sources[3] similarities may be drawn with the positivist tradition of attempting to quantify the natural world. This is particularly apparent when considering processes attached to the *content analysis* of image-based materials. However, and to paraphrase Banks (2007), content analysis is in itself an enormous disciplinary topic that cannot be adequately condensed here into several short paragraphs that provide adequate representation.[4]

Nevertheless, to illustrate how content analysis may be applied to visual studies of cultural phenomena in attempts to make conclusive statements of the social world, one may refer to Robinson's (1976) visual study of men's facial hair and a similar inquiry of conditions noted within 'hospital' settings during the nineteenth century by Dowdall and Golden (1989). Both of these studies involved a retrospective analysis of photographs from which the respective authors were able to draw conclusions pertaining to particular cultural conditions as a result of quantifying visual consistencies and shared features observed within the relevant datasets. For example, Robinson (1976) conducted a content analysis of photographs published in the *Illustrated London News* during a 130-year period (1842–1972) in order to provide sociological comment on the frequency, style and appearance of men's facial hair in relation to fashion trends throughout various generations. One of the most remarkable conclusions from this study is that the length and style of beards (not moustaches) correlates with the length and style of women's skirts and dresses during different periods of history. From these findings, Robinson suggests that shared behavioural influences can have

---

3   In this context, primary sources include documents, images and artefacts gathered whilst in the field by the researcher but not actually recorded or produced by that researcher. Secondary sources include photographs, posters, images that have produced by other people and are subject to analysis by a researcher at a later date and by a researcher not responsible for their production.

4   Accordingly, this section serves only to introduce the analytical concept (in relation to visual research) to the readership. For more nuanced and in-depth considerations of content analysis see Ball and Smith (1992), Russell (2010) and Saldana (2009).

an impact upon culture (fashion); that similarities in trends operate in cultural 'waves' (that are not gender specific) and that there are historical and cultural associations between short skirts and short beards, and similarly, between longer skirts and longer beards. However, the positivist tradition here undoubtedly lies in the somewhat deterministic nature of these findings, in which no association or interpretation regarding the influence of culture (such as religion or faith) upon men's facial hair decisions is made apparent (Banks 2007).

A similar process may be noted in the content analysis conducted by Dowdall and Golden (1989) in their study of over 300 images taken within a 'mental institution' (namely, the Buffalo State Asylum for the Insane) (*sic*) during the late-nineteenth century (1880–90). This study involved multi-staged analyses of images as part of a contribution to the development of historical sociological inquiries of health care provision. More specifically, their analysis involved a visually-focused '-appraisal' (comparing images to historical texts associated with the 'asylum'); '-inquiry' (identifying themes within the visual dataset) and '-interpretation' (establishing judgements on thematic concordance). As a result of this process, Dowdall and Golden identified 'compelled activity' and 'enforced idleness' amongst 'residents' that were noted within the images and conclude that these were conditions and features of the disciplinary regime within the setting. From a *methodological* perspective however this study appears to be situated at a less fixed point on the positivist-interpretivist continuum described by Prosser and Loxley (2008). Instead this study appears to be a genuine attempt at combining positivist quantification with constructivist interpretation in regard to understanding mental health-care provision in one particular setting over one century ago.

In this study of street-based injecting drug use, content analysis of injecting environments visually recorded by the author *did* take place. However, this did not involve the objective enumeration of items within photographic images that typify content analysis *per se*. Instead, and as will be noted in Chapters 4–8, a methodological flexibility occurred that involved a more epistemological *quantification* (that prioritised the content analysis of physical features pertaining to socio-spatial, drug-related harm reduction/production) alongside ontological *interpretation* (critical realism and the relationship between structure/agency) of over 400 environments that were affected by regular episodes of street-based injecting drug use.

Researcher vs. Respondent-Generated Visual Data

In an effort to encapsulate the above accounts of how and why visual data may be generated by different people for different academic and applied purposes, one may refer to Marcus Banks' (2007) succinctly adroit statement on this matter. According to Banks, researcher generated data attempt to document ways of life and other experiences that are external to the life of that social researcher. In this way, visual data represent 'images to study society' (Banks 2007, 7). Conversely, data generated by research respondents and/or participants (or photographs that exist as secondary source materials) involve attempts to make a direct connection to a specific socio-cultural milieu from which the researcher is naturally *ex*cluded. In this way data analysis by the researcher becomes a 'sociological study of images' (ibid.).

In this study, although all data were physically generated by the researcher, some collaborative work with research respondents and participants did take place. For example, frontline service personnel provided access to a range of street-based injecting environments and provided advice and direction on how to best frame/compose images from the perspective of their employment (whether toilet attendant, security guard or other). Similarly, when visiting these settings with injecting drug users, the latter provided similar advice on how spatial appropriation took place and assisted in advising and directing how video could record their embodied experiences (without their presence on film). Accordingly, environmentally-situated experiences relating to the processes, practices and outcomes of street-based *injecting drug use* were obtained from etic (frontline service personnel 'looking in') and emic (injecting drug users 'looking out') perspectives. In this regard, this study may be defined as an example of the 'postmodern turn' (Banks 2007, 7) due to the combined generation of data by the researcher and relevant respondents as a suitable methodological design for theoretically and politically de-constructing 'otherness, difference and heterogeneity' (Best and Kellner 1997, 14) whilst simultaneously prioritising an epistemological position of harm reduction throughout.

Disciplinary Visuality ...

One aspect of visual research that appears to receive scarcely any attention (outside of anthropology) is an account of how particular academic disciplines claim to 'see the world' (and how *visual* research assists in this process). As Oldrup and Carstensen (2012) note, different academic disciplines within the social sciences (whether sociology, anthropology, geography, psychology etc.) have different ways of 'shaping how we see, what we see and what is (made) visible' (ibid., 224). This divergence has been termed 'disciplinary visuality' by Gillian Rose (2003) and the term provides a useful hermeneutic device when considering *applied* visual research (in relation to whatever discipline it may be grounded) and how the visual may assist with 'interpreting' the social world around us. That is, when considering visual research within a methodological design, the researcher should be conscious of how the relevant applied methods and resulting data may further inform (or advance) the ways in which a particular discipline (or relevant sub-discipline) constructs, de-constructs and/or understands the society, culture, or milieu concerned. For example, in the context of this study, disciplinary visuality relates to how this *applied* research may meaningfully inform (public health) intervention whilst simultaneously advance the discipline of sociology (and the sub-discipline of public health sociology). In short, disciplinary visuality relates to an appreciation and understanding of how the 'visual' may *provide new knowledge that is specific to particular academic disciplines.*

... in Geography

Rose (2003) appears to view the disciplinary visuality of geography as somewhat restricted despite the fact that the subject is characterised by visual representations from the physical and human world. Furthermore, Rose suggests that constructions of the 'visual' within this particular discipline are currently under-theorised from a methodological perspective, inferring detriment and loss to geography *per se*. In this regard, Oldrup and Carstensen (2012) appear in agreement with Rose and stress that geography's disciplinary visuality is dominated by the single concern of representation, that in turn 'affects the discipline's understanding of how things are made seeable and what visual methods are' (ibid., 224).

Psychology

Similar comments have been noted in how visuality is constructed within the discipline of psychology. For example, Paula Reavey (2011) similarly infers that visual research in qualitative psychology has failed to keep pace with anthropology and sociology in developing sophisticated visual methodologies over the last three decades. Instead, she comments that psychology has tended to focus upon images only as a communicative mechanism, (especially in research concerning young children), whilst also noting that communication is not restricted to language and cognition. For these reasons Reavey appears to confirm the view that the visual (within psychology) 'has traditionally been given the status of a naïve or more simplistic form of communication' (2011, xxvii). These views are confirmed in the same volume, in which Carla Willig (2011, i) states that until recently there has been 'a noticeable lack of accommodation of 'the visual' in contemporary qualitative psychology' (ibid.). With these limitations in mind, it should be noted that the vignette described in the Introduction of this book occurred within a psychology seminar in the relevant anonymous university setting (and perhaps assists in confirmation of the naïve and under-developed disciplinary visuality suggested above).

Anthropology

The disciplinary visuality of anthropology has been firmly established throughout the development of the subject since its 'origins' in the late nineteenth century (Hockings 1995, Parkin and Coomber 2009b). Indeed, the 'visual' possibly defines all aspects of archaeological, biological, evolutionary and social anthropology due to the discipline's central concerns in providing representations of culture, relationships and shared/individual cultural practice (Pink 2007b). Although the development of visual anthropology has been characterised by criticism and counter-criticism (see Pink 2007a, b) it is perhaps a fair assumption to note that Margaret Mead's (1995) concerns of a visual medium lost in a 'discipline of words' would now appear completely redundant. Instead, contemporary anthropology embraces visual media in which many researchers adhere to one of anthropology's original methodological dictates that the interplay of text and image should serve to emphasise 'the native's point of view, his relation to life, to realise *his* vision of *his* world' (Malinowski 1922, 25, original emphasis, [sic]).

As an illustration of the value brought to anthropology by disciplinary visuality one may refer to the exemplary and pioneering work conducted by Bateson and Mead (1942) in their photographic analysis of *Balinese Character*. Whilst at first sight this may appear as a collection of images recorded in a tribal setting or as an academic's fieldwork travelogue (Ball and Swan 1992), the accompanying text validates the visual component as a rigorous academic enterprise. More poignantly *Balinese Character* provides an account that explains how culture shapes individual and collective personality (Ball and Swan 1992, Becker 1996). This is achieved with visual and textual reference to a wide range of practice observed by Bateson and Mead, including Balinese constructions of the mundane (childcare, nurturing, toiletry), and Balinese constructions of the sacred (attitudes and values pertaining to witchcraft, fear and ceremonial rites).

In complete contrast, the more contemporaneous visual work by Bourgois and Schonberg (2009) is equally comparable to Malinowski's directive concerning the use of image and explanatory (interpretative) text. Bourgois and Schonberg are conscious that many of the images contained within *Righteous Dopefiend* may inadvertently perpetuate pejorative stereotypes of street-injectors or provide a form of 'voyeuristic pornography' (ibid., 9). Nevertheless, they further stress that all images should be viewed and considered in association with the various fieldnote attachments (that is, text) in which the images are embedded as a means to fully appreciate the social situations portrayed. Accordingly, Bourgois and Schonberg's account presents a master class in visual ethnography and a tome that is consistent with anthropological method and methodology. In addition, the book's overall disciplinary visuality deepens ethnographic understanding of social suffering in contemporary constructions of capitalist society (in the USA).

... And Sociology

The development of visual sociology has been a slow and laboured process and did not really gather pace until the 1960s when the discipline began to incorporate new technologies within studies of large-scale political and cultural change during that era (Becker 1974, 1996). Prior to that period, attempts at utilising the visual within the discipline were largely regarded as 'unscientific' and typically disconnected from sociology's reformist agenda (Becker 1974,

Parkin 2008). However, at the time of writing (2013) visual sociology enjoys a burgeoning and ever-expanding status within the social sciences. Indeed, this may be evidenced by the formation of interest groups such as the Visual Sociology Study Group of the British Sociological Association, the bi-annual International Visual Methods Conference and the ever-expanding literature and journals (such as *Visual Methodologies*, *Visual Sociology* and *Visual Studies*) dedicated to academic accounts of visual research.

Nevertheless, despite this rapid expansion, the criticisms outlined by Ball and Smith (1992) relating to the 'visual' in sociology remain valid over two decades after they were initially raised. Namely, photographic materials typically remain 'under-analysed, generally serving as little more than illustrative devices' (Ball and Smith 1992, 12). Within those studies that prioritise data as illustration, it could be argued that the disciplinary visuality of sociology has been overlooked in preference for work that may be comparable to a form of academic reportage or sociological-journalism (Becker 1996).

The author of this book contends that sociologists need to be more definitive and conclusive in any visual research agenda. Furthermore, sociology as a discipline should seek to emulate the ways in which photography and video are employed within anthropology as methods of reflecting the defining features of that academic discipline. Whereas anthropology is characteristically concerned with representation, experience and construction at a *cultural* level, sociology is more defined by an assortment of various social theories that seek to explain how society 'functions' and apprehend the organisation of human behaviour. Sociology is further concerned with theoretical inquiries of the inter-relationship between 'structure' (institutions, policy and 'power') and 'agency' (human actions and responses shaped by relationships with people and structure) at a *societal* level. That is, sociological precepts are essentially founded upon how aspects of and within society operate as a self-sustaining construct including the ways in which relationships may be patterned by social and institutionalised regularisation (Hughes 1971).

A disciplinary visuality of sociology would therefore aim to capture these academic precepts within all scholarly output and communication whilst also attempt to remain true to the original reformist character of the discipline (as determined by 'founding fathers' such as Emile Durkheim, Karl Marx, Max Weber etc.). As an illustration, Becker (1974, 13) states that the generation of the sociological photograph should be a reflexive, on-going process towards 'both confirming and disconfirming evidence relevant to … provisional ideas' – all of which are formulated in response to the methodological and theoretical frameworks attached to a particular line of inquiry. As a further aid, and in referencing the sociological precepts advocated by Hughes (1971), Becker provides a range of themes that would suitably characterise and guide the proposed disciplinary visuality of sociology. For example, visual data would aim to provide theoretically informed critiques of social role, cultural mores and expectations, in addition to similar constructs of conduct, cohesion, conflict, misconduct, resolution and restitution. The academic leitmotifs of sociology are therefore the guiding lights of its disciplinary visuality.

Whereas sociology originally developed from an interest in social reform and social justice, related research only genuinely becomes *applied* when it is conducted for external bodies with an actual agenda committed to social change. In its purist form, the author's advocacy of an applied visual sociology is therefore aligned to each of the aforementioned academic traditions in which disciplinary visuality is also focused specifically upon 'change'; challenging inequality, promoting social justice and preventing the abuse of power as part of a demonstration of Pierre Bourdieu's model of an 'activist science' (Wacquant 2008, 262).

As will be made more explicit in later chapters, an ethnographic methodology and ethnographic method attached to this research were integral to the disciplinary visuality of this study of street-based injecting drug use. Similarly, photographic engagement within environments affected by injecting episodes and physical attachment to the main protagonists within these places served to demonstrate that:

> the closer one gets to the actual world of the addict [*sic*] as *he* experiences it (as opposed to the worlds of institutions), the more rational and reasonable *his* behaviour becomes, and the more inappropriate the sick, retreatist, and maladaptive explanations of *most professionals become*. (Waldorf and Reinarman 1975, 48 emphasis added)

As well as demonstrating compatibility with Malinowski's vision of ethnographic research, the disciplinary visuality of this study is consistent with generating data that would challenge mainstream opinion of street-based injecting drug use and provide evidence to advocate meaningful (harm reduction) intervention. These particular goals are implied in this book's subtitle: as the relevant dataset essentialised and totalised 'picturing harm reduction' (as both a process and as an ideal).

Polysemicity and Interpretation of the Ethnographic Photograph

As noted throughout this chapter thus far, visual data may prove problematic for any intended interpretation. This is due to the polysemic and ambiguous qualities that can accompany almost any image (whether moving or still). These dilemmas of mixed-meaning have been described as reflecting various 'sites' (Rose 2001) in the construction of visual data involving 'production' 'image' and 'audiencing' – in which disputes regarding interpretation typically relate to various (mis) understandings of these particular methodological constructs (ibid.). Accordingly, in any study of social phenomena there is a need for the relevant researcher(s) to validate and explicate the methodological qualities attached to any visual data so that image and meaning are concordant with the intended and specified interpretation of the research(er(s)).

Several scholars (Banks 2007, Ball and Swan 1992, Pink 2007b, Pole 2004, Prosser and Schwarz 2004, Schembri and Boyle 2011, Schwarz 1997) have commented that visual data obtained from fieldwork primarily represents a visual record that authenticates a particular period of data generation. Similarly, each have in varying degrees agreed with the principle that the deployment of visual research (and related data) typically provides *ethnographic access* to particular people and places. This ethnographic access subsequently attempts to demonstrate and explain how social relationships may be constructed, defined, experienced and made significant by particular socio-spatial interaction and overlap. However, beyond the immediate research environment and interpretative agenda, the relevant data may be equally misread and/or inadvertently re-constructed towards alternative (potentially antithetical) meanings and agendas. Accordingly, in order to reduce these misrepresentations, the broadcasting and/or publication of visual data should include some 'expository discourse' (Bal 1996, cited in Prosser and Schwarz 2004) which has clear parallels with the explanatory (textual) accompaniments described above associated with 'disciplinary visuality'.

More specifically, there is a fundamental necessity for the visual researcher to be able to demonstrate and articulate the 'site of production' (Rose 2001, 20) concerning the overall 'context' and the contextualisation of image (Becker 1974). That is, explanations should prioritise how and why images are constructed during data generation, and similarly how and why they are subsequently disseminated to wider audiences following analysis. That is, in order to avoid misrepresentation, the ethnographic veracity and interpretive context of (any) data need to be made clear and evident to the audiences that view the relevant text/images.

However, the short response to the question 'what makes an image ethnographic?' is that there is actually no definitive or simplistic answer that would concretise this aspect of authenticity (Pink 2007b, 22–3). For these reasons, the inherent polysemic, amorphous and ambiguous qualities of researcher-generated images need to be contained, checked and regulated by a rigorous prioritisation of all ethnographic *context* and *interpretation* in order to confirm ethnographic and methodological credentials. Or, more simply, 'what makes a photograph ethnographic is not necessarily the intention of its production *but how it is used to inform viewers ethnographically*' (Scherer 1995, 201 emphasis added).

The polysemicity and interpretation of image as discussed above may be further understood with the assistance of two illustrations. The first provides an example of the way in which visual images may be misinterpreted and distorted to validate a particular (political) position. The second provides an exemplary demonstration of the way in which sensitive and provocative visual material may be ethnographically contextualised within a particular methodological, theoretical and interpretative framework.

When 'West' Talks About 'East'

In 2013 the author attended a bi-annual international conference that is dedicated exclusively to the issues of drug use, harm reduction and associated issues (such as policy, advocacy and intervention). In one session (consisting of four speakers from Western settings), a paper was delivered regarding the development of a network of advocacy projects dedicated to sex work/ers on an international scale. Throughout this presentation the speaker referred many times to the ways in which sex workers throughout the world are subject to various forms of structural control and stigmatised as a result of their labour. These references included the presentation of an assortment of images that comprised various punitive responses by authorities in several international locations. However, it was not clear if the speaker had personally recorded all (or any) the images – or if they had been obtained from/supplied by secondary sources with an advocacy interest in 'rights' for sex workers. However, all images presented were used to provide *illustrations* of the structural control of women's bodies and to support the advocacy campaign of the speaker concerned. Nevertheless, one such image depicted a so-called 'naming and shaming' ritual by statutory authorities in China and appeared to show female sex workers on 'public display' with their heads covered (and possibly their hands bound) in a municipal location of an unnamed city.

Whilst the events portrayed in the photograph from China are consistent with *western* definitions of stigmatisation, it should not necessarily be assumed that such interpretations are regarded as culturally unacceptable practices across all global societies. Indeed, the visual contextualisation and interpretation of Asian 'naming and shaming' strategies within a western (and capitalist) framework of analysis (at a non-eastern conference setting) is perhaps as inappropriate as it is inaccurate. More specifically, the 'ethnographicness' of the image and data do not exist. In order to comprehend this methodological paradox, one perhaps needs reminding that the interpretation of the relevant visual data involved a *western* speaker discussing and critiquing culturally situated activity located in an *eastern* setting. Accordingly, the so-called 'naming and shaming' responses were situated within the speaker's own western, philosophical and cultural tradition in which the actions were viewed ethnocentrically, logocentrically and from an antithetical cultural viewpoint to those women whose heads had been covered as part of a shaming ritual. Whilst western views (that adopt a specifically neo-liberal, feminist, advocacy agenda) may be valid and appropriate when applied to western settings, to assume philosophical equity across heterogeneous cultural settings is *not* entirely valid. In fact, holding such assumptions may serve to mis-represent and distort observations of cross-cultural practice to the extent that it denigrates other societies from a privileged position of self-imposed western righteousness.

This seemingly harsh criticism may be validated when the relevant 'shaming rituals' portrayed are *contextualised* within the society from which they originate. For example, what the speaker failed to add was that 'naming and shaming' rituals are not unique to sex workers in south-east/east Asian society. In fact, throughout this geographic area there is widespread practice and acceptance of broadcasting 'unacceptable' images (Winn 2009) of those who commit acts deemed anti-social, criminal and/or culturally objectionable (including traffickers, poachers, illegal immigrants, sex workers, drug users, thieves, murderers, rapists, corrupt officials). That is, the specific purpose of public humiliation (and stigmatisation) is exactly that. The humiliation is intended, it is made explicit and completely overt as – *from a cultural relativist perspective* – it may be *interpreted* as a universally shared and accepted process that serves to establish cultural boundaries and social regulation within that particular society. In short, humiliation may be interpreted as an accepted form of social control.

Accordingly, to view the deliberate and overt humiliation of others through the lens of Socratic (western) philosophy, instead of the Confucian (eastern) tradition in which such actions are set, serves only to perpetuate particular assumptions and traditions associated with western hegemony and its intellectual and epistemological imperatives. As an explanation, Lloyd (1996) emphasises that Confucian-based knowledge is essentially based upon transmission and cultural spread in which its proponents seek to stand on shared, intellectual, common ground. Within this tradition (Confucianism), knowledge is regarded as a 'lineage' and as a cultural artefact that establishes collective links and connections that form 'a relationship between masters and disciples over several generations' (Lloyd 1996, 32). Accordingly, this lineage is a means of preserving knowledge, tradition, compliance and cultural order. In absolute contrast to these values however, are those that characterise the philosophical traditions upon which western society is founded. Lloyd describes this western (Socratic) tradition as one that is purposely oppositional and is embroiled in a constant cycle of critical and adversarial challenge. In this tradition, knowledge and wisdom (and their producers) are open to challenge, subject to change and are topics of never-ending debate and/or contestation. Indeed, as Lloyd notes, the requisite of argument (and being able to defend a particular view in the face of hostile challenge) within this tradition seeks to enhance 'prestige' (not 'respect') of an individual's academic/philosophical stance within a particular 'school' of thought.

It is due to these diametrically opposed philosophical traditions associated with western and eastern cultures, that visual data from the latter cannot necessarily be used to contextualise and interpret culturally-similar phenomena situated in the former. Accordingly in this example, the ethnographicness, contextualisations and analytical interpretations of polysemic images (presented in a conference paper) are methodologically inconsistent and – essentially – flawed.

The Cultural Relativism of Suffering

The second illustration of the 'ethnographicness' of image revisits the aforementioned study of injecting drug use and homelessness in San Francisco conducted by Bourgois and Schonberg (2009). *Righteous Dopefiend* is a text that contains a dataset of over 70 images, some of which may be regarded as providing extremely graphic representations of injecting drug use, related injury and social suffering. For example, images of peer injecting (pp. 7, 243) accompany photographs of abscesses (p. 101) skin grafts (pp. 97, 105) and necrotising fasciitis (p. 104) that in turn are embedded within written accounts of poverty, homelessness, trauma, violence, viral infection, despair and death. In addition, Bourgois and Schonberg contextualise words with images (and images with words) from a view that prioritises the cultural relativism of urban deprivation within a capitalist setting. Accordingly, their work does not necessarily conform to a particular structural hegemony or political ideology that serves to punish, criminalise or further stigmatise an already marginalised population. Instead, the interplay of words with image provides relativist context and interpretation that in turn is intended to reflect the lived experience of structural inequality in contemporary America.

Whilst the methodological foundations and theoretical frameworks that underlie *Righteous Dopefiend* are informed by orthodox anthropological inquiry, the explanations provided by the researchers regarding the use of emotive, provocative and challenging images (and thus polysemic) in their work is slightly less conventional. For example, in an account of their images prior to the publication of *Righteous Dopefiend*, Schonberg and Bourgois (2002) express a reluctance to 'sanitise' their ethnographic photographs. This decision was taken purposely to avoid 'collusion with the conspiracy of apathetic silence around extreme social suffering' and that any self-censorship in this regard would perpetuate the obfuscation of 'an already confusing inaccessible social setting' (2002, 392). Similarly, Philippe Bourgois (2011) further claims that the written accounts associated with the book's images serve to 'prevent a pathologizing gaze by alerting readers to the logic for injecting in the midst of filth' (2011, 7), adding that the photographs' content emphasise how contemporary structural and economic forces engender street-level decisions to become complicit in drug-related harm production. Finally, and perhaps most salient from an applied perspective, Bourgois states (ibid.) that the ethnographic images aim to portray 'the disjunction between hypersanitary HIV-prevention outreach messages and the reality of street-level addiction' (*sic*).

In conclusion, the polysemic nature of ethnographic images may be reduced if the visual researcher adopts a position (commencing during data generation) that emphasises ethnographic intimacy, analytic engagement and reflexive analysis. Similarly, the dissemination of image-based material should also attribute ethnographically-founded *interpretations* to those particular social and environmental *contexts* directly relevant to fieldwork. This is particularly relevant, as noted by Schwartz (1997), when the generation of visual data may have involved collaborative interaction (as in this study) in which the meaning of the image is filtered through a range of experiences and perceptions held by those assisting and/or conducting the research. Failure to consider such fundamental academic practice may only generate material suitable for illustration and/or *mis*-representation.

Ethics and Visual Research

A final point to consider in *any* sociological study relates to the ethical design of a proposed research project and the ethical conduct of the researcher whilst working in the field with respondents/participants. This consideration therefore extends to the design of any 'visual' sociology, in addition to orthodox sociology (both qualitative and quantitative) and whether (or not) the relevant study is for applied or academic purposes. That said, ethical frameworks for all sociological research will differ throughout each individual project and will probably differ even further within and between those projects with a specifically applied research agenda (as a result of bespoke constraints and regulations imposed by organisations and/or institutions that are external, and additional, to the academy's Research Ethics Committees[5]).

Due to the variation in ethical considerations per individual project, it would be inappropriate for this author to provide a suggested template that outlines an apposite ethical code of conduct for an applied visual sociology. Such guidance would, by design and implication, fail to recognise the diversity within (and situated-nature of) all qualitative research. For these reasons, the following introduction to ethical concerns as part of an applied visual sociology discusses the key issues that should be addressed as priorities in any proposed study that includes visual-focused data generation. Accordingly, in an attempt to inform practice attached to an *applied visual sociology* that involves *researcher-led data generation*, the following guidelines provide only the most rudimentary of requirements that are considered necessary for visual research.

As an immediate starting point, the reader is recommended to become familiar with the statement of ethical practice issued by the Visual Sociology Study Group of the British Sociological Association (VSSG-BSA 2006). This document outlines universally recognised ethical standards regarding researchers' overall conduct during the course of their studies as well as informs, educates and raises awareness of ethical expectations whilst conducting visually-focused fieldwork. Issues covered by VSSG-BSA relate mainly to professional integrity (for example, knowledge acquisition that is not exploitative or deceptive), legal considerations of recording visual material (such as documenting illegal and/or harmful actions, dissemination of visual material that may be subject to copyright) and the main responsibilities towards research respondents/participants (including duty of care, cultural sensitivities, issues of vulnerability and taboo). However, each of the 69 points contained within the VSSG-BSA (2006) statement on ethical standards may be arranged into one of three broad categories. These categories also represent the *core* issues of ethical concern in all (visual) research; namely anonymity, confidentiality and consent (Wiles et al. 2008).

---

5 For example, such as those required within the UK's National Health Service (NHS)

Anonymity

As with conventional research, the visual identity of all research participants in visual sociological research should essentially remain anonymous, particularly in applied studies that may focus upon sensitive issues (such as drug use, political conflict, sex work etc.). Unless there is a specific rationale that validates, permits and requires the visual representation of people encountered and places visited during fieldwork, then the visual researcher would be best advised to follow Bourdieu's (1965, 24) assumption that 'nothing may be photographed apart from that which must be photographed'. This is particularly noteworthy when considering the generation/ use of images involving young children, buildings of political significance (such as bridges and other important communication centres), cultural events (such as funerals) and/or people involved in activities deemed harmful and/or illegal (Banks 2007, Bourdieu 1965, VSSG-BSA 2006, Wiles et al. 2008).

Similarly, the use of *covert* visual methods (recording images in 'secret') is generally regarded as antithetical and unethical practice throughout the social sciences particularly if/when this involves recording other *people*. Covert research activity not only resembles 'surveillance' but demonstrates a fundamental unawareness of ethical procedures attached to the conduct of research. Furthermore, if the 'covert researcher' is noted by those being photographed whilst in the field, then the opportunity for physical harm becomes significantly amplified. Correspondingly, decisions attached to the *overt* photographic recording of 'places' (such as those documented in this book) should be implemented with immense care and ethical consideration (from the perspectives of researcher safety and implications of the image taken). For example, one may consider the political and legal implications that may emerge from noting the author taking photographs within sites of public convenience (namely, male and/or female toilets). Although such street-based settings characterise injecting environments described later in this book, decisions how and why they were photographed need to be considered from legal, ethical and pragmatic perspectives. Similarly, researchers should be aware of any consequences in disseminating material that contains images of 'controversial' issues that remain unresolved by the relevant authorities (such as any active, on-going issues connected to street-based drug using environments) and how the revelation of this information (via the dissemination of pictures/film of recognisable public toilets) may influence positive or negative responses by opposing *structural* forces (for example: police surveillance or harm reduction intervention in a street-based public toilet that regularly contain episodes of injecting drug use).

Confidentiality

Parallel to the above are issues of *confidentiality* that should also be regarded as pre-requisite for any applied sociological study of social problems. As with textual data, visual data should aim to maintain the discretion and privacy of all research participants. Indeed, if visual research methods intentionally or inadvertently breach this requirement (as a result of their design and application) then a reappraisal of the validity of this form of research should take place without delay. In such circumstances it is highly probable that the visual approach may not necessarily be the most appropriate form of data generation.

The underlying rationale for adhering to research confidentiality (especially in sensitive issues) is to provide respect and dignity to the relevant participants. Concomitantly, applied visual sociological inquiry premises the generation of new knowledge for positive intervention and does not aim to visually identify individuals – or provide image-based material – that will lead to penalty, prosecution or persecution of research respondents/participants.

Consent

The final core strand of ethical consideration for an applied visual sociology relates to the rationale and process for acquiring informed consent from all relevant research participants. As indicated elsewhere (Pink 2007b, c, VSSG-BSA 2006) the purpose of obtaining research consent *per se* is to establish recognised boundaries that are mutually shared, applied and observed by researcher and research participants. This may be interpreted as the design of a set of research-related 'rights and responsibilities' in which the researcher purposely demonstrates an awareness of social, moral and ethical accountability to research participants as well as to the 'academic community'.

The process of obtaining consent within an applied visual sociology should therefore emulate conventional consent procedures. That is, the researcher makes explicit the research agenda (aims, objectives, purpose and intended outcomes) as well as any criteria involving the use, reuse and dissemination of visual data generated that directly involves participation from (or representation of) the respondent. In an applied visual sociology the provision of a verbal/written statement that outlines the above obligations, expectations and requirements of the researcher/respondent will also characterise this aspect of 'obtaining consent'.

Other issues of consent to consider may include the 'longevity' of the visual data, negotiations on the reproduction of image and the actual 'ownership' of all visual materials generated during the research. The latter point is particularly salient in terms of applied research, in which there is possibly a need for greater discussion regarding whether all visual data become materials owned by the researcher, the research-participant, the research-commissioner or co-owned as part of a commitment to a joint-venture enterprise of the research collaboration.

In short, the processes attached to obtaining informed consent (whether verbally or written) serves to strengthen the overall credibility, integrity and rigour of the research *and the researcher*. Furthermore, adherence to these elementary ethical considerations will steer the researcher through all stages of research design, delivery and dissemination.

Considering an Applied Visual Sociology

In considering a research project that may be dedicated to an applied visual sociology of a given issue, this chapter has outlined a suggested framework of priority issues that may be included in the initial stages of research design. In essence, this framework consists of:

- A need to consider the actual purpose of adopting a visual approach to applied sociological research. The researcher needs to be able to validate how and why visual data will further inform a particular study and to explain the way in which visual data may complement more orthodox forms of data generation.
- Accordingly, the researcher needs to situate any visual-oriented study within an academic paradigm that is appropriate and compatible with specific ontological and epistemological orientation. Failure to follow these academic pre-requisites will undoubtedly generate material suitable only for illustrative purposes (or generate mis-representation).
- The latter point is made more significant given the polysemic nature of almost all visual material. The researcher should therefore aim to situate their own visual data within a subjective and interpretivist framework that prioritises the relevant academic paradigm adopted for applied purposes. Failure to follow this tradition will generate ambiguous material that may be more damaging than constructive to the applied intervention concerned.
- The polysemic nature of images may be reduced if the researcher adopts an interpretative position that emphasises ethnographic intimacy, analytic engagement and reflexive analysis.
- The design of an academically and methodologically robust visual research project should generate data that has *applied* value when translated to real world settings (and academic value when considered for those purposes).
- Researchers should be aware of disciplinary visuality. Within an applied visual sociology, this relates to how applied research may meaningfully inform intervention whilst simultaneously advance the discipline of sociology.
- Disciplinary visuality relates to an appreciation and understanding of what the 'visual' may offer both forms of inquiry (that is, academic and applied).
- The academic leitmotifs of sociology are the guiding lights of its disciplinary visuality in an applied visual sociology.
- Disciplinary visuality can be significantly affected by the chosen form of visual data generation. Researchers should therefore consider which is the most appropriate visual methodology for a given study (whether respondent or researcher driven). More specifically, is the intent to produce 'images to study society' or inform the 'sociological study of images' (Banks 2007)?
- All research within an applied visual sociology should be conducted in a manner that is ethically approved and ethically robust (as with 'conventional' social science research).

- Although ethical concerns are typically dictated by the specificity of individual studies. The core elements of anonymity, confidentiality and consent should not be overlooked or understated due to the universality of these issues in social research.
- The statement of ethical practice issued by the Visual Sociology Study Group of the British Sociological Association (VSSG-BSA 2006) is *essential* and *required* reading for any person considering an applied visual sociology.
- Applied visual sociology concerns the generation of new knowledge for positive intervention and does not aim to visually identify individuals – or provide image-based material – that will lead to penalty, prosecution or persecution of any research respondent/participant.
- As Bourdieu notes, 'nothing may be photographed apart from that which must be photographed' (1965, 24). An individual engaged in applied visual sociology should therefore not assume that the taking of images is validated and justified by their position (as 'researcher').
- An applied visual sociology is an attempt to bridge academic traditions with applied intervention in which the relevant and respective conclusions may be translated to (and shared with) the relevant and respective audiences.

This book provides an applied visual sociology of street-based injecting drug use and harm reduction intervention. In order to guide the readership through the epistemological (and thus methodological) design of this study, the following chapter seeks to summarise the core issues of harm reduction and injecting-related harm. Comprehension of these issues will facilitate the applied interpretation of images displayed throughout this book and further contextualise considerations that underlie the notion of an 'applied visual sociology'.

Chapter 2
Harm Reduction and Injecting Drug Use

The following chapter is concerned exclusively with the topic of harm reduction. This summary has been included in recognition that the readership of this text may not necessarily be completely *au fait* with the politics of harm reduction, especially within the field of injecting drug use. As such, this chapter aims to introduce the reader to some of the key issues that form the underlying, and central, tenets of harm reduction as applied intervention in 'real world' settings. In the following sections, harm reduction is defined and its rationale, practice and principles are made explicit. Other sections summarise the political origins of harm reduction and the various modes of standardised, often internationally recognised, intervention. Perhaps most significantly (in the context of this study of street-based injecting environments), this chapter concludes with an overview of what constitutes 'safer' injecting drug use from a harm reduction perspective.

Harm Reduction Defined

Throughout this book, the term 'harm reduction' follows the definitions provided by the World Health Organisation (WHO 2005) and the International Harm Reduction Association (IHRA 2010). Namely:

> In public health, harm reduction is used to describe a concept aiming to *prevent* or *reduce negative health consequences* associated with certain behaviours. In relation to *drug injecting* harm reduction components of *comprehensive interventions* aim to *prevent transmission of HIV and other infections* that occur through the *sharing* of *non-sterile injection equipment* and *drug preparations*. (WHO 2005, 5, emphases added)

Similarly, harm reduction as defined within an IHRA Position Statement (2013) notes that:

> Harm reduction refers to *policies, programmes and practices* that aim primarily *to reduce the adverse* health, social and economic *consequences* of the use of legal and illegal psychoactive drugs *without* necessarily *reducing drug consumption*. Harm reduction *benefits people who use drugs, their families and the community*. (IHRA, 2010, emphases added)

Whilst these defining statements on harm reduction (above) may appear almost identical at first glance, there are subtle differences that may be noted on subsequent readings. In each statement, the defining features of harm reduction in the context of injecting drug use have been placed in italics. As such, one may note that both institutions (each venerable in the field of public health) consider the reduction, prevention and minimisation of opportunities for the transmission of harm (relating specifically to blood borne viruses) as the key operational component within such frameworks. Similarly, both organisations either explicitly (WHO) or implicitly (IHRA) prioritise the reduction of shared injecting paraphernalia (needles, syringes, cookers, swabs, filters and drug solute) in order to prevent viral transmission (but also includes bacterial infection and a wide range of other injecting related harm and injury). Furthermore, both bodies generally advocate achieving these particular aims with a range of related and relevant intervention. However, significant and meaningful differences between the two definitions may be noted in the use of the term 'comprehensive interventions' by WHO. Whilst this term may be open to wider subjective interpretation, this author interprets this to include 'treatment' options for drug dependency. In contrast, and as noted by IHRA (2013), 'the majority of people who use drugs do not need treatment'. As such, harm reduction intervention is designed to provide *options* that will reduce the risk of potential or actual harm and essentially aims to assist with keeping people 'safe' and 'well' in relation to drug consumption. Harm reduction is therefore not necessarily concerned with the medicalisation of an individual's drug use – but makes allowances for this route should it be needed.

Perhaps a more succinct definition of harm reduction may be noted in the following declaration by Wodak and McLeod (2008) that encapsulates the entire content of the two definitions presented above. Namely, with harm reduction approaches to substance use 'drug related harm is accorded an even higher priority than the reduction of drug consumption' (Wodak and McLeod 2008, S81). Indeed, this definition resonates with the formal recommendation made by the Advisory Council on the Misuse of Drugs (ACMD) in a report *two decades earlier* to the UK government following an inquiry into injecting drug use and the transmission of the human immuno-deficiency virus (HIV). Namely:

> the spread of HIV is a greater danger to individual and public health than drug misuse (ACMD 1988, 17)

Indeed, the oft-cited opening words of the ACMD statement (above) has been regarded as *the* sentence that radically transformed drug policy and practice (including public health intervention) in UK settings (McKeganey 2011). Similarly, the legacy of the ACMD statement is that harm reduction has become firmly embedded within successive National Drug Strategies of all British government administrations since 1988 (Conservative Party, Labour and the Conservative-Liberal Democrat Coalition). More accurately, harm reduction has become one of four central pillars (in addition to 'enforcement', 'education' and 'prevention') upon which national (and international) drug policy and practice typically rests (McCann 2008, Single 1995). Accordingly, the introduction of needle exchange programmes and opioid substitution therapy (OST) for drug dependency form the cornerstone upon which current harm reduction intervention throughout the UK is built upon (in addition to various educative and outreach programmes).

However, although harm reduction has only a relatively short history of formal institutionalisation (Smith 2012) by many governments throughout the developed and developing world (see below), the concept is actually 'culturally-richer' than the above references may infer. In the following section, the origins of harm reduction (in the context of injecting drug use) are presented in order to provide a more qualitative insight and understanding of the issue – as well as provide an (albeit limited) historic perspective of contemporary (and controversial) public health policy in UK settings.

The Origins of Harm Reduction

The HIV pandemic noted during the 1980s undoubtedly had a significant impact upon global policy pertaining to public health and injecting drug use. However, as noted by many scholars (MacDonald and Patterson 1991, Riley and Pates 2012, Rhodes and Hedrich 2010, Royal College of Physicians (RCP) 2000), harm reduction as a concept, as practice and as a paradigm within the field of *substance use* had existed for decades prior to the advent of HIV.

Perhaps the most notable example of this form of intervention was the British government's inquiry into the role of prescribing morphine to treat opiate dependency almost *one century ago* in 1923 (Rhodes and Hedrich 2010, Riley et al. 2012). The findings from this study, often termed the Rolleston Report (1926), defined what has become known as the 'British System' for addressing drug dependency (Strang and Gossop 2005a, b). In fact, the Rolleston Report established suitable medical interventions regarding the prescribed use of morphine/heroin as a legitimate treatment option (Riley et al. 2012). Indeed, the terms and conditions of treatment outlined in the Rolleston Report appear almost identical to those of contemporary policy regarding the prescription of methadone. A further illustration of this form of harm reduction may be observed in the 'methadone clinics' established throughout New York during the mid-1960s (op. cit., ibid.). The latter were introduced as a response to widespread opiate dependency and have been cited as a health intervention model upon which the 'British System' emulated two decades later (O'Hare et al. 1992, Strang and Gossop 2005a, b).

It should also be noted that each of the 'harm reduction' approaches to substance use noted above are premised upon *institutionalised* and *structural* responses to injecting drug use or opiate dependency. Furthermore, these responses may illustrate a 'top-down' (Smith 2012) approach to public health concerns in which a particular (health-based/government-based) authority attempts to minimise negative, harmful effects associated with a particular substance (whether licit or illicit). Current international drug policy, which prioritises reducing drug-related harm associated with HIV transmission, therefore mirrors this historical formalised and institutionalised approach to protecting public health – at an aggregate and individual level.

Grassroots Activism

However, in the context of *street-based* injecting drug use, contemporary harm reduction intervention also has a parallel history that reflects health-related intervention and activism at a more grassroots level *by drug users for other drug users*. Furthermore, this activism within peer and social networks of injecting drug users equally predates the advent of HIV *and* the Hepatitis C virus (HCV) – the latter of which was 'identified' as recently as 1989 (Fraser and Seear 2011, O'Shea 2010).

Perhaps the most renowned of these activist groups (or at least, the most described in the relevant literature) is the Netherlands-based Rotterdam Junkiebond (RJB) or 'Junkie Union' (Grund 1993). This collective was formed in 1977, (Hunt et al. 2010) and was established as a localised response by drug users to issues such as enforced detoxification by authorities; reducing stigma associated with substance use and to provide a platform to lobby for the legalisation of illicit drugs (Friedman et al. 2007, Hunt et al. 2010). However, perhaps most significantly, the Dutch-based drug user activist groups are also credited for establishing 'the world's first needle exchange programme … in *1984*' (Hunt et al. 2010, 334 emphasis added).

Furthermore, by 1985, 35 Junkiebonden existed in 28 Dutch cities in which most had established informal needle and syringe programmes in response to growing concerns surrounding Hepatitis B (HBV). The organisations' core activists also provided an informal advice service (regarding injecting technique) and produced a newsletter that aimed to politicise injecting drug use and mobilise support for continued grassroots activism by other injecting drug users (Friedman et al. 1988, 2007, Grund 1993, Marks et al. 2005).

It is also perhaps necessary to recognise that other groups/individuals, in other countries, during the same time period, were also involved in similar intervention. For example, Friedman et al. (2004) refer to drug user activities in New York City, Brazil and Central Asia, in which they contend that autonomous (and illegal) acts of harm reduction may have assisted in limiting the spread of HIV. For these reasons, Friedman et al. term street-based harm reduction activities as a form of 'peer intravention', in which 'prevention activities are conducted by and sustained through ongoing actions of members of communities at risk' (of harm) (Friedman et al. 2004, 250). Similarly a number of initiatives based in the UK, and contemporaneous with the Dutch Junkiebonden model, may be equally termed as exemplars of peer intravention, grassroots activism and/or public health-focused direct action *by* drug users *for* other drug users.

Harm Reduction in the UK

In order to contextualise 'radical interventions' employed by 'ideological renegades' (McDermott 2005, 149) during the 1980s, it is also necessary to acknowledge that many towns/cities experienced post-industrial recession, large scale unemployment and epidemic heroin use that, in turn, influenced a growth in injecting behaviour (Parker et al. 1988, Pearson 1987). At this time, HIV-awareness was widespread and various national epidemics had been identified that were associated specifically with transmission via injecting drug use (Berridge 1994, Robertson 1990). For example, by the mid-1980s, HIV-seropositivity amongst injecting drug users in Edinburgh (Scotland) was noted *in excess of 50 per cent* of that particular injecting population (Pearson 1992). Edinburgh was also a setting where individuals could be arrested for possession of injecting paraphernalia at that point in time (Pearson 1992).

Indeed, as both Pat O'Hare (1992) and Peter McDermott (2005) each note, it was due to similar structural/health concerns associated with HIV, coupled with the prevalence of injecting drug use in areas of Merseyside, that demanded an *immediate* response in the city of Liverpool. However this call for statutory intervention was seemingly frustrated, as existing policies and strategies (to adequately and appropriately address the large scale uptake of injecting drug use) appeared to mirror the Scottish experience noted above. Namely, structural forces appeared to exacerbate – rather than ameliorate – drug related harm and associated pressures (O'Hare 1992). McDermott's (2005) reflection of these times is slightly less diplomatic than O'Hare's commentary however – in which the former critically describes the British System (relating to drug policy) as one 'moribund', 'bankrupt' and unable to manage the spread of injecting drug use/HIV at that particular time.

Nevertheless, the two colliding pressures of escalating injecting drug use and government inaction inspired – what is generally regarded as – the genesis of harm reduction in the UK. This is made evident in the work of both McDermott (2005) and O'Hare (1992, 2007) who provide insights of the development of informal needle and syringe provision made available in the city of Liverpool during this time.

The initiation of harm reduction interventions in Merseyside were modelled upon the Dutch 'Junkiebondon' activities and strategies described above. As such, O'Hare (1992) remarks that the first attempts at distributing needle and syringes in UK settings were designed and managed by drug users for drug users and not by policy makers. In addition, as the 'project' developed and grew, O'Hare (ibid.) further reflects that the initiative received support by the local police constabulary. Perhaps more significantly, premises providing needle and syringes were not placed under surveillance by police as a method of identifying and arresting known drug users. Instead, the Merseyside police constabulary was to eventually initiate a system of referring injecting drug users to appropriate services following arrest (and is a model that has since been adopted throughout the UK). It is also noteworthy that one of the first static needle and syringe exchange schemes made available in Liverpool during this time (1986) was established within a converted toilet (O'Hare 2007, 142).

In addition to the Mersey project above, Southall (2009) and Millar (2009) each provide similar retrospective and historic accounts of 'underground', peer-based, injecting-related intervention in areas of England and Scotland respectively. In each of these settings, drug users were also actively involved in the distribution of injecting equipment in response to the identification of HIV in particular communities. Similarly, as with the Mersey project, many of these street-based activities pre-dated the formal piloting and/or introduction of state-sanctioned needle and syringe programmes in England and Scotland.

Indeed, it was not until *1987* that experimental schemes for needle and syringe projects were commissioned by the Department of Health and Social Security (England) and the Scottish Home and Health Department (Scotland) (Sheridan 2005, Stimson 1988).

Mainstreaming the Radical

Regardless of geographical location, each of the examples presented above demonstrate that direct action by community activists with a harm reduction agenda (pertaining specifically to injecting drug use) typically pre-dates the formal introduction of needle/syringe programmes (NSP) sanctioned by various statutory bodies in the relevant settings. Furthermore, these informal (and possibly illegal) responses to viral infection may be regarded as street-based reactions to authorities that were unable (or unwilling) to respond to drug related harm in a manner other than enforcement, coercion and prohibition (O'Hare 1992, McDermott 2005). From more sociological and political perspectives however, these experiences of the development of harm reduction perhaps confirm the view that community activism can indeed influence (and/or hasten) change at a structural level in matters pertaining to public health (Tempalski et al. 2007). Similarly, these historic events *perhaps* consolidate the view (Smith 2012, McDermott 2005) that grassroots initiatives that originally encounter groundswell opposition by structural, political and social forces may eventually become institutionalised by 'the system' as a valid and recognised mode of intervention. In such circumstances, alternative visions and progressive agendas that initially challenge existing policy frameworks may become appropriated and reinterpreted by those in more powerful (structural, institutional) positions. That is to say, the radical becomes mainstream, 'bottom-up' approaches are made 'top-down' strategies and radical activism becomes accepted as legitimate and pragmatic government policy.

The Legacy of 'Grassroots' Radicalism

A legacy of grassroots activism and health-oriented direct action may also be noted in the union that has been made between practitioners and academics with a shared interest in harm reduction. More specifically, in 1989 the *Mersey Drugs*

Journal was transformed from a localised publication to become the *International Journal of Drug Policy*. The latter (in 2013) is a bi-monthly academic journal that provides a forum for researchers, practitioners and policy-makers on matters pertaining to licit and illicit drug use and associated policy/practice. According to the journal's website, it is 'ranked 4th out of 22 journals in the substance abuse' category. In addition, the *Editors in Chief* of the journal are Professors Tim Rhodes and Gerry Stimson; both of whom are established and influential advocates of harm reduction as well as eminent public health sociologists in their respective fields of research.

Similarly, in 1990, the first international conference dedicated to the issue of reducing drug related harm was staged in the city of Liverpool. This event was organised by those that had been directly responsible for introducing harm reduction to the Mersey region (O'Hare 2007). From this conference, the International Harm Reduction Association (IHRA) was born, and in 2013 the latter body presented the *23rd* international conference dedicated to reducing drug related harm was staged in the city of Vilnius (Lithuania).

(Indeed, many of the images included in the following chapters were displayed at the IHRA 2013 conference in Vilnius as part of an exhibition associated with this book. At this event the author discussed the exhibition images within an interactive 'Dialogue Space' (Parkin 2013b) in the context of the conference theme (namely, *The Value[s] of Harm Reduction*). In addition, the photography exhibition in Vilnius (and this book) can be traced to an oral paper delivered by the author at IHRA's *20th* International Conference in Bangkok (Thailand) regarding the use of use of applied visual methods as harm reduction intervention (Parkin 2009d). As such, the author can perhaps confirm, from personal experience and responses to contributions at these events, that IHRA's International Conference does indeed provide 'a global village for the exchange of knowledge and practice of harm reduction' (Stimson 2007, 68).

A further legacy of grassroots activism may be noted in the level of academic interest in harm reduction. This may be illustrated with a Scopus search of peer reviewed journal articles that contain 'harm reduction' and 'drugs' within the title, abstract or keywords. In June 2013, this search provided a reading list of exactly 2,620 items. However, the earliest item on this topic was published in 1982 when only one journal paper dedicated to drug-related harm reduction was noted (Casswell et al. 1982). It is not until 1989 – a period of seven years – that the 'second' peer-reviewed paper on 'harm reduction/drugs' features in the Scopus database (Engelsman 1989). These single items rise to six in 1990, 27 in 1995, 78 in 2000, 172 in 2005, 234 in 2010 and a further 234 in 2012. Accordingly, in the three decades that harm reduction has formally appeared on the world stage as institutionalised public health policy (c.1984), there has been an incredible two thousand-fold increase (that is, rising from one publication in 1982 to over 2,600 in 2013) in academic publications dedicated to this particular issue. (These figures, of course, do not include all publications and reports relating to drug-related research commissioned specifically by statutory, regional, local authorities and third sector organisations as part of various needs assessments and/or service evaluations).

The Principles of Harm Reduction

Harm reduction approaches to substance use typically focus upon public health, the wider social environment and typically do not seek to criminalise drug use/rs (Buning 1990, Hathaway 2006). Instead, the operational principles of harm reduction seek to minimise the harmful and/or negative effects of drug use upon individuals (and the societies in which they reside) rather than prevent or eliminate drug use from occurring *per se* (Newcombe 1992). In tandem with this philosophical approach is a morally neutral stance and accepts that society cannot be completely drug-free regardless of punitive legislation or coercive control (Fraser and Moore 2011, International Federation of Red Cross and Red Crescent Societies (IFRC) 2003).

In addition to the above framework are the generally accepted principles that harm reduction is the antithesis of abstentionism, contrasts with medical models that favour 'addiction' as 'disease' and challenges notions of paternalism (O'Hare 1992, Newcombe 1992, MacDonald and Patterson 1991). Proponents of harm reduction typically regard each of the aforementioned constructs of substance use as unhelpful, unsupportive and unrealistic measures for reducing the social and physical harms associated with injecting drug use. Similarly, the principles of harm reduction typically prioritise the notion of informed choice, in which individual decisions regarding drug-using episodes aim to maximise a process of enablement. In more simplistic terms, this principle refers to individual autonomy, free will and independent decision-making regarding reductions in drug-related harm to self, others and wider community members.

As further noted by several authors (Erickson 1995, MacDonald and Patterson 1991, Single 1995), more medical/abstinence-oriented approaches to substance use typically minimise (or completely remove) the process of enablement and individual decision-making (regarding drug consumption) in the pursuit of idealised goals and standards determined by others. In this approach, individuals become disempowered, as autonomy and choice are surrendered to those who may attempt to regulate, monitor and control drug-centred lifestyles. It is due to these conflicting approaches that harm reduction is further defined as prioritising a 'person-centred approach' (MacDonald and Patterson 1991) to individual drug consumption, in which practitioners and service users work together to design, mutually-determined goals and targets that are considered practical and not idealistic (Single 1995).

In addition, the principles of harm reduction accept that the goal of abstinence for some drug users is an unrealistic target. For these individuals, more short-term realisable goals may be more successful in a harm reduction approach to drug use (Single 1995). For these reasons, harm reduction may be regarded as a *hierarchical* paradigm as individual interventions 'vary in their propensity for decreasing negative effects of drug use' (Newcombe 1992, 1). Accordingly, initiatives such as needle syringe programmes and methadone prescribing purposely provide metaphorical safety nets as individuals attempt to ameliorate negative and adverse consequences of their drug use whilst their drug intake actually continues (Crofts 2012, Newcombe 1992, Single 1995).

Harm Reduction and Human Rights

As well as an overriding commitment to public health, a further principle of harm reduction is that which considers a 'human rights' approach to substance use issues (Barrett et al. 2009, Chen 2011, Csete and Cohen 2003, IHRA 2010, Stimson 2007). From this position those people who use illicit drugs are regarded *as equal* as those who do not. Furthermore, the 'human right' to health, social services, employment, education, liberty and dignity is not denied on the basis of whether an individual uses an illicit substance (or not). Concomitantly, proponents of harm reduction typically oppose policies and practice that may initiate drug-related harm, particularly in regard to drug control and coercive policing. These objections are premised upon grounds that such actions are discriminatory, exclusory or prejudicial responses and thus contrary to particular 'health' and/or 'human' rights.

As noted by Erickson (1995), these latter principles of harm reduction may be better understood if contextualised by punitive and coercive approaches that may emphasise punishment, incarceration and/or the augmentation of physical and actual harm. Perhaps the most extreme illustration of this regard may be the decisions made by the Thai government during 2003 to permit the extra judicial killings of over 2,000 suspected drug sellers/users in an attempt to create a 'drug-free Thailand' within a controlled period of enhanced enforcement (Cohen 2009). A less extreme illustration may be the ways in which public space is managed to purposely exclude those who are *known* to inject illicit drugs *because* they inject illicit drugs (Parkin 2013, Parkin and Coomber 2010).

It is often because of a commitment to these 'rights-based' reasons that many harm reduction academics may struggle with institutionalised Ethics Committees to obtain approval to conduct social science research involving cohorts of injecting drug users. For example, Research Ethics Committees may reject cash payments to drug users for participating in studies of injecting practices. These rejections are typically premised upon fears and concerns that the money provided may be regarded as coercive, as rewarding illicit behaviour or used to finance continued drug use (Fry and Dwyer 2001, McKeganey 2001, Parkin 2013, Seddon 2005). However, as others (for example, Seddon 2005, Parkin 2013) have argued convincingly, such righteous claims may be regarded as antithetical to a 'rights-based' approach to participation in academic research. Accordingly, all ethically-approved research that informed this book adopted a 'business framework' of participation (Seddon 2005) in which injecting drug users were not denied access to cash payment 'simply because of who they are' (ibid., 103).

Pragmatism and Humanism

In an earlier paragraph (above), harm reduction was described as one of 'four pillars' that typically supports contemporary drug policies on a global scale. In continuing this analogy, the reader should now imagine the pillar of harm reduction consisting of two inter-twining threads that form a double-helix design, similar to that used to represent the model for portraying DNA (Watson 1999). In a harm-reduction representation, the two interlocking strands that strengthen the pillar of harm reduction consist of *pragmatism* and *humanism*. Gerry Stimson (2007) once described these two characteristics as those that separate harm reduction from all other approaches that aim to resolve problems associated with substance use. Accordingly, it is contended by this author that these characteristics also define the *principles* of harm reduction. More specifically, in the above analogy of a harm reduction double-helix, the strand of *pragmatism* represents the libertarian, radical and pioneering attitude of harm reduction advocates and proponents, whilst simultaneously articulates the value of informed choice and the development of realistic goals relating to individual health care (determined with assistance from others). Similarly, the thread of pragmatism seeks to diminish the 'arbitrary moralism' (O'Hare 1992, xv) generally afforded to drug use/rs and simultaneously challenges constructs created by stigma/stigmatisation from a position that aims to be morally-neutral.

Pragmatism is consolidated by the second strand within the harm reduction double-helix. That is, the thread of *humanistic* approaches to those affected by drug dependency and injecting drug use. This position emphasises respect for others, dignity for humanity; it values a rights-based approach to public health and confronts the harmful consequences of policies and practice that establish (or perpetuate) drug-related harm. Similarly, a humanistic approach to drug-related problems equally values empowerment and enablement, whilst providing safety-nets for some of society's most vulnerable and marginalised people. In this regard, the humanistic principles of harm reduction become 'co-contingent with humanity' and are inextricably linked to the state of being human whilst equally reflecting individual compassion and empathy for others (Crofts 2012, x).

The Practice of Harm Reduction

Whereas the principles of harm reduction reflect a more theoretical orientation of such intervention, the practice (and practise) of harm reduction here refers to the ways and means of how (and where) intervention is made operational on a day-to-day basis. As noted above, harm reduction is not necessarily concerned with achieving total abstinence amongst people who use (or inject) drugs. However, harm reduction services do typically emphasise the need to decrease potential and actual drug-related harm that individuals may do to themselves and/or their immediate/wider social and physical environment (Buning et al. 1992).

Harm Reducing Intervention for Injecting Drug Use

With specific regard to injecting drug user populations, a wide variety of health-focused interventions and services currently exist on a global scale that have the universal goal of reducing drug related harm. Perhaps the most widely recognised of these interventions are needle and syringe programmes (NSP) and opioid substitution therapy (OST). NSP typically provide access to sterile injecting paraphernalia (cookers, filters, syringes and needles), low threshold intervention with service providers and serve as potential gateways to treatment options. However, OST often involves the prescription of a synthetic opioid (such as methadone or buprenorphine) to replace the use of street-based opiates (heroin) as part of programme of stabilisation, maintenance or reduction in which (long, medium and/or short term) goals are often associated with recovery from drug dependency.

In addition to these standardised interventions are those that vary between nations – and even within nations (that is, available in some cities/towns, but not in others). This international range of service delivery includes:

- residential rehabilitation/detoxification programmes.
- prison-based NSP.
- prison based OST.
- drug consumption rooms – state-sanctioned, medically supervised, hygienic environments used for the preparation and consumption of illicit substances.
- diamorphine prescription programmes.
- the provision of emergency 'overdose kits' and/or peer-based training in the delivery of naloxone.
- peer-based outreach and education services.
- mobile services (NSP, OST, peer outreach).
- un/supervised OST consumption.
- varying availability of swabs, filters, cookers, water ampoules and citric acid with injecting paraphernalia from NSP.
- the availability of aluminium foil from NSP.
- the availability of 'crack' pipes from NSP.
- Hepatitis B vaccinations.
- HIV/HCV screening.
- wound care facilities (relating to abscesses, injecting injury etc.).
- on-site pill testing (for analysis of content in substances such as 'ecstasy').

It should also be stressed at this point that the provision of all harm reduction services in the above outline exist in varying degrees of availability (or *unavailability*) in practice settings across the globe. However, regardless of the variation of harm reduction services available within a given geographic location (whether city, country or continent), all intervention is typically universal in attempting to affect some form of behaviour change within a health-oriented framework.

From a more 'operational perspective', the planning of harm reduction services in the 21st century (such as those listed above) continue to follow the conceptual framework described by Pat O'Hare and Russell Newcombe in their respective chapters within *The Reduction of Drug Related Harm* (1992). In this model, 'consequences' of drug use (harm and benefits) are considered from two distinct positions ('type' and 'level'). 'Type' of consequence relates to whether drug related harms and benefits impact upon *health*, *societal* issues or *economic* circumstances. 'Level' of consequence however pertains to whether these harms and benefits impact specifically upon *individuals*, *communities* or entire *societies*. Underlying this grid-like matrix of 'consequence' is a secondary framework that 'considers the behaviour patterns associated with particular outcomes' (O'Hare 1992, xvii); or more simply, *drug-related risks*. In this regard, harm reduction practice provides a classificatory system that prioritises quantitative dimensions (such as dosage, potency and frequency of use) alongside qualitative components of an individual's drug use (such as access to drugs, preparation, route of administration, poly-drug use, role of others present and the impact of place/environment). Accordingly, when applied at an operational level, the cross-consideration of 'consequence' with 'risk' by service provider and service user would aim to identify and reduce harmful drug use whilst constructing a programme of appropriate intervention.

The above conceptual framework may be further simplified in the guidance provided by MacDonald and Patterson (1991) in their *Handbook of Drug Training*, which presents a manual for 'learning about drugs and working with drug users'. In this practitioner-focused text, MacDonald and Patterson demonstrate that the goals of harm reduction exist at both 'individual' and 'environmental' levels. More specifically, 'behaviour change' may be noted as an aspect of all the services listed above that aim to reduce drug-related harm associated with 'individual' health and allied lifestyles (general health, physical and psychological well-being) of drug users and all/any significant others (parents, partners, children, friends). Similarly, each of the services above attempt to reduce harm caused by actual/potential participation in the legal-justice system (and may include the reduction of convictions, arrest, prosecution, prolific/recidivist offending and the harms caused by a lifelong 'criminal' record for drug-related offences). Other 'individual' level benefits of harm reduction aim to counter more personal and negative consequences that may accompany a drug-centred lifestyle (such as vulnerability, stigma, social exclusion, and marginalisation from work, school and other social arenas). At a more 'environmental' level, harm reduction practice also seeks to ameliorate hazard associated with street-based -injecting drug use, -drug-related litter, (drug-related) -violence, -theft, -acquisitive crime, -sex-work, in addition to preventative public health programmes dedicated to blood borne viruses (HIV, hepatitis), as well as reduce the financial costs (via taxation) associated with the policing and imprisonment of drug users.

Other texts written specifically for *applied* audiences (Blume et al. 2001, Coombs 2001) typically highlight the importance of the relationship between providers and 'clients' in harm reduction settings. For example, Blume et al.'s (2001) account of harm reduction programming stress that the goal of such intervention is to improve an overall quality of life by reducing harm associated with substance use, in which practitioners negotiate an appropriate *recovery of health* plan via collaboration and pragmatic responses. Similarly, a more medically-oriented account of harm reduction, provided by the Royal College of Physicians (RCP 2000, 31), emphasises that related intervention involves the 'minimising of suffering and ill health indefinitely or until such time as the condition, if curable, is cured'. This latter vision of harm reduction clearly emphasises drug use as a 'disease' construct (that can be 'cured') and perhaps illustrates that harm reduction can be generally interpreted as existing across a spectrum of intervention.

Indeed, this interpretation may be further strengthened with Gerry Stimson's (1992) view that harm reduction is about recognising and establishing culturally-relevant cultural-controls within milieux that may inject illicit drugs. More precisely, Stimson advocates a more nuanced understanding of the etiquette and customs of drug user lifestyles as they occur *within* drug-using cliques and networks in an attempt to identify and promote less harmful injecting/drug using techniques.

Harm Reduction on a Global Scale?

The global state of harm reduction issued by the International Harm Reduction Association (IHRA 2013) provides a precise and accurate overview of harm reduction policies noted in international settings. For example, IHRA notes that of 158 nations where injecting drug use has been reported, more than half had adopted some form of harm reduction practice. Furthermore for the year 2010 IHRA (ibid.) reports that:

- 93 countries support harm reduction in policy or practice.
- 82 countries have needle and syringe exchange.
- 74 countries have opioid substitution therapy.
- 39 countries have opioid substitution therapy in prisons.
- 10 countries have needle and syringe exchange in prisons.
- 8 countries have drug consumption rooms.

Much of this variation may be explained by inconsistencies in national drug policies and/or associated legislation that often make it illegal for health and social services to provide or distribute particular items of paraphernalia, and/or prevent/restrict the delivery of other internationally recognised services. For example, in the UK (in 2013) drug consumption rooms are prohibited on political and legal grounds; similarly NSP are prohibited in many cities of the USA and the distribution of water, citric and aluminium foil (as a method of making route transitions from injecting to smoking drugs) from services is highly contested in many countries – regardless of whether other paraphernalia is distributed for injecting drug use from the same sources. As such, the global practice of harm reduction is made inconsistent by political/legal frameworks in which the reduction of drug-related harm may be frustrated by micro-level structural forces (that perhaps favour less radical, more abstinent and/or more coercive forms of intervention).

Nevertheless, at first glance, the summary statistics regarding the global state of harm reduction (above) appear somewhat optimistic. However, when IHRA (2013) further notify its audience of the global scale of injecting-drug use (including estimates of 11–20 million injectors), injecting-related HIV (affecting an estimated 3–6 million injecting drug users worldwide) and hepatitis (affecting people often living with HIV co-infection) these statistics actually present much more pessimistic reading.

What becomes further evident is that in those countries where harm reduction policies have been long-established, there appears to be a correlation of reduced HIV prevalence. For example, according to the Health Protection Agency (HPA 2012) amongst people who inject drugs in the UK, approximately 50 per cent live with hepatitis C and around one per cent has been infected with HIV. Whilst the prevalence of hepatitis C is clearly a concern in this setting, the low rates of HIV suggest that the epidemics of 30 years previous have been controlled (if not reversed).

However, the significance and relevance of harm reduction becomes more apparent (and urgent) when these data are compared to those nations where the interventions and policies listed above are less developed or are resisted and/or rejected by government. This may be substantiated with reference once more to the IHRA international profile (2013) that highlights a comparative HIV prevalence rate of over *40 per cent* amongst injecting drug users in eight countries where harm reduction is less influential (that is, Argentina, Brazil, Estonia, Indonesia, Kenya, Myanmar, Nepal and Thailand).

Similarly, in those eight countries (Australia, Canada, Germany, Luxembourg, the Netherlands, Norway, Spain and Switzerland) where harm reduction is arguably at its most advanced level, the global state of harm reduction becomes remarkably insignificant and somewhat disheartening from a public health perspective. Whilst the provision of state-sanctioned drug consumption rooms perhaps reflects progressive and innovative intervention in the field of HIV prevention and harm reduction, when one further considers that only 87 of these facilities operate throughout a mere 58 cities in only 8 nations of the entire world (Shatz and Nougier 2012, 5–6), then the global state of harm reduction appears somewhat inadequate?

Reclaiming Harm Reduction in the UK

As noted in Chapter 1, this book is only one component of an academic triptych that is, in part, an attempt at resituating and reclaiming the role of harm reduction paradigm in contemporary drug policy (in the UK). The companion text to the book, *Habitus and Drug Using Environments* and a visual exposition titled *Frontline: A Photo-Ethnography of Drug Using Environments* complete this harm reduction triumvirate. Individually, and collectively, these three works do not seek to glorify or demonise injecting drug use/rs. Instead, they each aim to portray the environmental settings associated with drug dependency and homelessness from a variety of perspectives (empirically, practically, theoretically and visually). It is further anticipated that these three works will collectively 'make visible' a range of 'invisible' environments associated with street-based injecting drug use and reflect the physical conditions in which drug-related harm can (and does) occur in British settings. Finally, images of these environments are presented within all of three of the above outputs with the specific intent of stimulating political debate, public engagement and to emphasise the continued need to sustain an appropriate harm reduction response to this particular public health issue. This political stance, *in support of* and *in solidarity with* harm reduction, is articulated and explained in further detail in Chapter 3 (regarding the *epistemological* approach underlying all research). However, prior to that particular account is a harm reduction guide to 'safer' injecting drug use.

A Harm Reduction Guide to 'Safer' Injecting Drug Use'

This section provides a summary of the optimal conditions, recommended equipment and desirable practice required for the safer preparation and safer injection of illicit drugs (with particular reference to heroin). This potentially controversial account has been included in this text in recognition that most publications dedicated to the issue of injecting drug use typically assume that the readership is fully aware of how illicit drugs *should* be prepared and injected. However, as will be evident from the summary below, the ideal conditions attached to injecting drug use typically involve a meticulous adherence to hygienic procedures, environmental management, spatial awareness and corporeal conduct. As will be made further apparent in later chapters the settings and socio-spatial qualities attached to street-based injecting often make adherence to these ideal injecting requirements problematic (if not impossible). Accordingly, if the readership of this text is to fully appreciate the circumstances of street-based injecting drug use then it is essential that a comparative benchmark is provided in order to facilitate comprehension of the harm production-reduction dichotomy that relates to street-based injecting environments (as described in later chapters). For these reasons, this chapter is written from a perspective that continues to prioritise the principles and practice of harm reduction.

The following harm reduction guide to 'safer' injecting practice has been informed by four key texts which are fully referenced in Box 2.1 below. All of these texts were written by academics, practitioners and/or clinicians with an applied and qualified understanding of injecting drug use. As such, the summary below may be regarded as an accurate and professionally informed account of how illicit drugs may be best prepared for injection.

However for additional information, *The Safer Injecting Briefing* (Derricott, Preston and Hunt 1999), provides anatomical and physiological information on injecting practise in both graphic and textual formats. The second and third reference texts are the relevant chapters contained within *Injecting Illicit Drugs*

(Pates, McBride and Arnold 2005) by Jennifer Scott (2005) and Helen Williams and Mark Norman (2005). Scott's chapter provides an account of the pharmaceutical aspects of injecting and includes useful information on injecting environments, the role of acidifiers, water and routes of drug administration. Williams and Norman however provide a step-by-step guide to drug preparation, the injecting process and the optimal (social and environmental) conditions required for safer injecting drug use. The final text that has informed this chapter is that by Strang, Griffiths and Gossop (2005) regarding different types of heroin historically made available in the UK and the significance of this variation upon administration (including injecting). As such, the guide presented below has been constructed by collating key issues from each of these texts and are deemed relevant when considering *street-based* injecting. However, for reasons relating brevity, this guide is presented mainly in a series of annotated 'bullet' points. (For these reasons, should additional information be required on any of the complex issues associated with injecting drug use, readers are advised to seek the relevant documents cited below in Box 2.1).

Derricott, J., Preston, A. and Hunt, N., 1999. *The Safer Injecting Briefing: An Easy to Use Comprehensive Reference Guide to Promoting Safer Injecting*. Liverpool: HIT.

Scott, J., 2005. Pharmaceutical aspects of injecting, in *Injecting Illicit Drugs*, edited by R. Partes, A. McBride and K. Arnold. Oxford: Blackwell Publishing (Addiction Press), pp. 33–46.

Strang, J., Griffiths, P. and Gossop, M., 2005. Different types of heroin in the UK: What significance and what relationship to different routes of administration, in *Heroin Addiction and the British System: Volume 1 Origins and Evolution*, edited by J. Strang and M. Gossop. Routledge, Abingdon, pp. 157–69.

Williams, H. and Norman, M., 2005. Safer injecting: individual harm reduction advice, in *Injecting Illicit Drugs. Blackwell Publishing*, edited by R. Partes, A. McBride and K. Arnold. Oxford: Blackwell Publishing (Addiction Press), pp. 135–59.

Box 2.1   References Relevant to 'Safer' Injecting Drug Use

A Visual Guide to Injecting Paraphernalia

The following photographs (Figures 2.1–2.3) depict the various paraphernalia central to injecting drug use. These images are accompanied by explanatory *Keys* that identify all equipment and, where necessary, provide short descriptions of function, purpose and role in the injecting process. The inclusion of these images is considered a useful pedagogic method for familiarising the readership with the type of equipment that is cited throughout this book and are terms/items that may be not be used in everyday speech/actions of all readers.

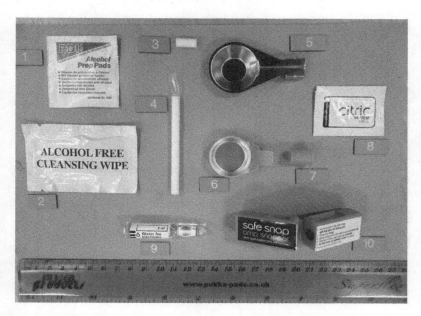

Figure 2.1 Paraphernalia Associated with Injecting Drug Use

Key to Figure 2.1

Item

1. Alcohol-based cleansing wipe (swab).
2. Alcohol free cleansing wipe (swab).
3. Single filter (designed for use with hand-rolling tobacco; less fibrous than cigarette filters and cotton wool).
4. Pack of filters (taken from box of filters for use with hand rolling tobacco).
5. Sterile spoon (also known as 'cooker' and used for 'cooking' drugs; regarded more hygienic than using a kitchen spoon or adapted metal cans [such as those used for carbonated drinks]). Note lengthy handle to permit holding and prevent burning fingers when 'cooking' drugs.
6. An earlier spoon design by Steri-cup® with shorter handle than Item 5 (now withdrawn from supply).
7. A Steri-cup® handle-cap (without this item attached greater opportunities arise for minor burns to occur).
8. Citric (used to mix with *brown* heroin and water in order to assist dissolving the former; citric does not need to be added to white heroin).
9. Glass water ampoule (containing 2ml of sterile water).
10. Ampoule snapper (used to avoid glass related injury when opening Item 9 above).

An Applied Visual Sociology: Picturing Harm Reduction

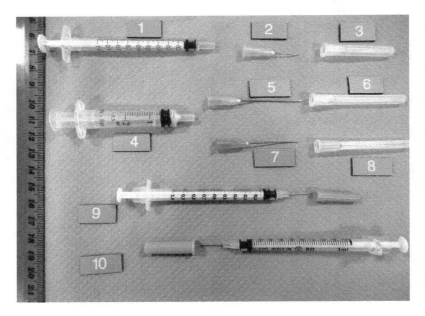

Figure 2.2 Needles and Syringes Used for Injecting Drug Use

Key to Figure 2.2

Item
1. 1 ml syringe barrel without needle attachment (Items 2, 5, and/or 7 may be attached).
2. 'Orange' needle attachment (often used for injecting into smaller veins in hands or feet). 25G 5/8" (see below).
3. Protective cap (for when not in use) for Item 2.
4. 2 ml syringe barrel without needle attachment (Item 5 and/or 7 may be attached). Often associated with femoral (groin) injecting
5. 'Green' needle attachment. Often associated with femoral (groin) injecting. 21G 1½" (see below).
6. Protective cap (for when not in use) for Item 5.
7. 'Blue' needle attachment. Often associated with femoral (groin) injecting. 23G 1¼" (see below).
8. Protective cap (for when not in use) for Item 7.
9. 1 ml syringe barrel with fixed needle attachment and protective cap (made available as single item in sealed pack). G29, 12.7mm (see below).
10. Variation of Item 9 with bolder calibration. Often termed as 'insulin syringe' due to associations with diabetes and insulin injections (and labelling on syringe barrel). Syringe, needle and cap made available as a single item in a sealed pack G29, 12.7mm (see below).

A Note on Needle and Syringe Identification[1]

- Needles used for injection are colour coded and universally identified by a 'G' number followed by a second numerical listing. For example, Item 2 = 25G 5/8".
- The 'G' number refers to the needle *gauge* and determines how thick/thin the needle is in diameter. Higher 'G' numbers are thinner needles; lower 'G' numbers are thicker needles.
- The second figure relates to the length of the needle in inches (") or millimetres (mm). Item 2 is therefore five-eighths of an inch in length. Injecting drug users typically refer to needle attachments by their colour-code (for example, 'greens' or 'blues').
- In Figure 2.2, Item 2 represents the thinnest needle on display in this set.
- As a rough guide, intravenous (into veins) injections and subcutaneous (below the skin) injections require a G number of 25–29. Intramuscular injections (buttocks, groin) require thicker needles with a G number of 21–23.
- Syringes are labelled in terms of the volume of liquid they can hold, usually in millilitres (mils). 1 cubic centimetre = 1 millilitre (1cc = 1 mil).
- Injecting drug users generally refer to needles by the appropriate colour-code (for example, 'I use green needles ... ') and syringes by their specified volume (' ... with 2mil syringes').

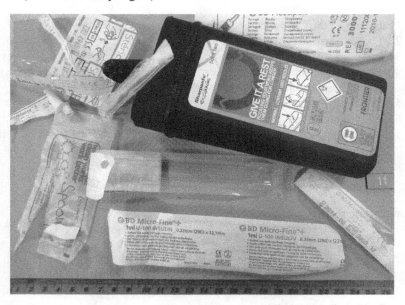

Figure 2.3   Drug-related Litter Associated with Injecting Drug Use

---

1   This account is based upon observational fieldwork conducted by the author within NSP at various settings throughout the south of England during 2006–2011 (see Parkin 2013).

Key to Figure 2.3

Item 11: A portable sharps container for depositing used equipment and paraphernalia (also known as a sharps box and/or 'cin bin [from in*cin*eration, not – as many may believe – from '*sin*'])

- Item 11 is surrounded by various seals and wrappers for containing needles and other paraphernalia contained in Figure 2.1 and 2.2. Litter such as these may serve as an indicator of locations used for street-based injecting.

A Harm Reduction Guide to 'Safer' Injecting Drug Use

The following section consists of five sub-sections that correlate to various stages associated with safer injecting drug use. These concern 'pre-injection' preparations and 'preparation of injecting environment' (pertaining to selecting/organising body and space within a particular environmental setting), followed by guidance on 'preparing to inject', and 'preparation of drug of solute'. The final section is concerned with the actual steps required to conduct an individual 'safer injecting' episode.

Pre-Injection

1. Locate a familiar environment for preparing and injecting drugs.
2. Environment should be safe from interruption and unexpected disturbances.
3. Environment should be quiet, relaxed and warm.
4. Environment should provide access to sterile water – or facilities to permit the boiling of water and space to allow it to cool.
5. Environment should be well-lit.
6. Environment should be hygienic and clean.
7. Always attend an injecting environment with another who can be relied upon to provide emergency assistance if needed.
8. Never inject alone.

Preparation of Injecting Environment

1. Avoid dirty/unclean surfaces.
2. Create a preparation space, preferably with a plastic tray, wiped with an alcohol swab or anti-bacterial gel.
3. If a plastic tray is not available, a newspaper or magazine will provide a temporary alternative.
4. Place all injecting paraphernalia – and drugs to be injected – onto the clean preparation surface.

5. Select preferred/required needles and syringes with appropriate gauge, length and volume for relevant injection site (on body).
6. Always use the most appropriate needle: thinner needles will reduce needle trauma to veins but thicker needles are needed for intramuscular injecting.
7. All injecting paraphernalia should be contained within their original seals. Avoid using equipment if it is not contained within the relevant wrappers (or if the seals are broken).
8. Safely store any excess equipment (remove from preparation surface).
9. Always have a sharps bin nearby at all times.
10. Never share any equipment. This includes water, filters, swabs, cookers, tourniquets and especially needles and syringes.

Preparing to Inject

1. Remove all jewellery attached near to injecting site (on body) – especially those items worn on the wrist and fingers (if injecting in those areas).
2. Wash hands and intended injecting area thoroughly with hot water and soap.
3. (If soap/water is unavailable for washing, improvise using alcohol swabs).
4. Dry hands with a clean towel.
5. (If using alcohol swabs, allow alcohol to dry on skin. If the alcohol is still wet then sterilisation of skin-site has not occurred).
6. (Preferred injecting locations are in the crook of the elbow. Veins in the hand and feet are fragile and easy to rupture. Always avoid injecting in the neck, groin, armpit, penis and breasts).
7. Remove seals from injecting equipment.
8. Preparation of drug solute
9. Place drug into clean, unused cooker.
10. If using *brown* heroin, add a small amount of citric.
11. (Do not use citric bought from supermarkets or grocery stores.)
12. If using *white* heroin, no citric is needed.
13. Add water from ampoule (being mindful how *glass* ampoules may be opened and discarded).
14. Stir liquid using needle cap until both substances are completely dissolved.
15. If necessary add more citric to assist further dissolving if solute appears granular or 'lumpy' (be aware that too much citric can create burning sensations when injected)
16. Once dissolved, heat the mixture, but do not boil.
17. Stir once more with the needle cap after removing heat source.
18. Place filter into the liquid.
19. Using both hands carefully place the tip of the needle onto the surface of the filter
20. (Avoid contact between needle tip and base of the spoon).

21. The needle aperture should be facing down when placed upon the filter so as to assist 'drawing up' solute into the syringe barrel.
22. When the solute is completely 'drawn up', expel air from syringe by moving the plunger towards the level of solute in the barrel.
23. (When air has been expelled, a small droplet of solute may appear on the needle tip. Do not lick this droplet).
24. Allow the solute to cool in the syringe.
25. As solute is cooling, clear up any seals and used equipment. Place all items into the sharps bin.

Safer Injecting

1. Avoid standing.
2. Avoid injecting into damaged veins, scar tissue, existing wounds, or swollen skin.
3. Avoid rolling veins between fingers.
4. Avoid arteries.
5. Do not insert the needle too deep or too shallow (as this will 'miss' the vein).
6. Do not push the plunger too quickly and too fast once the needle is in the vein (this can burst veins and/or initiate hypoxia).
7. When seated comfortably, raise a vein for injecting purposes by tapping the relevant vein area.
8. (Towels soaked in warm water can be used to help raise a vein when wrapped around the desired area).
9. If using a tourniquet do not fasten too tight (to allow for quick release).
10. Using appropriate needle, make sure the aperture is facing up (so as the point can pierce the skin surface).
11. Place tip of needle onto injection site with needle pointing towards the heart.
12. (If subcutaneous injecting, syringe needs to be 15–30 degrees to injecting site (body)).
13. (If intravenous injecting, syringe needs to be 15–45 degrees to injecting site (body)).
14. (If intramuscular injecting, syringe needs to be 45 degrees to injecting site (body)).
15. Slowly insert needle, insert only partially.
16. Feel for reduced resistance and cease inserting when resistance is complete.
17. Draw back the plunger.
18. (If intravenous injecting look at the blood colour entering the syringe; remember the adage, 'if it's red, go ahead, if it's pink, STOP and think').
19. Release tourniquet (if used).
20. Slowly push plunger towards needle.
21. If there is any pain, STOP injecting and withdraw the needle slowly.
22. Injection is complete when the syringe plunger is fully inserted into the barrel.

23. At this point, remove needle and syringe slowly from the injecting site.
24. Use clean tissue to stem any blood flow.
25. Immediately deposit used needle and syringe into the sharps box.
26. Never share (provide or receive) any equipment.

Critique of Safer Injecting Recommendations when Applied to Street-based Settings

From the above harm reduction guidelines one may note that there are a total of 68 key messages to remember and apply when injecting a particular substance. This is no easy task. (As an illustration of the complexities of this requirement, the reader is now requested to recall (without review or reference) as much as possible of the process described above). Nevertheless, no matter how familiar one may be with injecting behaviour, the above advice clearly prioritises individuals who may reside in safe, secure accommodation complete with appropriate furnishings and access to amenities such as running water and electricity. There is also the assumption that illicit drugs can be prepared and injected in a relatively relaxed atmosphere in which there is little chance of disturbance or interruption from others (whether hostile or friendly).

Essentially, the above guidelines represent an *idealist* and *optimistic* view of the preparation and injection of controlled substances. One should attempt to consider how the above guidelines may be undertaken by a street-based sex worker, a hostel resident (who may be evicted for possessing injecting paraphernalia), a homeless/roofless person and/or a parent who does not want to expose their family to (or reveal participation in) injecting drug use. Similarly, the above guidelines do not appropriately consider the social nature of drug use, such as acquiring money to buy drugs *together*, sharing drugs *together*, sharing resources as part of reciprocal or intimate partner *relationships* (Parkin 2013).

In the context of street-based injecting many of those guidelines above are made null and void due to the socio-spatial circumstances that many of those who inject in public locations find themselves in (see Chapters 5–7). Similarly, the various environments appropriated during street-based injecting do not provide naturally-occurring sanitised surfaces, adequate lighting, comfortable seating areas where jewellery can be removed without fear of loss. Nor do they contain relaxed, ambient atmospheres that facilitate careful, considered and meticulously efficient injecting technique and hygienic (hand washing) procedures. Instead, as will be made evident in later chapters, street-based injecting is characterised by perpetual haste, hurriedness and swift actions; all of which are strategies used to avoid detection, interruption and a loss of liberty whilst situated within public environments. In such locations, it would be almost impossible to perform all 68 of the above guidelines without some form of interruption or disturbance from a member of the public – or by a police officer. From a street-based perspective, the above 68-point formula for safer injecting becomes condensed into the following 5-point charter:

1. Identify suitable environment.
2. Prepare solute as quickly as possible.
3. Draw solute into syringe.
4. Inject rapidly.
5. Exit setting as quickly as one entered.

Due to the idealistic and optimistic expectations associated with injecting drug use, Bourgois et al. (1997) are of the view that in the context of street-based injecting such guidance may be interpreted as the provision of 'hypersanitary ... messages'. Furthermore, these messages 'exemplify how the medical establishment morally rebukes street addicts by promoting unrealistic slogans ... that relegate street addicts to the category of self-destructive other' (Bourgois et al. 1997, 160–1) (*sic*). In short, these criticisms echo those outlined above (as they concur with the harmful socio-spatial circumstances surrounding street-based injecting and relate to the reciprocal and reciprocating lived experiences associated with a drug-centred lifestyle).

Chapters 1 and 2 have summarised the topics of inquiry that frame this study and provided an introductory overview of issues relating to visual methods, harm reduction and injecting drug use. The remainder of this book now focuses upon a *visually*-focused, *theoretically*-driven, *empirical* account of street-based injecting drug use in four British settings throughout the south of England. This account commences in the following chapter in which the methodology and methods of inquiry underlying the five-year study are presented.

PART II
Empiricism

Chapter 3
Methodology and Methods

Thus far, Part I of this book has provided a review of visual research and provided an introductory overview of harm reduction. What has emerged from these initial chapters is that although there appears to be meaningful and significant academic overlap between visual methods and harm reduction, there has been less of a concerted effort to advance the notion of an 'applied visual sociology' in the field of substance use. Part II of this book therefore attempts to address this disciplinary paucity in providing an account of a specific research design applied to the study of street-based injecting. The intent of this Chapter (and the remainder of this book) is to establish and promote flexible guidelines for conducting methodologically-driven and applied visual research for use across the social sciences (and especially within sociology).

Although the title of this book advocates *visual* research in the discipline of sociology, it should be stressed that the work described throughout this text included the combined use of qualitative approaches in a multi-site, longitudinal study of street-based injecting drug use. Indeed, it is more accurate to state that video and/or photography in the relevant fieldwork settings were employed as methods to support and enrich more orthodox measures of data collection (such as interviews, observation, fieldnotes).

In *Habitus and Drug Using Environments* (Parkin 2013) the author provides a more *theoretical* account of street-based injecting drug use based upon analyses of more traditional 'language-based' datasets (interview transcripts, reflexive fieldnotes, analytic memos etc.). *This* book is also concerned with the same six-year period of research described in *Habitus and Drug Using Environments*, but extends focus upon the various accounts of *visual methods* employed throughout the study in order to emphasise the impact afforded by these procedures in aiding the identification of drug-related harm. As such, it is important the reader recognises that the use of visual methods throughout the various studies was only one aspect of a suite of qualitative methods employed throughout the relevant period. Similarly, the overall rationale for including visual methods within the qualitative research design was to purposely synthesise 'academic' and 'applied' sociology. More precisely, it was envisaged that the inclusion of visual methods would inform the academy of a particular 'research method' whilst simultaneously generate meaningful knowledge for service intervention at local, national and, possibly, international levels.

This chapter therefore represents an amended and edited version of the corresponding section that appears in *Habitus and Drug Using Environment*. Whereas the latter work focuses almost entirely upon the *theoretical* framework underlying this research,[1] this book prioritises the *epistemological* positioning of all research conducted by the author during 2006–2011 (that is, relating to a harm reduction approach to public injecting drug use). As such, this 'methods' chapter consists of a reworked version of that contained within *Habitus and Drug Using Environments*, in which the initial section is concerned with the overall research philosophy (*Methodology*) and a second section provides an account of the processes conducted during all fieldwork (*Methods*). Due to the methodological innovation attached to this study (relating to the deployment of visual methods to inform harm reduction), this chapter is followed by an 'additional' methodological concern not previously included in *Habitus and Drug Using Environments* and summarises the analytical processes conducted throughout this study (see Chapter 4).

In order to proceed, it is perhaps necessary to provide a 'purpose statement' (Cresswell 2003) that encapsulates the overall design of the research underlying the empirical study described within this book. According to Cresswell (ibid.) the inclusion of purpose statements prior to undertaking of any social research represents good practice and academic rigour. Similarly, the design of such a statement is useful for maintaining a fundamental research focus – not only for the researcher(s) concerned but also for the audience and/or readership of the eventual findings.

Purpose Statement

This *qualitative research* is designed to articulate the essence of public (that is, street-based) injecting in *four* urban settings within the UK. The research follows *interpretive and ethnographic traditions*, which are applied in settings that have been directly affected by the issue or experiences of street-based injecting drug use. These qualitative modes of inquiry are *ontologically* located within a *critical realist* paradigm, in which all research is *epistemologically* informed by the practice and principles of *harm reduction*. Finally, all data analysis is anchored within particular schools of thought (that of applied harm reduction and Pierre Bourdieu's critical theory) as a means of interrogating the role of *structure* and *agency* in the context of injecting drug use.

The *aim* of the study however, is to identify the way in which 'place' (that is, environments located in street-based settings) may affect episodes of injecting drug use. Accordingly, this research aims to cross-examine the way in which different environments may influence harm (whether environmentally, socially and spatially) within the lived-experience of injecting drug use from the *theoretical* and *applied* perspectives of habitus and harm reduction respectively. Similarly, the research aims to *visualise* the lived-experiences of public injecting drug use and

---

1 In which the author presents an empirical assessment of Pierre Bourdieu's theoretical construct of *habitus* in the context of public injecting drug use.

the environments that influence the embodiment of a particular logic of practice in which the latter may produce and reproduce drug-related harm.

Methodology

The above 'purpose statement' outlines the key methodological principles (in italics) attached to this study. In the following account, the reader is guided through the ontological and epistemological positions that characterise the methodological stance of this study. Each of these aspects are summarised below in order to provide further clarification of the overall research design and rationale attached to this work.

Ontological Positioning: Realism

As noted in Chapter 1, a social science interest in ontology relates to the nature of existence, the state of being and how this is unpacked via academic inquiry. The specific ontological position of this study however is one that accepts all knowledge exists as apprehendable realities and independent of individual social worlds (Guba and Lincoln 2004). That is, this research employs a 'realist' ontology in which other realities exist beyond subject social worlds and that these worlds can be made comprehensible by means of rational abstraction (Becker and Bryman 2004, Guba and Lincoln 2004). This view stands in contrast to a positivist tradition that assumes reality is objective and can be made comprehensible by measurement, observation and testing, in which researchers are able to remain objective and detached from the field of inquiry (Banks 2007, Guba and Lincoln 2004).

The nature of relationships and behaviour within these realities is a further defining feature of ontology (Bhaskar 1989, Stanley and Wise 1993), in which a 'realist' paradigm seeks to identify causal mechanisms resulting in specific outcomes. Critical realism further posits that the world is stratified by social structures, relationships and interaction that is characterised by power (and powerlessness), each of which are capable of producing and reproducing associative knowledge and behaviour as a response (Guba and Lincoln 2004, May 1997). Bhaskar refers to this often concealed symbiotic relationship as 'generative mechanisms' that may 'endure (whilst) inactive and act where ... there is no one-to-one relationship' (Bhaskar 1978, 48–51). Sayer (2000) advocates a realist research design aims to uncover these mechanisms and to determine how they may have been activated. Consequently, a realist research agenda is predominantly 'context-dependant' as it is premised upon the nature of social worlds relating to the cause and effect of behaviour within structures. Sayer furthers this view in adding that realism is also concerned with 'concept-dependence' (Sayer 2000, 18) in which individual reasons for meaningful action may extend beyond the physical setting and become constructs that simultaneously shape behaviour.

A study of social action informed by a realist ontology is both concept and context dependant. Research within realist ontology therefore seeks to uncover social worlds extraneous to the researcher in an attempt to explain behaviour, beliefs and attitudes by reference to the 'conditions in which they (are) situated' (Sayer 2000, 24). Such explanations are made possible by the employment of qualitative methods located in 'natural' settings. Such practice essentially involves 'getting closer' to the realities under investigation, as a pragmatic way of accessing and understanding respondents' social worlds and associated knowledge.

A 'realist' research design would appear entirely appropriate when applied to an empirical assessment of street-based drug using environments upon harm reduction (and harm production) due to the interaction of structure, agency, context and concept. From this perspective, the employment of interview strategies therefore seeks to document the experience of others as 'meaningful properties' (Mason 2002, 63) whereas ethnographic observation aims to represent 'faithfully the true nature of social phenomena' (Hammersly 1992, 44). The use of visual methods however, seek to further explicate the relevant findings and demonstrate the applied value of photography/video by informing 'harm reduction' service development and/or intervention.

Visual Methodology and Realism

The application of a visual-oriented methodology is deployed in this study as a means of facilitating the 'realist' inquiry of the social and environmental arenas of injecting drug use. In this research, visual methodology refers to the *applied* use of photography and video as a means of 'capturing' particular social and physical realities associated with street-based injecting.[2]

Whilst Ball and Smith (1992) acknowledge that some researchers may question the credibility of attempts at realist representations of cultural phenomena with visual images, they equally infer similar criticisms may be attached to qualitative inquiry *per se*. As such, attempts at visualising 'realism' in this study concur with the view that documentary photography (and video) can provide an adequate, albeit tentative, method for reflecting 'how the world is and the way it works' (Ball and Smith 1992, 17). Indeed, the aforementioned caution regarding realist representations is echoed here, in that *all* ethnographic data are ultimately the craft of the individual responsible for collecting such information.

---

2 To reiterate, this 'visual methodology' complemented and emulated the more orthodox methodological approach described throughout this chapter. That is, the visual methodology should not necessarily be regarded as a framework that existed outwith the overall methodological design of the study.

As such, in the context of visual data, cameras *can* lie and pictures can paint a thousand *lies* (Schonberg and Bourgois 2002, 388) due to the ambiguous and polysemic content of 'naked images' (that is, those without explanatory text or other detail). As emphasised in Chapter 1, the basis of such ambiguity often rests upon a viewers' own 'ethnocentric judgements, social affiliations' (Ball and Smith 1992, 20), subjectivity, prejudices, values and beliefs. Accordingly, it is the visual researcher's challenge to re-present all data in a manner that facilitates comprehension whilst being compatible with the overall methodological (ontological and epistemological) design of the study.

For these reasons, this research provides a demonstration of the aforementioned challenge in which all visual images of injecting environments are accompanied by interpretative accounts that situate content, referent and context of image as authentic evidence of the relevant ontological, epistemological, theoretical and applied assumptions attached to this study. Without the language-based explanations accompanying the visual datasets, it is entirely probable that images of injecting environments contained in this work would be viewed differently by other professions, academic disciplines and possibly initiate conflicting (and valid) interpretations to those of the author.

Visual data in this study have been collected, collated and represented in a manner to reflect not only the social and physical organisation of injecting environments, (from individual and collective perspectives) but also the structural and societal level responses/circumstances that initiate/perpetuate drug-related harm and hazard. Visual methodologies in this context aim to identify the way in which harm may be produced within street-based environments and to make the *invisible* hazards associated with public injecting environments more *visible* to harm reduction intervention in an almost literal manner.

Visual Methods and Realism

In addition to the above, the actual *methods* of visual data generation also seek to synthesise the methodological orientations of this work. More specifically, taking photographs of injecting environments (that are informed by frontline service personnel[3]) coupled with video-recordings of these settings (informed by injecting drug users) introduces polysemic representations of shared public space to the research project as a whole. Data generated by the above mixed visual methods, used in conjunction with wider ethnographic inquiry, seeks to determine the social organisation of injecting environments and assist in identifying drug-related harm within the affected public settings encountered during all fieldwork.

---

3   This term is used throughout this book to describe various forms of street-based employment. This term is an all-encompassing expression that includes police officers, security guards, toilet attendants, drugs workers, outreach staff, social workers, refuse collectors and those employed by statutory, non-statutory and third-sector bodies.

Representations of social phenomena accrued in a visual manner typically involve 'engaging in a *process* through which knowledge is produced' (Pink 2007b, 105, original emphasis) in the particular social world under investigation. In this regard, the methodological value of photography/video-making aims to consolidate authentic experience in providing opportunities for the author to physically engage with, and better understand, street-based injecting environments through a process of actually 'doing' data collection. Visual data obtained in this manner seeks to strengthen the ontological positioning as it aims to 'visualise' verbal accounts of respondents' experiences of street-based injecting as well as the structural circumstances underlying the phenomenon.

Furthermore, the overall methodological design aims to generate data that inform realist representations of street-based injecting drug use; to 'visualise' verbal accounts and 'verbalise' visual representations of these environments. Cumulatively, and from an *ontological perspective*, this multi-faceted qualitative research design seeks to provide authenticity with the generation of assorted 'thicker descriptions' of lived-experiences of street-based injecting drug use from a variety of contradictory and corresponding perspectives. Such authenticity emerges from an analysis of the inter-relationship between local structures (including social policy, practice and law enforcement procedures); social agency (of injecting drug users and frontline service personnel) and through an engagement with specific public environments affected by injecting drug use. The challenge of the study is to situate these *oppositional* experiences and perspectives within an epistemological (and analytical) framework that usefully informs the practice and principles of harm reduction.

Finally, the visual methods attached to this work (described below) aim to portray the social, political and cultural contexts (Keller et al. 2008) of street-based injecting drug use and *assist* (not illustrate) in elucidating a range of harm associated with street-based drug use. From a *methodological* perspective, the collection of visual data aims to concretise the reliability, credibility, validity and generalisability of findings relating to *longitudinal* studies of public injecting drug use. Accordingly, the combined application of visual and non-visual *methods* facilitate a process of data triangulation (Quine and Taylor 1998) towards the identification of harm and hazard associated with a *public injecting habitus* (Parkin 2013). This triangulation process is further assisted by the interrogation of the diverse, yet constituent, aspects of street-based injecting drug use that are observed and encountered in four different geographic locations in the south of England.[4]

---

4 These settings are Barking, Dagenham (both Outer London), Plymouth (Devon), and Southend-on-Sea (Essex). All locations are described at length in this book's 'companion' text, *Habitus and Drug Using Environments* (Parkin 2013).

Epistemological Stance

Epistemology is concerned with theories of knowledge, its production and how individuals assume to know what they claim to know. As with ontology, epistemology is a foundational and integral component of any research design within the social sciences. It is these methodological traditions that provide the bases for constructing – and *de*constructing – academic discourse, debate and argument. These methodological principles equally inform applied research as they may facilitate and validate advocacy, transformation and restitution within particular fields of practice (for example, health-care). Epistemological and ontological groundings are therefore not only the prerequisite 'nuts and bolts' within a researcher's toolbox, they are also the metaphorical compasses that guide the vessel that is 'social science'.

Epistemology #1: Research is Political

The epistemological positioning of the author is twofold. The first epistemological stance adopted in this study is that research objectivity within the social sciences is an artificial and implausible construct (see Schostak and Schostak (2008) for a more detailed account of this claim). As Mills (1959) notes, social scientists are often located *within*, and not separate from, the societies and cultures they study. Accordingly, and as noted by Letherby (2003), social researchers are *complicit* in the worlds they study; in which their own subjectivity, political persuasion and associated values may consciously and/or unconsciously influence the design, delivery and outcome of research agendas. Due to this potential for subjective bias, whether conscious or unconscious, it has been claimed that 'hygienic research is a myth' (Letherby 2003, 68), with the implication that research objectivity is an unrealistic pursuit (or one that may serve to simplify and/or obscure findings). Furthermore, as a result of the social and economic structures that influence, direct and determine individual lives on a daily basis (Mills 1959), the author contends that research subjectivity is generally *politically*-orientated. Accordingly, a related contention is that *all* research is unavoidably political; in terms of funding, design, delivery and dissemination of findings. Such a claim is not unique within sociological research and is by no means a declaration of radical intent. Indeed, 'Bourdieu has said repeatedly that the production of scientific texts is a political act' (LiPuma 1993, 15), and his sociological analyses have been described as 'a mode of *political intervention*' (Swartz 1997, 12, original emphasis). Similarly, others have discussed research as a component of institutionalised power, or describe unequal power relations that may exist between researchers and the researched (Bourgois 2000, Bourgois and Schonberg 2009, Fitzgerald 1996, Hammersley 1995, Rhodes and Fitzgerald 2006).

Indeed, it is perhaps difficult to dispute this particular politically-constructed contention given that the collated body of research summarised within this book was funded by the Economic and Social Research Council of Great Britain (2006–2009), Plymouth Drug and Alcohol Action Team (DAAT) (2006–2009), and subsequently commissioned by Barking and Dagenham DAAT (2010) and Southend-on-Sea DAAT (2010–2011) as part of a (post-doctoral) research initiative based at the University of Plymouth (Parkin, Coomber and Wallace 2010). *All* of these bodies and organisations receive funding and direction from central government. As such, the epistemological stance adopted throughout this study is that research cannot be apolitical and that there must *always* be an underlying political agenda associated with social research.

It is for these reasons that the following sentence is included in the above Purpose Statement: *all data analysis is anchored within particular schools of thought (that of applied harm reduction and Pierre Bourdieu's critical theory) as a means of interrogating the role of structure and agency in the context of injecting drug use.* That is to say, critical theory has been considered as an ontological framework for deconstructing and challenging the political and individual circumstances that surround injecting drug use in street-based settings. This however is not intended to be mis/interpreted as a statement of personal ideology on behalf of the author. Instead it should be considered as a legitimate sociological and epistemological challenge that seeks to interrogate structural forces that influence (whether positively or negatively) the lives of those that inject illicit drugs. Additionally, this epistemological stance follows a disciplinary tradition within sociology, established by 'founding fathers' (such as Karl Marx, Emile Durheim, and Talcott Parsons), regarding a drive towards social reform, transformation and emancipation in which social scientists purposely engage in addressing social issues (Becker 1967, Bloor 1997, Scheper-Hughes 1995, Schostak and Schostak 2008). As Kincheloe and McLaren (1994) note:

> (c)ritical research can be best understood in the context of the empowerment of individuals. Inquiry that aspires to the name *critical* must be connected to an attempt to confront the injustice of a particular society or sphere within the society. Research thus becomes a transformative endeavour unembarrassed by the label 'political' and unafraid to consummate a relationship with an emancipatory consciousness. (Kincheloe and McLaren 1994, 140, original emphasis)

As such, this research is openly 'critical', in which the author unashamedly seeks to emulate the above sentiments in providing research findings of practicable value to support the principles of a *harm reduction* approach to drug-related hazards. This is the second epistemological stance adopted throughout this research.

Epistemology #2: Harm Reduction Advocacy

In addition to the above political stance is also an interpretative epistemology brought to the research as a result of the author's previous professional and experiential training in drug-related issues. More specifically, prior to embarking upon this large-scale, multi-site study of street-based injecting, the author had previously provided assistance on several qualitative, substance use-related research projects during 1995–2005 (for example, Barnard 2006, Forsyth 2013, McKeganey, Neale, Parkin and Mills 2004, Parkin and McKeganey 2000, Walker et al. 2011). Most of these studies were located throughout Scotland and/or the north of England, but most required an awareness of current drug and alcohol policy, including a general awareness of harm reduction, drug treatment and law enforcement procedures throughout the UK. Accordingly, the author had accumulated almost one-decade of applied harm reduction awareness at the onset of commencing a doctoral study of street-centred injecting drug use in 2006 (in Plymouth, Devon). For these reasons, it would not have been possible to become removed and/or completely detached from these professional influences and associated *knowledge* in a study that directly concerned policy, practice and injecting drug use. As such, the author's conscious and unconscious awareness of harm reduction approaches to drug use were purposely embraced and advocated throughout all research concerning street-based injecting drug use.

As described in Chapter 2, harm reduction approaches to drug use typically shift an emphasis from the criminalisation of drug use/rs towards a reform of public health intervention and the wider social environment (Buning 1990, Hathaway 2006). In adopting an epistemology that acknowledges these values in harm reduction, the research becomes dedicated to unpacking meaning, motive and lived-experiences of drug use that are spatially, culturally and contextually bound. Consequently, the findings described throughout this work may be defined as 'value mediated' (Guba and Lincoln 2004, 26) as the research, researcher and researched are linked by a common cause, (that is, the reduction of drug-related harm in public places).

Converging Epistemology

The two epistemological positions described above converge when considered in the applied context of this study. For example, if service development in the field of harm reduction is denied on the basis of activities considered illegal and illegitimate (that is, possessing/injecting illicit drugs) then such reactions may be described as contravening individual health rights (Barret et al. 2009, Turner 1993) and access to health-care. Accordingly, this research seeks to 'consummate a relationship' (methodologically and politically) with harm reduction approaches to drug use in providing findings that explicate place-specific hazard to injecting drug users and to inform and/or advocate intervention that seeks to minimise these harms. Such an epistemological convergence may be regarded as an illustration of the way in which 'researchers ... should be laying the groundwork for citizen resistance rather than fostering the extension and effectiveness of expert power' (Bloor 1997, 319). In adopting such an approach to sociological inquiry, an academic allegiance may be further drawn with Bourdieu's own brand of 'activist science' (Wacquant 2008, 262) or the advocacy of the 'transformative intellectual' (Guba and Lincoln 2004, 29) concerning attempts within the academy at challenging inequality, promoting social justice, preventing the abuse of power and 'disseminat(ing) weapons for resistance to symbolic domination' (Wacquant 2008 276).

Despite conceding that this text is a politically-orientated study, it should be further reiterated that these concerns are *not* premised upon any ideology or structural subversion that may have been improperly attached to the harm reduction movement (for example, cf. Smith 2012). Similarly, whilst concurring with the false promise of objectivity, attempts have been made to ensure that any author bias throughout all fieldwork/analysis was monitored by means of 'theorised subjectivity' (Letherby 2003, 71–2); in which researcher subjectivity is accepted but regulated by a process of reflexivity.

On Reflexivity

Qualitative research is typically physically-situated in the social world, in which researchers are typically 'outsiders' within the relevant milieu they choose to study. This 'marginal' status of the researcher has potential to establish problems relating to subjectivity, bias and political persuasion (Hammersley and Atkinson 1995) that in turn may affect the findings obtained. Consequently, there is a need for constant critical awareness whilst engaged in social research, (of the self and of the data collected), and for a need to develop a reflexive approach to all aspects of fieldwork. Bourdieu refers to this process as 'epistemological vigilance' (cited in Webb et al. 2002: xii) and involves developing an ability to shift between understanding data and the way it is collected by means of detached self-scrutiny (Hertz 1997). In applying such introspection the researcher seeks to establish a dialogue with the self that is intended to provide a 'reconstructed logic of inquiry' (Hammersley and Atkinson 1995) and simultaneously provide awareness of the relevant research setting. Such systematic practice is intended to enrich data collection and the analytical process that subsequently contribute to the credibility and validity of research findings (ibid.).

Qualitative Research

The use of verbal and physical communication between researchers and research respondents is employed throughout the social sciences as a key method of symbolically accessing the social worlds of others (Parkin 2013). As such, in this study, the 'sociological interview' (with frontline service personnel and drug users) is employed as the initial point of entry to the physical places used for injecting drug use and as a meaningful way of generating knowledge relating to place-based experiences of drug-using environments. However, as this knowledge acquisition typically relies upon research respondents' overall ability to adequately recall and verbalise the experiences subject to study, the research interview *per se* may not necessarily be completely reliable if used as the sole method of data collection. Accordingly, given that this study prioritises '*place*-based *experiences*' of injecting drug use, the sociological interview is complemented by other qualitative modes of inquiry; namely *ethnographic observation* and *visual methods* (that is, street-based photography and video recording).

A qualitative research design is applied in this study in order to obtain 'thick description' (Geertz 1973) of the social and environmental experiences attached to street-based injecting drug use. Furthermore, a critical and interpretive framework of inquiry is applied to the study to further explain collective and conflicting accounts of the relevant drug-using environments. This is facilitated by extensive contact with those affected by public injecting environments (whether injecting drug users or frontline service personnel) and aims to provide an account of public injecting that is verbally and visually informed by their respective experiences and perspectives. In adopting such methodological assumption, the 'meaning' of place-based injecting practice emerges from data analysis whilst simultaneously informs the practice of harm reduction at an applied level.

Ethnography

Various researchers (Emerson, Fretz and Shaw 1995, Mason 2002) have described ethnography as a valuable means of gaining appreciation of others' social realities, of comprehending the fluctuating nature of social life including its associated uncertainties and complexities. Such commendations essentially relate to *ontology*, regarding the philosophical study of the way in which others exist. This is due to the premise that ethnographic observations and assumptions are premised upon how the social world *per se* is organised and negotiated from other perspectives. In the context of 'place-orientated' research such as this, the joint-application of phenomenological and ethnographic traditions seek to interrogate the social and environmental contexts of injecting environments, whilst simultaneously 'capturing the actors' point of view' (Schwandt 1994, 121).

Ethnographic fieldwork is incorporated into the research design as a means of observing public injecting sites in 'naturalistic' settings in order to acquire an environmental and spatial appreciation of these locations. This mode of inquiry specifically aims to provide important detail of the environmental circumstances attached to particular settings that may escape the more formal interview process. Furthermore, as noted by Pink (2007b), ethnographic knowledge does not necessarily rely upon observation alone and may incorporate a multitude of encounters that are material, physical, sensory and social. As a means of capturing this experiential diversity, this study implements a *visual*-orientated ethnography in order to purposely generate applied output that aims to provide solution-focused responses to 'real world' problems relating to injecting drug use (see below).

Serial Triangulation

Although triangulation strategies are frequent within social research, the process has typically relied upon mixing qualitative and quantitative methods. For example, surveys and questionnaires may be used simultaneously to inform/validate semi-structured interview schedules (and/or vice versa). However, in this study, visual data contributes to triangulation processes in a genuinely innovative manner. This is because visual methods facilitate the cross-examination of all language-based data during on-going and final analyses. Similarly, by incorporating visual data collection alongside other facets of qualitative research in *four consecutive* and *four different* geographic locations, the assorted findings are subject to a process of continuous and on-going testing, confirmation and corroboration. This valid*ation* and valid*ating* process, conducted in a linear process across several geographic settings, is here termed *serial triangulation* (Parkin 2013).

Serial triangulation therefore refers to the multi-site context of empirically tested research and specifically in regard to the topics of street-based injecting and harm reduction. Accordingly, serial triangulation can only provide increased credibility and validity to the research conclusions, in which observed regularities and consistencies within the findings may assist the overall 'generalisability' of qualitative research regarding street-based injecting issues (cf. Pearson, Parkin and Coomber 2011)

To close this section on methodological orientation, it is perhaps necessary to reiterate the paradigms and traditions associated with this study of street-based injecting. In short, what follows is an account that is guided by paradigm of critical theory, that follows an ontology of critical realism with an epistemology that prioritises the practice and principles of harm reduction (see Chapter 2). In order to interpret street-based injecting environments within this disciplinary vision the appropriate approach would involve transactional, communicative, dialogical and dialectical research methods (Guba and Lincoln 2004) that permit the subjective and reflexive reconstruction of 'other' multiple realities. The methods used in this study to satisfy this methodological requirement are summarised below. As will be further noted, these methods were all *qualitative* in design and application in order to reflect the interpretive and dialectical bases of the study.

Methods: Serial Triangulation Explained

Whereas the previous section concerned the methodology underlying this study, the following presents a summary of the methods that were applied in the four geographic settings where fieldwork was physically located. If a research methodology may be compared to the spine of a body representing the core of its being, then the methods of research, following this corporeal analogy, may be regarded as the way in which this body is 'fleshed out'. Similarly, methods of research represent the way in which the overall research design becomes *embodied* by the researcher and become manifest in the way in which data are collected.

As noted above, this is a *second* book founded upon research that took place in four English towns/cities during the period 2006–2011. The initial phase of the study was based in the south-west of England, in the city of Plymouth (2006–2009). This stage of the study was the author's doctoral research completed as a studentship granted by the Economic and Social Research Council (ESRC) of Great Britain (Parkin 2009a). More significantly, this was also a study completed as part of the ESRC's Collaborative Award in Science and Engineering (CASE) scheme. This is significant to the epistemological and applied design described above, as CASE studentships involved the award of finances (from the ESRC) to an academic institution (following the submission of a successful research application) to conduct social science research in partnership with a non-academic institution. In this instance the non-academic institution was Plymouth Drug and Alcohol Action Team (DAAT), (a local-level, statutory body responsible for overseeing and implementing the national government's drug and alcohol strategy) and the academic partner was the University of Plymouth. Although the CASE studentship scheme has now been discontinued by the ESRC, this award was an early example of the way in which the ESRC continues to facilitate the academy and industry in developing collaborative and applied research to inform policy and practice. The initial study of public injecting was located in the city of Plymouth, commenced in October 2006 and concluded in August 2009 with the submission of the author's doctoral thesis.

Upon completion of the above doctoral research, the author assisted in the development of a research initiative at the University of Plymouth, known as the Public Injecting Rapid Appraisal Service (PIRAS). This project offered the public injecting-related research conducted throughout Plymouth as a 'service' available for commission and was aimed specifically at those with an interest in local drug and alcohol issues (Parkin, Coomber and Wallace 2010). PIRAS was subsequently commissioned by two more DAAT during 2010–11. These research commissioners were located in the London Borough of Barking and Dagenham and the Essex town of Southend-on-Sea. Whereas the initial study of street-based injecting took a period of three years to complete (as a result of the academic and doctoral focus), the two commissioned studies were completed in two consecutive six-month periods in which the author was responsible for all data collection, analysis and writing-up. The Barking and Dagenham study took place in 2010 (April–October) and was followed by further research located in Southend (November 2010–May 2011).

Although some variation in research methods did exist during all fieldwork, it should be stressed that this relates almost entirely to the time that was available to complete the original study (three years). For example, the doctoral research provided opportunities to include more lengthy periods of ethnographic research, greater attachment within various street-based settings and some analysis of relevant quantitative data. However, in the commissioned studies, this period of fieldwork was intensified and condensed into two eight-week periods (four months) in which the author physically relocated to the sites in question. As such, the commissioned studies were genuine attempts at the *rapid appraisal* method incorporated into the PI*RA*S moniker.

Rapid Appraisal

Rapid appraisal methods (McKeganey 2000, Murray et al. 1994, Ong et al. 1991, Parkin and Coomber 2011, Rhodes et al. 2000, Stimson et al. 1998) may be regarded as a means to gather suitable data regarding a particular issue as quickly and efficiently as possible in order to accelerate and implement an equally swift response by the relevant stakeholder organisations. As such, the array of qualitative methods used in the author's doctoral study of public injecting (Parkin 2009a) were subsequently adopted, adapted and re-applied in three further settings albeit in a more rapid and condensed format. Similarly, despite some variation in the time/completion ratios between the funded and commissioned studies, the qualitative methods attached to each study were consistent across all four geographic locations.[5]

Described below is a summary of the shared methods that were applied by the author throughout all studies of street-based injecting drug use in four English settings. Although these studies were conducted specifically for particular organisations, they are nevertheless *thematically* and *theoretically* connected. Similarly, as all research was conducted by the author in a linear process, the various findings obtained from the application of the same methods produces a rigorous process of continuous and on-going testing, confirmation and corroboration of the emergent findings. As such, the work described in this book has been subject to a process of on-going validation and validating, in which the theoretical and applied (harm reduction) arguments have been empirically-tested on *four* occasions! This process is here termed *serial triangulation* and relates to the overall credibility and veracity of the research findings. However, the *techniques* of serial triangulation relate to the methods of research applied during data collection. As such, the remainder of this chapter focuses upon those methods.

---

5   Barking, Dagenham, Plymouth and Southend-on-Sea.

Table 3.1 Methods of Research within a Methodological Framework

Method	Function	Methodological Value
Ethnography and Observation	1. To obtain thick-descriptions of drug-related issues events in community settings 2. To directly observe wider community issues 3. To observe settings attended by drug users and the relationship with key staff	Ontology of experience; rational abstraction of others' social realities Epistemology of harm reduction
Environmental Visual Assessments	1. To visit and observe the varied environmental conditions used for injecting drug use in public settings 2. To familiarise the researcher with the physical settings used for injecting episodes and to assess these locations from a harm reduction perspective 3. To elicit the views of non-drug users (community residents/various employees) affected by public injecting 4. To observe and note how public injecting is policed and managed from a harm reduction perspective 5. To compare interview data with environmental setting and identify constants/discrepancies 6. To photograph sites of public injecting drug use	Ontology of experience; rational abstraction of others' social realities Epistemology of harm reduction
Semi-structured interviews with 169 frontline service personnel	1. To appreciate public injecting from a range of experiences 2. To note how/where/when public injecting immediately impacts upon 'workplaces' and/or community settings 3. To consider official responses to public injecting issues from a harm reduction perspective 4. To discuss matters relating to drug-related litter and identify associated concerns 5. To identify structural barriers to local harm reduction intervention	Ontology of experience; rational abstraction of others' social realities Epistemology of harm reduction
Semi-structured interviews with 71 injecting drug users	1. To discuss the lived-experience of public injecting 2. To consider the effect of place upon injecting practice 3. To discuss injecting-related harms and hazards associated with public injecting 4. To assist in identifying a range of public settings frequented for the purpose of injecting 5 To empirically test the public injecting habitus concept	Ontology of experience; rational abstraction of others' social realities Epistemology of harm reduction

Serial Triangulation Illustrated

The qualitative research methods employed during all studies of public injecting drug use involved ethnography and participant observation; semi-structured interviews, visual methods (photography and video) and environmental visual assessments (EVA) of street-based settings used for injecting drug use. These methods are described in further detail below and have been summarised in Table 3.1 (which also indicates the methodological value of each approach). Each of the aforementioned methods were conducted in all four geographic settings of the study and involved interviews with a cumulative cohort of 169 frontline personnel, 71 injecting drug users and visits to over 400 sites affected by regular episodes of injecting drug use.[6] Table 3.2 collapses this dataset and depicts the number of research respondents that participated in the study per location. In addition to these data were also the various *visual* databases generated throughout the study, in which over 1,000 digital images and over one-hour of video footage were accrued for visual data analysis.

Table 3.2 The Collapsed Dataset

Location	Injecting Drug Users	Frontline Service Personnel	Total	Year
Plymouth	31	33	64	2006–2009
Barking & Dagenham	20	63	83	2010
Southend on Sea	20	73	93	2010–2011
Total	71	169	240	

Negotiating Access

Several potential problems were identified prior to the commencement of any fieldwork in each of the four locations. Primarily, injecting drug use typically involves the use of illicit drugs (such as heroin, crack-cocaine) and consequently is an activity one may not openly disclose, and probably less-so when part of another's research agenda. Furthermore, all related research aimed to recruit a cohort of drug users with recent experience of injecting substances in public settings (such as car parks, toilets). This potentially problematised recruitment procedures as previous research notes stigma and shame associated with public injecting (Rhodes et al. 2007, 2008). These issues thus raised concerns of a

---

6 In which 'regular' is defined as 'on-going and within the last month'.

possible reluctance to 'double disclose' sensitive information to the author in the relevant research settings.

A second potential difficulty related to gaining access to injecting sites and how the author would negotiate this in a manner that would be considered ethically sound for all concerned. It is perhaps due to similar considerations that there is a general lack of research from the United Kingdom regarding the social organisation of so-called 'safe-houses' (aka crack-houses, shooting galleries) used for drug-taking purposes. In such situations, research ethics committees may not be satisfied that the safety of those involved in potentially dangerous research environments can be guaranteed (Pearson 2009). Indeed, Dan Briggs' study of London-based crack-users was conducted in a somewhat unconventional manner as 'two university ethics committees … indicated the work was 'too risky' and would not support it' (Briggs 2011, 33). As such, Briggs conducted his study without conventional academic approval and he should be applauded for his commendable response to the restrictions imposed upon social research(ers) by ethics committees. However, both Briggs' actions and the restrictions of ethics committees also appear somewhat incongruous (from a research perspective) given the sizeable body of ethnographic research, mainly from North America that documents precisely these settings (for example, Carlson 2000). Consequently, fieldwork design for this study of *street-based* public injecting had to consider the way in the author (alongside visual and audio recording equipment) could access drug-using environments with appropriate academic and ethical approval, given the illegal nature of drug use; the clandestine settings in which it occurred and the potential for various field-related health and safety concerns (Singer et al. 2001, Williams et al. 1992).

Each of these issues was resolved with the assistance of the various Drug and Alcohol Action Teams (DAAT) involved in each respective study. As noted above, DAATs are local bodies that oversee the organisation and management of the government's National Drug Strategy, as well as commission most drug and alcohol services in the relevant area of statutory authority.[7] As such, all three DAATs in this research acted as 'gatekeepers' of considerable importance throughout the entire study. For example, each DAAT facilitated and *formalised* the author's attachment to various drug and alcohol services where opportunistic/ organised contact with service-users/clients could occur. Similarly each DAAT expedited contact with other professional bodies within the statutory authority that may have been directly or indirectly affected by public injecting drug use. In such circumstances, the author could access the relevant department by a process of formal and informal referral originating from each DAAT. Indeed, with hindsight, each DAAT attached to this study perhaps established credibility and trust by default upon the research/er by matter of association.

---

7   In April 2013 the introduction of Public Health England involved large scale restructuring and reorganising of Drug and Alcohol Teams. Roberts (2013) provides a full account of these structural changes and how such services are currently organised.

Environmental Visual Assessments

The term environmental visual assessment (EVA) is used to describe visits to settings of public injecting drug use whilst alone; accompanied by a representative from a frontline service, or with an injecting drug user participating in the study. EVA were conducted primarily to assist the author in becoming familiar with a wide range environments appropriated for injecting purposes and, more significantly, to consider these locations from a harm reduction perspective. Similarly, EVA are a relatively simple means of acquiring first-hand appreciation of the environmental qualities and social activity that are located within or adjacent these sites of drug use. EVA also provided opportunities to obtain the views of various employees (and even community residents) affected by public injecting episodes and to observe the way in which these settings were physically managed by the relevant personnel/community members. During every EVA session, photographs were taken of injecting sites known to frontline services, as well as of any evidence of drug-related litter in street-based settings. Images of the latter were taken as confirmation that sites were used for injecting and/or discarding purposes and used as clarification of any so-called 'anecdotal evidence' associated with particular locations.

Tripartite Research

All research, regardless of location, was organised into three distinct stages. This design aimed to address the overall lack of data typically available in each setting concerning the actual locations, prevalence and incidence of public injecting drug use *per se*. As such, the original research format established in Plymouth (Parkin 2009a) provided the foundational and organisational bases of each of the subsequent studies conducted during 2010–2011. This tripartite system of research established a pattern that involved:

- Stage 1 EVA: street-based research and interviews with frontline service personnel to assist in the mapping and photographing of known public injecting sites.
- Stage 2: intensive interviews with drug users regarding experiences of street-based injecting episodes.
- Stage 3 EVA: a second phase of street-based research to visit/photograph/film any additional injecting environments not visited during Stage 1 fieldwork. This stage involved some collaboration and participation with injecting drug users in attempts to video record how injecting episodes are conducted in the relevant street-based settings.

Each aspect of these three stages is discussed in further detail below.

Stage 1

The first stage of all fieldwork involved identifying the extent of public injecting in the given locations and mapping any street-based settings that contained higher concentrations of drug-using environments. This was achieved with the assistance of a variety of frontline service personnel with direct contact and/or experience of public injecting episodes (and/or contact with drug-related litter as part of their employment). This mapping exercise typically involved informal, unrecorded interviews with statutory officials, municipal council employees, street workers, outreach workers, police officers and those employed in the private sector (such as retail outlets, security companies and shopping malls). In addition, these interviews often took place *in situ* of the public injecting sites concerned and occurred as part of EVA conducted by the author in tandem with the relevant frontline personnel. During these field visits to known public injecting sites, photographs were taken in order to compile a database of environments affected by drug use. All locations were photographed from a variety of spatial perspectives, each directly informed by the experiences of the relevant frontline service personnel, in which the environmental setting was given priority (for example, levels of hygiene, physical location, points of access/exit etc.). This method generated views and experiences of public injecting in street-based environments in which the relevant accounts were provided by non-injecting drug users. Accordingly, the assorted data gathered during this process – and especially that of visual images – provided 'etic' (Pike 1954) re-presentations of injecting environments. That is to say, these data provided environmental accounts from the viewpoint of the 'outsider looking in' (Parkin 2009c) with regard to socio-spatial management and the use of injecting space from a harm reduction perspective.

A further rationale for photographing street-based injecting environments sites was to enable the author to become familiar with the various settings from an epistemological (*harm reduction*) perspective. However, these images were integral in the subsequent design of all semi-structured interview schedules designed for application with respective injecting drug user cohorts. Indeed, this particular research design was influenced by Suchar's (1997) 'shooting scripts' model for conducting street-based *visual* methods.

Inverted 'Shooting Scripts'

As part of a study of urban gentrification in a North American city, Charles Suchar (1997) advanced an established visual method for integrating research into sociological analyses of socio-cultural phenomena. Central to Suchar's study was a procedure that involved the formulation of questions he wanted to answer with photographic images, as part of an established method in 'visual sociology' termed 'shooting scripts'. Such scripts, according to Suchar, can assist 'sociological sight' by means of interrogating patterns that may emerge from visual data. As such, 'shooting scripts' provide informative guidelines for both photographic and sociological inquiry, and facilitate academic structure and focus to the relevant study. More specifically:

> shooting scripts involve the creation of a series of categories of photographic evidence to be collected and questions to be explored (Suchar 1997, 36)

In this study of public injecting, Suchar's generic guidelines for developing 'shooting scripts' were purposely and deliberately *inverted*. Namely, photographs of environments gathered during Stage 1 EVA were taken in order *to inform the questions* to be asked of injecting drug users during Stage 2 interviews. In compiling pictures of injecting environments from each particular research setting (prior to any interview with any drug user about injecting episodes in street-based settings), the author was able to identify numerous themes (or 'patterns') requiring further clarification from a harm reduction perspective (such as environmental access, cleanliness, dirt, seclusion, obstacles and contact with others). Such themes/patterns therefore informed and guided the central interview schedule in which there was a direct correlation between questions and images. At no point during these procedures did interview respondents view the images taken by the author. Similarly, the author did not reveal awareness of, or previous attendance at, any public injecting site discussed during interview.

Other 'Stage 1' data that contributed to the identification of public injecting sites included local newspaper stories reporting on drug-related events in the local community. These data were obtained via online searches of the relevant provincial newspapers and typically provided valuable indicators of where and when street-based injecting drug use was a local issue. More importantly, such stories also have a tendency to identify particular *places* in the relevant community that are affected by sex-work, drug-related litter, drug-related arrests, drug use in public places and drug-related crime.

A final component of the Stage 1 'mapping exercise' involved accessing quantitative data, where possible, from the relevant authorities regarding the volume and locations of drug-related litter collections/deposits.

Stage 2

'Stage 2' commenced on completion of the above mapping exercise in which the author had become more familiar with the locations and frequency of public injecting in the relevant geographic locations. Stage 2 therefore focused upon obtaining drug users' experience (and perspectives) of the injecting environments identified during 'Stage 1' mapping procedures. These experiences were obtained by a period of semi-structured interviewing that typically took place within needle/ syringe programmes (NSP) or other services accessed by injecting drug users (including various open access, drop-in centres as well as hostel accommodation).

Semi-Structured Interviews

Semi-structured interviews were held with 71 injecting drug users throughout the entire project. The primary entry criterion for participation in the research was that respondents were to have had recent experience of public injecting drug use (that is, *in the last month*). Consequently, recruitment involved the use of a non-random, purposive sampling strategy (Green and Thorogood 2004). Such selective recruitment to the study was necessary in order to provide insights of the 'lived-experience' of the effects of injecting drugs in environments located in the public sphere. Whereas such selective sampling procedures have previously been questioned (Berg 1998, Maher 1997) for a perceived lack of representation amongst a given milieu (in this instance, of injecting drug users *per se*), they have also been commended (Maher 1997, Taylor 1993) as a useful process for including more 'hidden' populations that have particular insights of a given phenomenon (in this instance, injecting drug use in public settings). Furthermore, an over-emphasis upon 'representativeness' may 'obscure what the anomalous or the marginal can reveal about the centre', (Maher 1997, 29). As such, the selective recruitment strategy adopted in this study appears legitimate as it relates to the recruitment of a cohort of injecting drug users considered 'harder-to-reach' and engaged in behaviour that may not necessarily typify that of the wider injecting fraternity within a given location (*street*-based injecting).

Semi-Structured Interviews within Service Settings

Stage 1 fieldwork in each setting consistently identified several services with an explicit 'substance use' remit that would provide relevant opportunities for recruiting injecting drug users into the research project. Sites of recruitment in all four locations were primarily within local, open access, NSP. Other recruitment sites included various drop-in centres (all locations) and local hostel accommodation (Plymouth only). All services fully-supported the research agenda and all provided private office space in which interviews with respondents could be conducted in confidence and anonymity. This arrangement suitably addressed the problems involved in maintaining contact with hard-to-reach populations and facilitated interviews to take place *in situ* at the time of initial contact.

Making Contact with Injecting Drug Users

Having secured the support of the relevant points of access (often facilitated by the relevant DAAT), the author was able to attend each service on a regular basis at pre-arranged times to make contact with respective service users. The contact procedures employed varied slightly within each setting and involved a system of semi-referral (drop-in centres), direct referral (hostels) and opportunistic contact (NSP).

The process of 'semi-referral' involved frontline service staff (or keyworkers) identifying individuals with known injecting careers as they accessed the drop-in facility. These individuals were approached by their keyworker who explained the research and asked if they would be interested in participating in the study. If the response was positive, they were introduced to the author, who provided a verbal account of an ethically-approved Respondent Information Sheet attached to the research.

A system of direct referral took place in a hostel setting as keyworkers identified 'new' clients seeking accommodation who also disclosed injecting drug use histories. These individuals were informed of the research via the aforementioned Respondent Information Sheet. If these individuals agreed to participate, an appointment was made for the author to visit the client in the hostel at a designated time. Interviews in such settings were conducted in private (in a room that provided health care intervention by visiting health professionals).

Opportunistic contact involved the author making face-to-face 'cold' contact with individuals as and when they visited the relevant NSP for various injecting paraphernalia.

Opportunistic Contact and Question Threat

Due to the informal service typically provided by NSP, service users are generally 'unknown' and officially 'anonymous' to the frontline staff that provide access to injecting equipment. As such, throughout this study (regardless of geographic location) consideration had to be given to the way in which the issue of *public* injecting episodes was raised with service users, given such experiences are typically framed by stigma and shame (Rhodes et al. 2007). This concern related to a need to recruit the desired respondents into the study, but also to be mindful of avoiding offense when raising the issue of street-based injecting experience. To meet this objective, the following protocol was employed within all needle and syringe programmes to which the author was attached.

1. As service users entered the facility, they were introduced to the author who explained the purpose of the research and his temporary attachment to the relevant service (in order to allay any fears of breaching confidentiality)
2. The service user was provided with their requested paraphernalia by the relevant personnel present
3. Once the exchange/supply was complete, the author approached the service user with the following 'screening questions':
    While you are here, do you mind if I ask you a quick, confidential, research question about your injecting?

> If the service user disagreed to this question being asked, no further contact was made. If the service user agreed, they were subsequently asked:
>
> In the last month, have you injected in a public place?

During initial pilot sessions of this protocol, this approach to research recruitment did not produce any positive responses amongst service users. Indeed, almost all were negative, almost *vehement* denials of injecting in a public place. As a consequence, the final screening question was deemed to be confrontational and possibly loaded with 'question threat' (Foddy 1993, 112). As such the 'screening question' was subsequently reworded to 'decrease the *specificity* of the information called for' (ibid., emphasis added), to become the following, less threatening, question:

> In the last month, have you ever injected in a place such as a toilet, car-park or somewhere outside?

The slight amendment to this critical question proved more conducive to opportunistic respondent recruitment, as the following fieldnote illustrates:

> I explained my research at an opportune moment and asked if they had ever 'used (injected) outside in a car park or the like?' The male replied, 'Yeah, we're just about to!' nodding towards the door (suggesting the car park opposite). He was immediately told to '*Sshhh*' by his girlfriend. (Postscript: both subsequently agreed to be interviewed). (*Fieldnotes*)

Interview Procedure

Once contact procedures had been established, subsequent interview procedures followed a standardised protocol that took place in private rooms. Namely, respondents were initially briefed on the nature and purpose of the research; including their role and expectations within the study if they agreed to be interviewed. Informed consent was obtained through the author's verbal recital of an ethically approved Respondent Information Sheet. At this stage, respondents were informed they:

- could leave the interview at any time.
- did not have to answer 'uncomfortable' questions.
- would not be personally identified in the research (or any subsequent text)
- all responses would be confidential and audio-recorded for research purposes only.
- would be given a cash payment of £10 for completing the interview.

Verbal Informed Consent

Once briefed, respondents were asked to confirm on a digital voice recorder that they had understood the nature of the research, were willing to participate and had understood the content of the Respondent Information Sheet read out *verbatim* by the author. Such *verbal* informed consent replaced the more conventional *written* informed consent in order to avoid identifying individuals and their participation in an illegal activity (namely, their previous involvement in buying/possessing illicit substances). Written consent from respondents who are engaged in such activity on a daily basis is perhaps ethically *inappropriate*, as it fails to protect individual identities and actually has the effect of forcing respondents to admit criminal activity in writing. Verbal informed consent has become regarded as acceptable ethical conduct, especially when concerned with sensitive research topics. This is because it is regarded as a means of protecting the identity and confidentiality of research respondents who may prefer to remain 'anonymous' for reasons of personal safety and/or avoid litigation (Coomber 2002). The respondent Information Sheet read-out *verbatim* during all research was similarly approved by the relevant ethical reviews attached to each respective study.

Following the provision of verbal informed consent, respondents answered a short questionnaire (also read-out *verbatim* by the author) that aimed to establish a demographic profile of the cohort that was specific to each geographic location. This was followed by the semi-structured interview that focused on place-specific experience, health and social behaviour, injecting-practice, -technique and – hygiene within all drug using environments discussed.

All 71 injecting drug user interviews were recorded using a digital voice recorder, with each interview lasting, on average, approximately 35 minutes (range 16–55 minutes). All interviews were transcribed verbatim and subject to analysis assisted by qualitative software programme (NVivo versions 7, 8 and 10).

On Socially Desirable Responses

Sutton and Farrall (2005) define socially desirable responses (SDR) as attempts by research respondents to create favourable impressions of themselves with interview responses that have been positively 'shaped' to suit the nature of interaction. Throughout all semi-structured interviews there was a need for the author to be constantly vigilant of any 'interviewer effect' when discussing the sensitive issue of *street-based* injecting drug use with all respondents. Such responses were anticipated in sensitive matters relating to public injecting *per se*, but also extended to associative themes, including sharing paraphernalia (injecting equipment), blood borne viruses and the discarding strategies of needles/syringes (that is, littering in public places). Previous studies (Beynon et al. 2010, Latkin et al. 1993, Rhodes and Treloar 2008) have highlighted the under-reporting of specific harmful behaviours in drug-related research, in which respondents may provide SDR to avoid any concomitant stigma associated with blood borne virus status/transmission (such as HIV and HCV). Various strategies have been used to counter SDR; such as computer-assisted interviewing (Des Jarlais et al. 1999) and so-called 'lie-scales' (Sutton and Farrell 2005) that seek to provide more candid responses to sensitive topics. In the present setting however, such methods were considered impracticable and were generally not compatible with the methodological orientation of this *qualitative* study.

Accordingly, throughout all relevant data collection procedures, the issue of SDR was addressed in a more reflexive manner that was considered non-threatening to all respondents. This was achieved by the repetition and reframing of particular questions regarding sensitive issues as a means of cross-checking earlier responses.

Ethnographic Observation

Opportunities to conduct ethnographic observations were made possible in all four sites of the study. In each setting, the author physically re-located to the relevant town/city in order to complete the relevant fieldwork. The cumulative period of time dedicated to ethnographic data collection consisted of 14-months fieldwork, in which all research was conducted during a total period of 56 months (October 2006–June 2011).

Within each geographic setting, the author was primarily attached to the relevant location's main needle and syringe programme (NSP). Ethnographic observations located within four NSP throughout the study noted the way in which service users interacted with frontline personnel (and *vice versa*) and the type of injecting paraphernalia requested per visit per individual. In observing the range of paraphernalia requested by service users, it was possible to make an informed assessment of *where* an individual chose to inject, both physically and spatially. (For example, requests for longer needles suggested 'deeper' injecting practices such groin injecting whereas requests for water ampoules may infer homelessness: each of which were used as *indicators* of potential episodes of, and participation in, public injecting prior to the screening question). Similarly, observations within various open access, drop-in centres were considered a useful means of experiencing the spatial dimensions and social realities of homelessness alongside the utility such places (extraneous to injecting drug use) provided to those affected by rooflessness, poverty, unemployment and domestic/violence.

Research attachment to various street-based outreach teams also provided useful insights of the social and physical conditions surrounding rough sleeping and drug use throughout the four locations. For example, temporary and occasional attachment with various housing services, street-cleansing teams, outreach workers (targeting young people, sex workers, homeless, street drinkers), police officers, youth workers, toilet attendants, car-park security, and concierges each provided thick description and experiential accounts of the social and physical environments affected by, poverty, social exclusion and economic marginalisation. Harm and hazard relating to rooflessness and substance use were frequently reported by these respondents as regular/daily features within these particular urban landscapes.

Stage 3

The final stage of fieldwork involved a second period of EVA in which injecting environments discussed by drug user respondents (during Stage 2 interviews) were visited by the author. This was primarily an exercise in validating interview content with environmental context. The aim of such rigour was to identify any place-based hazards not noted during Stage 1 EVA (and possibly raised during the relevant interview) in order to confirm or refute environmentally-influenced experiences reported during individual interviews.

Consolidation of Experience with Video Data

A further aspect of 'Stage 3' EVA exclusive to one site (Plymouth) was the additional collection of video data that aimed to provide 'thicker description' and explanation of the photographs gathered during Stage 1 fieldwork. In addition, this method of data generation aimed to reflect the lived experience of street-based injecting specifically from the perspective of injecting drug users.

Inclusion in this aspect of the study was assessed during Stage 2 interviews and was further informed by each individual's lifetime experience of public injecting and the range of street-based injecting environments known and/or articulated by the relevant interview respondents. If considered as suitable *participants* in the visual research, respondents were informed of the visual study and invited to contribute at the conclusion of their interview. If they agreed, an ethically approved Participant Information Sheet was provided and telephone contacts exchanged for future reference.

At this point it is perhaps necessary to make a clear distinction between 'respondents' and 'participants' within this study. That is, *respondent* is the term used to describe individuals (frontline service staff and injecting drug users) that took part in semi-structured interviews only. *Participants*, however, were injecting drug users that were interviewed *and* made meaningful contributions to the visual aspect of the study. This particular definition is necessary as it reflects the level of involvement in the study, whereby 'respondent' refers to the nature of interaction during interviews and 'participant' reflects the physical contributions made towards data collection (Letherby 2003).

A total of 14 individuals agreed to take part in the video component of the study. However, due to the difficulties involved in maintaining telephone contact with homeless individuals (who may be subject to police detention, imprisonment, geographic relocation and/or drug-related fatality), meetings with only 8 individuals subsequently took place as arranged/agreed. It was also possibly due to the lengthy time span between these meetings (up to 12 weeks in one instance), that contact was lost with six individuals, reducing the original 'video cohort' from 14 to 8 respondents. Nevertheless, eight injecting drug users assisted in the direction and compilation of video material pertaining to 50 street-based environments. In all environments, the relevant participants had previously completed injecting episodes of illicit drugs on multiple occasions.

This second tranche of EVA, accompanied by injecting drug users, involved visits to a number of public injecting sites that had not necessarily been reported to the research by frontline personnel. Similarly, as with 'Stage '1 EVA, these visits to injecting environments provided opportunities to visually record (with photographs and/or video) the sites in question from the lived experience and perspectives of those present in the field. This latter aspect of visual data collection aimed to record environments used for drug injecting episodes in an attempt to specifically identify environmental opportunities for influencing drug-related harm, based upon the injecting drug users' intimate knowledge of the sites involved.

Environmental Visual Assessments and Recreations of Injecting Episodes

The collation of *video* data as part of field-based EVA with injecting drug users involved more systematic and controlled procedures than that described above concerning the collection of photographs during 'Stage 1' mapping procedures. More specifically, during each individual video session, all participants were requested to select up to six 'favoured' sites they had previously accessed for street-based injecting episodes.

As each site was visited, participants were asked to explain how, why and when these locations were chosen, accessed and exited; to describe the measures used to manage personal safety and, finally, to recreate the processes of drug preparation and injecting episodes[8] specific to each location. These verbal responses were *audio*-recorded *in situ*.

Following this verbal evaluation of the injecting setting, the immediate environment was video-recorded from the physical position participants demonstrated the process of drug preparation and injection. From these positional perspectives, each injecting environment was recorded in a 360° arc-sweep (where possible) in an attempt to fully 'capture' the immediate physical surroundings and associated qualities of places appropriated for street-based injecting episodes. In this approach to gathering visual data, an attempt was made to instantiate the 'skilled vision' (Grasseni 2004) of drug users regarding environmental settings considered 'appropriate' for injecting drug use. This process facilitated the phenomenological representation of injecting environments as the 'skilled vision' of participants

---

8 No drugs or injecting paraphernalia were used or were present during this *mimed* exercise and *verbal* account of recreating injecting episodes.

(advice and direction on appropriate camera positions for recording the sites visited) generated 'sociological vision' for the author (regarding theoretical an applied [harm reduction] interpretations). In addition to this instruction, the author also gained a systematic appreciation of behaviour associated with street-based injecting. For example, the repeated wide-ranging sensory and spatial experiences encountered during visual data collection were features of the phenomena that had been only briefly discussed in the semi-structured interview process of Stage 2. Illustrations here may include the overpowering stench of urine, excrement and vomit noted in some locations, compared to the challenging negotiation of claustrophobic, cramped and confined settings in others.

In this respect, visual methods engage with the practice of 'observant-participation' (Wacquant 2004, 2005). This process involves 'learning-by-doing' and is situated within the particular field of inquiry. In this study, the process of generating visual data involved experiencing drug using environments in a manner similar to those that directly informed the study (frontline service personnel and injecting drug users). As such, the application of visual methods provided opportunities for the author to conduct ethnographic 'observant-participation' as a means to fully appreciate and understand the various environments affected by injecting drug use *from a variety of countering-perspectives*.

As with the photography of Stage 1, the process of video-recording recreations of injecting episodes by drug users served to further reinforce the methodological principles attached to the study. More particularly, these visual and verbal data related to injecting drug user views, experiences and demonstrations of injecting episodes situated within street-based environments. Accordingly, the assorted data gathered during this aspect of fieldwork – and especially that relating to the collection of video-based images – provided distinctly 'emic' (Pike 1954) re-presentations of injecting environments. That is to say, these data from injecting drug users typically provided nuanced environmental and experiential accounts of the 'insider looking out' (Parkin 2009c) with regard to socio-spatial management and the use of injecting space from the lived experience of public injecting perspectives.

Ethical Code of Conduct (Visual Methods with Injecting Drug Users)

Prior to any visual research conducted with all relevant injecting drug users in public, street-based settings, each participant was reminded of the nature and purpose of recording drug using environments (as part of research to inform local services of the conditions and harms associated with outdoor injecting sites). Similarly, all participants were reminded of their role and expectations within this aspect of the study and that their visual image would not be recorded at any point during data collection proceedings. All injecting drug user participants were subsequently verbally informed (in addition to the provision of a Participant Information Sheet):

- they could leave the field at any time (especially if they encountered other individuals at sites in order to avoid identification as a drug-user/research participant).
- they would be asked to accompany the author to several injecting environments and to explain the procedures of drug preparation/injection in these settings.
- they would be accompanied by a drugs worker throughout the session in order to oversee an ethical code of conduct; provide care and support in the event of any drug-related crisis and to ensure that the researcher-participant relationship remained mutually non-coercive.
- did not have to answer 'uncomfortable' questions.
- they would not be personally identified in the video recordings (or any subsequent text).
- they would be given a further cash payment of £20 for completing the session (based upon the principles of reciprocity and participation in 'work' related tasks described below).
- any verbal responses collected were confidential and recorded off-camera (on separate recording devices) for research purposes only.

Informed consent procedures followed the same protocol described above concerning semi-structured interview.

Wider Field-related Concerns

Several issues were identified prior to, and during, fieldwork that may have problematised the progress of the study had they not been addressed in an appropriate matter. These issues related to the dilemmas associated with providing cash payments to injecting drug user respondents, taking visual images of public setting and addressing place-based cravings with injecting drug users. These are discussed further below.

Cash for Questions?

Decisions to provide cash payments in health-related research often prove controversial, and this is particularly apparent in drug-related research. Criticisms for such practice typically relate to the perception that cash for participation may be coercive and subsequently unethical practice (Seddon 2005). Similarly cash 'incentives' may be regarded as legitimising and rewarding 'illegal' behaviour, in which there is the potential for researchers to inadvertently promote socially desirable responses or even finance drug use (Fry and Dwyer 2001, McKeganey 2001, Seddon 2005). The provision of non-cash alternatives (for example, shopping vouchers) has been equally criticised as it is considered that such currency will be subsequently sold at rates lower than their face-value (McKeganey 2000).

Despite these concerns, cash payments to respondents have become common practice in qualitative studies of drug-use. Examples of such ethically approved 'payments' include McKeganey and Barnard's (1992) ethnography of street-based sex work, Simmonds and Coomber's (2009) study of injecting-related stigma and Rhodes et al.'s (2006) visual ethnography of street-based injecting practices. Each of these studies legitimised cash payments as reflecting *reciprocal relationships* that were situated within the research design; in which respondents and researchers are mutual beneficiaries of the fiscal exchange. Indeed, several researchers have found that although *some* injecting drug user motivations for research participation may be related to economic gain, they equally relate to citizenship, altruism and drug user activism (Fry and Dwyer 2000).

Finances were made available from each respective DAAT to cover the costs of injecting drug user participation. At £10 and £20 per respondent interview and participant video, these payments were considered non-coercive and did not necessarily compel individuals to become involved in the study. Instead, all contributions by drug users were considered as a form of employment (Seddon 2005), in which respondents/participants were compensated for the provision of time, expertise and 'labour'.

'Shooting' in Public?

As Moon (2000) has previously observed, the lexicon of photography has appropriated vocabulary synonymous with militarism and may be thus compared with the language of warfare and/or conflict. Moon clarifies this potentially controversial point of view with the following illustration:

> *Shoot* and *shot* are obvious examples of this. A *snapshot* was a shot fired quickly, and without careful *aim*. Cameras have *triggers* or *firing* mechanisms, though button and shutter (release) are less antiquated and less militaristic terms. People *load* cameras with *cartridges* or *magazines* of film; they *cock* shutters, and they *fire off* films. .... . deep metaphor can be extended ... in images of someone *pointing* his or her camera at someone else and *aiming* it, or of someone being the *target* of paparazzi, or of cameras being wielded, carried or slung over one's shoulder, like *weapons*. (Moon 2000, all emphases added)

It is perhaps due to such symbolic value, coupled with the potentially *intrusive* quality of the visual medium, that street-based photography may invoke curiosity and suspicion amongst the 'general public' (Coleman 1987). Indeed, the global ubiquity of digital hardware appears to have intensified this intrusion in which suspicion and avoidance of cameras (and other mobile devices) may appear more commonplace in contemporary society than ever before. In some situations, this suspicion can provoke hostile responses, that in turn may be viewed by wider audiences (not directly involved in the relevant events) using online, video-based, social networking media.[9] Perhaps more serious are the concerns expressed by Louie Palu (Coomes 2012) who wrote the following statement regarding efforts to minimise the threat of intrusion and identification raised by cameras in hostile and violent drug using/selling environments:

> I have conversations with many people there and walk around the neighbourhood with my camera on my shoulder, but rarely use it. I do this continually so locals see me around frequently, letting them know I am not a threat. (Location) is *the kind of place where if you are not thoughtful about your activities someone could cause you serious harm*. (Coomes 2012, 2 emphasis added)

Concerns relating to street-based visual methods were pre-empted prior to commencing fieldwork. Indeed it was envisaged that the visual recording of car-parks, parkland and public toilets may be perceived (by those not directly involved in the studies) as suspicious behaviour; or in the very least be regarded as somewhat 'odd' and 'unusual' conduct. As such, all DAAT involved in the study provided the author with a 'comfort letter'. This formal document acknowledged an awareness of the visual methods attached to the study of street-based injecting. This document was counter-signed by several senior representatives of the relevant local authorities (including police officers) and was presented *in situ* on at least *nine* occasions when the research/er was challenged by official bodies in particular locations (security officers). In presenting complainants with the 'comfort letter', concerns were immediately appeased, and whereas the document did not necessarily *condone* the presence of cameras in certain settings, it did appear to *validate* this presence.

Place-based Drug Cravings

A further ethical consideration in conducting drug-related, place-based, visual research concerned the need to provide appropriate health care to all injecting drug users that participated in Stage 3 EVA. This was particularly pertinent as drug users were requested to provide access to injecting sites where they had previously (or currently) injected drugs. Such environmental stimuli may initiate cravings for drug use (especially heroin) amongst those seeking abstinence or recovery and may contribute towards drug-related relapse (Zinberg 1984, Clark 2006). For these reasons, it was necessary to ensure that all relevant participants were not attempting to be 'drug-free' at the time of video-based fieldwork, as the average

---

9   As an example, threats of violence and police intervention towards an amateur film-maker may be noted in a home-produced video-clip titled '*Madness at Toni's chip shop in Wishaw*' (http://www.youtube.com/watch?v=fOX-pXTRsWA).

time between initial interview and second contact was approximately six weeks. Consequently, when individuals were re-contacted to arrange a date/time for their visual participation, they were initially asked of their current drug using status. This process was repeated immediately prior to commencing street-based EVA and details of their last injecting episode were requested. Such measures ensured that the research would not place individuals into a coercive or vulnerable situation and impinge on any attempts towards 'recovery', abstinence or other measures of drug-related self-regulation. Furthermore, all EVA with injecting drug users was assisted by the presence of an experienced drugs worker who would have been better able to identify negative experiences associated with these environmental settings and intervene accordingly. However, during all EVA with injecting drug users, the professional worker did not have to intervene or advise in any capacity with regard to place-based cravings or drug-related health concerns.

Ethical Approval

Ethical approval for each aspect of the study was sought and obtained from the relevant Faculty Research Ethics Committees within the University of Plymouth as well as from a Local National Health Service (NHS) Research Ethics Committee (REC). These committees approved all research conducted during 2006–2009. For the period 2010–2011, and due to a restructuring of ethical procedures attached qualitative research within NHS (and associated) settings, approval for all PIRAS related studies was granted by the relevant committee within (the renamed) Plymouth University.

Data Collected

As with *Habitus and Drug Using Environments*, this book has been informed by three separate (but related) studies of street-based injecting drug use that were located in four geographic settings throughout the south of England. All research took place between October 2006 and June 2011 and involved over one-year (14 months) of street-based, ethnographic, fieldwork. Due to the large volume of qualitative data (textual and visual) generated from this study and due to the theoretical and applied priorities attached to the research (relating to 'habitus' and 'harm reduction' respectively), it is perhaps necessary to include detail of data analyses also attached to this work. The following chapter provides a more comprehensive account of the methods of qualitative *data analysis* employed to produce findings of academic and applied value.

Chapter 4
Analysis

In her invaluable text regarding *Qualitative Data Analysis with NVivo*, Patricia Bazeley succinctly observes that when it comes to their management, 'qualitative data are voluminous and messy' (Bazeley 2007, 131). This remark is likely to be regarded with indifference and/or ambivalence amongst those with little experience of conducting qualitative research. Similarly, those with experience are likely to view this remark with a wry smile of recognition or possibly provide a mischievous rejoinder that includes the word 'understatement'! For example, to illustrate the 'voluminous mess' upon which this text is based, the following data were generated during 56 months (October 2006–June 2011) of research regarding street-based injecting drug use:

- 169 informal, annotated ('gist'), semi-structured interviews with frontline service personnel.
- 71 semi-structured, audio-recorded, interviews with injecting drug users.
- 3 separate Field Journals documenting 14 months of ethnographic observation and reflexive fieldnotes.
- textual and visual accounts of over 400 environmental visual assessments at public injecting sites (spread across four research settings).
- over 1,000 digital photographs of street-based injecting sites.
- over one hour of video footage recorded within public environments.

Due to the volume of these collected data, the following chapter aims to provide an account of the way in which one may make 'academic sense' and provide 'applied value' to the various documents generated from studies of equal (as well as lesser and/or greater) qualitative depth. Although a similar account was briefly included in *Habitus and Drug Using Environments*, (Parkin 2013), it has been expanded in this volume in an attempt to underscore the 'applied visual sociology' of this book's title and to explicate the analytical procedures attached to the process of 'picturing harm reduction'. However, as noted in the previous chapter, the underlying research was informed by a combination of various qualitative methods that generated language- and image-based data. As such, the methods of analysis described below apply to both forms of data (text and visual) but should be read in the context of *visual data* in order to fully appreciate the applied value of visual methods.

Establishing Baseline Analytics

All *language-based* data generated throughout the entire study were subject to analysis using a popular qualitative software programme (NVivo versions 7, 8 and 10). The qualitative data entered into the programme consisted of the six different datasets listed above. Initial analyses involved categorising these various responses, observations and interpretations into themes relating to *habitus* and/or *harm reduction* in order to reflect the academic and applied nature of the study respectively.[1]

An identical analytical process to that described above was also applied to all *visual data* (photographs and video) and their related texts (fieldnotes and observations of injecting environments). All images/written accounts of drug using settings were ordered into common categorical 'themes' that prioritised the interpretative *epistemological* stance of harm reduction. In this respect, all image-based data of drug-using settings were visually compared to environments within medically-supervised 'safer injecting facilities' (for example, see Figure 4.1[2]). This process aimed to identify the extent street-based settings resembled or, perhaps more accurately, how much they differed from these 'gold standard' benchmarks of harm reduction intervention.

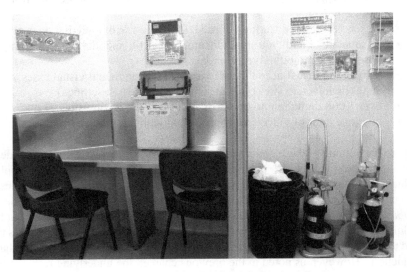

Figure 4.1 Inside the Medically Supervised Injecting Centre, Sydney (Australia)

---

1 All themes relating to 'habitus' are documented within *Habitus and Drug Using Environments* (Parkin 2013). Those pertaining to 'harm reduction' are contained within this volume.

2 Reproduced with kind permission from Mr. Rohan Glasgow at the Medically Supervised Injecting Centre, Sydney, Australia.

A second comparative benchmark used during all data analyses was an 'industry-based' harm reduction manual known as *The Safer Injecting Briefing* (Derricott, Preston and Hunt 1999). This text provides guidelines for promoting safer injecting procedures (technique and practice) and is audience-specific towards services and interventions with a substance use remit (such as needle and syringe programmes and associated service-users). As such, the guidance outlined by Derricott and colleagues (relating to the preparation of drug solute, injecting technique, routes of administration, overdose management and vein care) provided a similar, albeit textual, foundation upon which to compare drug user accounts of their injecting experiences in street-based environments.

From these two points of reference, applied (harm reduction) judgements could be made from images of (and related field accounts) of environments affected by injecting episodes in which the experiences of drug users were considered alongside the optimal conditions for applying 'safer' injecting procedures. Similarly, interview data, ethnographic observations and assorted images of drug using environments were also subject to triangulated analysis to determine how near/distant these experiences/environments were to/from the 'harm reduction ideal' of supervised settings and the guidance contained within the *Safer Injecting Briefing*.

Whereas the themes of habitus were informed by various theoretical models established by Pierre Bourdieu (for example, relating to 'practice', 'capital', 'field', 'symbolic violence' etc.) those concerning harm reduction were informed by 'real world' settings and health-related intervention (such as, 'drug preparation', 'injecting technique' etc.). Accordingly, secondary analyses of all data established a two-pronged hierarchical coding frame to create relevant 'sub-categories' within each the academic and applied themes. Cumulatively, these *deductive* and *empirical* processes, that jointly addressed sociological theory with applied intervention, established overlapping patterns of experience relating to particular places in public settings. This method of analysis also assisted in the *categorisation* (including explanations) of various harm associated with street-based injecting drug use.

Elaborating Analytical Procedures

Although the above section provides an adequate summary of how data analysis occurred throughout this study of street-based injecting, it perhaps lacks the sophistication required for a text proclaiming itself to be an 'applied visual sociology'. In the following section, a more detailed account of the underlying analytical process is provided in which the reader should regard visual data as the primary unit of data under discussion (although this account also applies to the analysis of all text-based data attached to the study). In short, this more 'sophisticated' account of data analysis aims to emphasise the importance and rigour of data coding (including categorising and classifying) attached to qualitative research throughout the social sciences *per se*.

Data Coding: An Understated Qualitative Skill

The centrality of data management and the analytical skills attached to creating 'coding frames' within qualitative research are undoubtedly understated – if not completely ignored – within the abundant literature dedicated to sociological research methods. Similarly, accounts of data *analysis* are largely absent from qualitative texts such as research monographs, journal articles and even doctoral theses. Indeed, during the course of a research career that spans almost two decades, this author has probably encountered more academics who openly disclose a general *in*ability to competently use data analysis packages (such as ATLAS, NVivo and EndNote) than those who claim proficiency and/or a working knowledge of such programmes. This lack of a particular set of skills in qualitative research has been noted at all levels throughout the academy, and includes newly enrolled doctoral students, established academics, senior teaching staff and – perhaps most concerning – research supervisors with records of successful 'completions'.

As an illustration of this concern, a senior academic known to the author once disclosed to postgraduate researchers that the use of 'highlighter pen and scraps of paper spread all over the floor' was their preferred form of qualitative data analysis. In the twenty-first century, when research is becoming increasingly dominated by mobile devices, computer software, online media and social networking sites, the notion of sitting on a floor amidst a mountain of highlighted paper cuttings, (possibly cut, pasted and copied from various documents), appears anachronistic and almost obsolete. Whilst some may contend that this view is unnecessarily overly critical (as each qualitative researcher has a preferred and established pattern of working), the countering line of defence would make reference to the relative ease of skill acquisition in this area of research (via online training, workshops and programme manuals) in an era in which the same software illiterate individuals are quite probably eager to embrace digital media (such as photography) as a form of social research.

In addition, a general lack of familiarity with key qualitative software programmes (such as those listed above) noted throughout the academy (especially at a professional level) perhaps further reflects an overall lack of importance placed upon the development of skills (at an individual, institutional and structural level) concerning *electronic* data coding, analysis and interpretation. This would appear somewhat incongruous given that several researchers have attempted to emphasise the prominence of academic rigour within all forms of research. For example, Bazeley (2007) argues that proficient qualitative researchers are adept at coding data in which the quality of the research output often reflects the quality of data coding and related analysis. Such a view echoes that made by Strauss who, two decades earlier, stated 'the excellence of the research rests in large on the excellence of coding' (cited in Bazely 2007, 66). As such, individual competence in programmes aimed to facilitate data management associated with large volumes of text (including coding/analytical processes) can only enrich qualitative research and related interpretations of social phenomena. Nonetheless, it is important to stress that computer-based programmes only facilitate analysis conducted by an individual able to manipulate the software. Such programmes do not miraculously produce bespoke results at the click of a mouse button – as many academics unfamiliar with the software would appear to assume (including those in senior, prominent positions)![3]

Codes, Nodes and First Cycle Analysis

Although other similar qualitative software packages do exist on the market, the preferred programme used throughout this research was various editions of QSR's NVivo series (versions 7, 8 and 10). The introduction of an interface to conduct analysis of photographs and other visual data within Version 8 of the programme, especially, facilitated a more enriched cross-examination of visual and textual data pertaining to drug using environments and related experiences.

Central to the analytical process within NVivo is the researcher's creation of a coding frame that contains individual codes. These individual codes 'are an abstract representation of an object or phenomenon ... a mnemonic device used to identify themes in a text' (Bazeley 2007, 66). As such, codes are generally informed by the data generated from the research (including literature reviewed, existing theoretical frameworks, and/or proposed hypothetical values) in which the range and volume of codes created reflects the analytical rigour of the researcher(s) involved in the relevant study. In this initial phase of data management, little differs from the analytical process inferred above using scissors and highlighter pens, as this method generally represents 'first cycle data coding' (Saldana 2009). However, whereas spreading papers and colourfully decorated cuttings across a wide surface area may prove difficult to physically manage, the creation of first cycle codes within an NVivo database provides equal opportunities to copy, cut *and* colour data into numerous files and folders that reflect an inventory of themes and issues central to the research question. As such, initial, first cycle analysis may generate codes that are descriptive, interpretative, analytical and/or theoretical in their design (Bazeley 2007) as the primary aim of such a process is to bring organisational order to the voluminous mess of qualitative data (Bazeley 2007, Saldana 2009).

As Bazeley (2007) notes, the generation of codes from initial analysis assist in making generalisations from a series of collected, specific, events in which codes link data to ideas and vice versa. In this study of street-based injecting, first cycle data coding initially identified and generated *descriptive, interpretative, analytical* and *theoretical* codes from language/image-based data relating to theory (habitus, field, capital, practice) and harm reduction (injecting –technique, -injury –hygiene etc.). Similarly, these initial codes served to identify and connect theoretical constructs of social agency to experiences of drug-related harm and *vice versa*.

---

3   This is a further personal observation made by the author within a number of academic institutions during 1995–2013.

An alternative term for code, especially when using NVivo software, is *node*. As with codes, nodes provide storage points for particular concepts and categories identified during the analytical process. Similarly, in the context of NVivo, nodes may be organised as 'free' or as part of a 'tree'. Whereas 'free nodes' represent an individual storage point for a form of data (whether text or visual), 'tree nodes' represent a hierarchical pattern that emerges from more sustained data analysis of individual nodes (Bazeley 2007). More specifically, tree nodes establish connections, relationships and associations between individual free nodes that in turn consolidate (and/or confirm) classificatory constructions and analytical frameworks.

In addition to 'tree' and 'free' nodes are those termed '*a priori*' and '*in vivo*' (Bazeley 2007, 73). *A priori* nodes may be defined as those that are linked specifically to the theoretical framework within which a particular study is located. In this instance, all related injecting data generated is subject to deductive *and* interpretative analysis simultaneously (as they are directed and informed by pre-existing sociological theories and the practice of harm reduction respectively). For example, some data may be organised within a framework containing tree nodes to reflect Pierre Bourdieu's theoretical constructs underlying this study. In this instance, interview and visual data are each coded to reflect evidence of *habitus* (such as embodied behaviour and action specific to public injecting), *capital* (social, economic, symbolic and economic relating to public injecting), *field* (local drug policy and practice and how these are made manifest in environmental design, employment procedures and injecting experience) and *practice* (how drugs are acquired, prepared and injected in street-based settings in addition to how environmental features of setting may impact upon such procedures).

In vivo nodes however represent codes from interview data that may be regarded as 'indigenous' terms of reference. *In vivo* codes therefore reflect the 'living voice' of the data as they connect directly to terms used by interview respondents and/or research participants. In this study of public injecting, examples of *in vivo* codes include 'blue lights', 'OD' (overdose), 'dirty hits' (drug solute containing environmental contaminants) and 'brown and white' (heroin and crack-cocaine respectively), 'gouching' (the desired effect of heroin intake) and 'rattling' (physical discomfort/pain associated with heroin withdrawal symptoms).

From an analytical perspective, the introduction of *a priori* and *in vivo* coding further seeks to consolidate the methodological principles attached to this study (as described in the previous chapter). For example, *a priori* coding seeks to identify specifically-grounded evidence of Bourdieu's generalised habitus construct, whereas *in vivo* coding provides a phenomenological framework for considering the lived experiences of public injecting. According to Bazeley (2007), indigenous typologies constructed from *in vivo* data coding assist in providing increased insight into a particular topic. In this study, a sociological vision of street-based injecting is further intensified due to the range of data (text and visual) generated from frontline service personnel, injecting drug users and ethnographic observation by the researcher.

These coding procedures are therefore appropriate in demonstrating the methodological protocol attached to this study. For example, *a priori* coding presents an *etic* mode of data analysis (that is, reflecting interpretations from the perspective of an 'outsider') in contrast to the more *emic*-aligned *in vivo* codes (reflecting the lived experience of events from the perspective of an 'insider'). Furthermore, the introduction and application of *in vivo* nodes during analysis of injecting experiences and drug using environments has been found by this author to be a useful method for disseminating research findings within 'applied' settings such as needle and syringe programmes and/or training sessions with health professionals (see Chapter 8). As such, the re-presentation of service relevant findings, obtained from the indigenous coding procedures attached to this study, aims to further emphasise the credibility and authenticity of the research in general.

Secondary Cycle Analysis

If first cycle data analysis may be compared to creating an elementary filing system relating to all the body parts of a particular organism gathered during fieldwork, then secondary cycle analysis may be equally compared to creating a system towards understanding how all the neatly filed components of that particular organism actually 'fit together'. Of the numerous coding procedures available to qualitative researchers, this study utilises elements of 'pattern coding', 'focused coding', 'theoretical coding' and 'axial coding' that are forwarded by Saldana (2009) in his *Coding Manual for Qualitative Researchers*. Each coding procedure and its relevance to the public injecting dataset is summarised below.

However, it should be reiterated that secondary stage analysis should only occur upon completion of first cycle coding. Without the availability of free nodes that establish and identify the components of a phenomenon under scrutiny (whether they are of *analytical, a priori, descriptive, interpretative, in vivo* or *theoretical* design), it is unlikely that the researcher would be able to establish connections, associations and patterns within the data. Accordingly, without completing first cycle coding procedures, analysis may thus fail to adequately unpack the metaphorical organism contained within the data and how it 'functions' as a 'social entity'.

More Sophisticated Coding for Applied Purposes

In 2006, noted qualitative researcher David Silverman commented pessimistically upon the proliferation of visual data to have emerged within the social sciences in recent times, believing that the inclusion of images (moving or still) as research had become a 'highly fashionable topic' (Silverman 2006, 264). Silverman expresses further reservations regarding 'the quality of analysis that passes as adequate in many areas of cultural studies' (ibid), inferring that visual data within the academy is used all too often for illustrative purposes. These criticisms of visual research emerged at a time when the author was commencing the initial study of street-based injecting as doctoral research which aimed to include video and photography in an ethnographic study of drug using environments (Parkin 2009a). For these reasons, the author's task was to consider the use of visual methods/data in a manner that did not conform to illustration; did not repeat the work of others, yet provided applied value and simultaneously made the relevant 'original contribution to knowledge' associated with doctoral research!

To address these assorted aims the author appeared to exist in a near-permanent state of reflexive, self-interrogation relating to the possible gratuitous use of visual methods/data. For example, whenever a photograph was taken, or a video-clip recorded, the author became guided by a single, over-riding question that essentially determined whether an image was recorded (or not) whilst in the field. This question being, '*how will this image inform harm reduction and related practitioners?*'

Definitive answers to this question were assisted by the analytical processes of visual data that occurred during the secondary coding cycle attached to this study. In order to fully appreciate the underlying rationale for secondary cycle coding procedures, the reader should refer once more to the methodological design of the research described in Chapter 3. However, as an *aide memoir* to this matter, the 'purpose statement' of this research concludes that 'all data analysis is anchored within particular schools of thought (that of Bourdieu's critical theory and applied harm reduction) as a means of interrogating the role of structure and agency in the context of public injecting' (see Chapter 3). Accordingly, due to the pre-determined theoretical and epistemological positions adopted at the onset of any fieldwork, all analyses (of image and text) were pre-situated within particular analytical frameworks by the author before any data was generated. To simplify this statement, in adopting this deductive position the author placed 'the theoretical horse before the analytical horse' (Ball and Smith 1992, 32). This is particularly pertinent to the epistemological stance of the study in which the author's previous experience of harm reduction (and related intervention) in other UK settings influenced the way in which drug using environments were visited, viewed, inspected and evaluated. Similarly all environmental settings, and associated injecting experiences described within, were subject to comparative analysis using equally pre-determined, baseline measures of 'gold-standard' intervention in the field of harm reduction.

With specific regard to *visual* data, first cycle coding established key 'free node' categories from which the 'naming' of 'body parts' for the 'qualitative autopsy' of street-based injecting environments could commence. The initial stage of the secondary coding cycle involved dividing, splitting and grouping these free-floating nodes into smaller, more compact collections of 'tree nodes' in order to establish recurring themes, constructs and categories located within the visual dataset. Saldana terms this process '*pattern coding*' (2009, 152) and suggests it is a form of coding used to identify 'rules, causes and explanations' within the relevant dataset (ibid). Analysis and the related pattern coding of visual images of settings used for drug-taking purposes sought to identify configurations of environmental similarity/divergence from a harm reduction perspective; identify the physical attributes that may produce/reproduce drug-related harm and categorize the various relationships within each setting noted to occur between place and 'people' (whether they were drug users or not).

Pattern Coding

The coding of visual data as 'patterns' provided almost instantaneous outcome with the emergence of a visual model termed the continuum of descending safety (Parkin 2009a). In this schematic representation of injecting environments, notions of safety/danger are determined from a harm reduction approach to substance use and relate to specific categorical settings located in public places. As such, this visually-oriented model presents a typology of street-based, drug-using environments in a manner that prioritises the practice and principles of harm reduction intervention. A summary of the analytical and hierarchical outcome associated with pattern coding follows in Chapter 5, in which over 400 injecting environments visited during fieldwork is abridged within an 'environmental template' consisting of only 15 images. This model is a direct result of organising and categorising over 1,000 images of injecting sites within a series of hierarchical patterns that reflect levels of parity/disparity with medically-oriented safer injecting facilities (as noted in Figure 4.1) and from environmental and spatial perspectives that prioritise the practice of safer injecting episodes. Furthermore, this hierarchical classificatory process additionally establishes a distinctive three-tier continuum that emphasises the potential for injecting-related harm and hazard to occur within each particular environmental category identified (based upon interview data with drug users and environmental divergence from the 'safer' injecting practice outline in Chapter 2). From this process of pattern coding, all street-based injecting environments may be positioned within a spectrum of actual danger premised upon the range of drug-related harm that characterises individual setting.

According to Saldana (2009), data arranged and managed by pattern coding provides interpretative opportunities that formulate empirically-grounded assertions to be made for the researcher. This author's experience of engaging with pattern coding during visual analysis confirms this claim. Indeed, the contention that drug-related harm is amplified in public places because of their environmental location (Parkin 2009a, 2013) emerged in conjunction with the development of the typology of descending safety. Furthermore, the relevant images of drug using environments within the model do not aim to *illustrate* drug-related harm but instead seek to complement language-based data that provides accounts of harmful experience. Similarly, the visualisation of generic drug-using settings contained within the continuum model presents a spectrum of *environmental settings* that may characterise harmful injecting episodes (as it is the *type of place* that matters and not necessarily *where* the photograph/video is taken).

Focused Coding

A further component of secondary cycle visual data analysis involved a process known as 'focused coding'. According to Saldana (2009, 155), 'the goal of this method is to develop categories without distracted attention ... to their properties and dimensions'. In essence, this form of coding requires the analyst not to become distracted by categorical overlap or thematic similarities within and between the data studied.

To illustrate this point, in the visual dataset attached to this study there are approximately one hundred images of public toilets. Furthermore, each image reflects the environmental conditions that may or may not facilitate safer injecting episodes. For example, one may compare the frequently sanitised, spacious setting of disabled-access toilets to those more characterised by pungent aromas of defecation where floor space is soiled with vomit, blood and/or urine. Both settings may then be further compared to public conveniences that are illuminated by fluorescent blue lighting in an attempt to prevent injecting drug use from occurring (Parkin 2013, Parkin and Coomber 2010). As such, the visual dataset of 'public toilets' in itself represents a sub-spectrum within the continuum model noted above, in which a descent from environmental hygiene to insanitation and injecting hazard may also be noted. In adopting Saldana's (2009) focused coding procedures, visual analysis therefore prioritised the environmental settings with shared function as a collective entity (for example, 'the *toilets*') rather attempt to individualise specific settings (for example, 'a particular *toilet*') accessed in street-based settings.

Focused coding therefore aims to identify how the collective settings of similar environments (for example, 'the toilets') were a feature situated within a public injecting habitus (Parkin 2009a, 2013) and how these range of locations produced/ reproduced drug-related harm. For these reasons, focused coding also follows Saldana's guidance in recognising information images *do not* contain as much as what they present to an audience. This aspect of coding identifies which harm reduction components are 'missing' from the relevant settings and whose presence may facilitate reducing drug-related harm. For example, analytical questions raised by images may include those such as 'is there access to clean, running water? Are the injecting areas spacious and well illuminated? Are there facilities nearby to dispose of sharps and other used paraphernalia? Are the premises open or secure?'

Focused coding therefore considers absent data within visual images as much as what is present. For this reason, this analytical procedure attempts to see the wood *with* the trees! In this study, focused coding of visual data aims to 'see beyond' the information presented in an image by noting the missing, the invisible and less obvious features of injecting environment from a harm reduction perspective. In this regard, 'less is more' (Saldana 2009, 160) as the codes that may emerge from such analysis provide quality – as well as quantity – of interpretation.

Axial Coding

A third component of data analysis with applied value attached to this study is termed 'axial coding' (Saldana 2009, 151). Axial coding involves the identification of (positive and negative) relationships within the data and how themes, issues, categories and sub-categories may be linked together. Axial coding would appear as a natural extension of focused and pattern coding as it seeks to refine previously determined categories (whether longitudinal or hierarchical) established by previous analysis. However, in Saldana's schema of coding proficiency, axial coding involves a further process of data analysis in which a category becomes further split and divided. In this respect, the category becomes an axis around which the emergent sub-categories form the wheel. To simplify axial coding further, if one refers once more to the three different examples of public convenience briefly described above, one may allocate 'toilet' as the axis, around which the three settings revolve. Add to this, supervised toilets, unsupervised toilets, bar room toilets, fast food restaurant toilets, shopping mall toilets and one may notice that the axis of analysis begins to cover a wider and richer circumference. In addition to expanding the spatially-oriented categories in this manner, the analyst also extends the social and physical characteristics of those places almost by default. For example, the social and physical differences between a supervised public convenience in a purpose built, out of town shopping mall and those within a small cubicle illuminated only with a fluorescent blue strip-light at a busy travel terminus will have various implications upon the way in which illicit drugs are prepared and injected in these particular public places.

Axial coding therefore aims to fully unpack the properties and dimensions of a particular category established in previous analysis. In this study of street-based injecting, axial coding was central to informing outcome relating to social behaviour (by injecting drug users and non-injecting drug users) located within, and characterised by, particular settings (see Chapter 5).

Theoretical Coding

The final component of data coding employed during this study of street-based injecting environments is termed 'theoretical coding' by Saldana (2009, 151). It is perhaps fair comment to state that this aspect of coding expands upon the allocation of *a priori* coding (Bazeley 2007) that occurs during first cycle analysis. However, whereas the latter aims to identify individual elements or components of a particular theory (or theories), the author of this work interprets the overall process of theoretical coding as the synthesis of these individual *a priori* codes towards a more holistic theoretical explanation of the research at hand. More specifically, the theoretical coding process attached to this study provided the dominant analytical framework under which pattern, focused and axial coding all took place. As such, the theoretical coding process prioritised Bourdieu's habitus construct (and is documented in full in Parkin 2013) and the applied study of harm reduction in street-based settings. When considered as a single, analytical, entity theoretical coding seeks to translate empirically-grounded data towards more theoretically- and epistemologically- oriented interpretations of the social phenomenon in question. In this analytical process, data and theory become intrinsically linked and reflect the researcher's methodological and empirical rigour. More simply, in this study, the process of theoretical coding demonstrates the deductive design attached to the analysis of all data. Whilst Saldana (2009) suggests that theoretical coding is a useful mechanism for *acquiring* explanations for particular research (*à la* 'grounded theory'), this particular study commenced with the prioritisation of particular theoretical and applied constructs (that is, habitus and harm reduction). As such, the relevant findings of this research did not 'emerge' from the data generated; instead they were 'arranged' via examination of empirically-grounded data in a multi-stage process of first and second cycle analyses.

Concluding Statement on Visual Analysis

Findings to emerge from the varied visual analyses discussed above are presented in Part II of this book (Chapters 5, 6 and 7). Throughout the following three chapters elements of the various coding procedures may be noted in the various accounts of street-based injecting. For example, aspects of pattern, focused and axial coding may be identified within the continuum of descending safety of Chapter 5. In Chapter 6, attention is placed upon the contentious issue of drug-related litter. This chapter has also been informed by elements of pattern, focused, and axial coding. Similarly, in Chapter 7, the environmental management of public settings affected by injecting drug use has been informed by pattern, focused and theoretical coding.

Finally, whilst the *Methods* section of Chapter 3 describes the physical processes attached to taking photographs and making videos whilst in the field (from methodological standpoints that reflect *emic/etic* perspectives of street-based injecting drug use), this chapter has provided a summary on the way in which more sophisticated coding techniques aim to re-present images of drug using environments in an *applied* manner (that is, meaningful to practitioners of harm reduction and related intervention) with *theoretical* value (that is, the academic rigour of sociology and the discipline's concern with structure and agency). Arguably, the overall methodological innovation associated with visual data generation, analysis and representation in this study should silence any criticisms similar to that noted above by Silverman regarding the preponderance of theory-lite visual research! Indeed, answers to the field question *how will this image inform harm reduction and related practitioners* will be made apparent in the subsequent chapters.

Chapter 5
Drug Using Environments as a 'Continuum of Descending Safety'

The following three chapters (5–7) present a summary of applied research findings relating to street-based (public) injecting drug use. Each of the three chapters incorporates visual data generated throughout the various studies of street-based injecting described in Chapter 3. Furthermore, each chapter is dedicated to particular themes, or 'outcomes', that were consistent in the four geographic areas of the research. In this particular chapter the theme relates to the environments and settings of street-based injecting; a theme which is perhaps fundamental to an inquiry concerning the relationship between 'health' and 'place'.

The *explicit* aim of this chapter however, is to demonstrate the utility and value of visual data in applied research especially when they are generated and analysed alongside more orthodox techniques that typify sociological studies (such as interviews, observation, reflexivity and analysis). The *inferred* aim of this chapter is to equally demonstrate the way in which research may utilise visual data in a process that extends beyond 'illustration'. Instead, this chapter seeks to emphasise the complementary and subtle symbiotic relationship that may exist between language-based and image-based data. Accordingly, the following section provides an account of the way in which visual data may facilitate and fortify harm reduction interpretations of environmental settings appropriated for purposes of injecting drug use. Similarly, it may be noted that the images used in this chapter have a particular pedagogic value. This is because each image provides a visual complement to verbal accounts of injecting-related harm reported by drug users interviewed throughout this study; a complement that *consolidates* and *reaffirms*, rather than illustrates, experience. Concomitantly, the visual material presented below (and throughout this book) may be used as *constituent* information to further appreciate the nature of harm reduction and harm production in certain drug using environments.

More briefly, the focus of this chapter is to provide an accessible account of how visual data may enrich understandings of drug-related harm that is made manifest within places that 'contain' specific practices. Furthermore, it is envisaged that presenting naturally-occurring 'thicker description' data (that is, photographs) alongside other qualitative findings (obtained from language-based data), the overall conclusions will be made more convincing, authentic and reliable.

Establishing a Typology of Street-Based Injecting Environments

Over 400 different sites of public injecting drug use were identified and visited during the three respective studies conducted during 2006–2011. Almost all of these street-based settings were photographed and/or video-recorded during fieldwork. Similarly, many of these places were discussed at length with frontline service personnel and injecting drug users during the various interview processes attached to the study. All injecting locations were located within a public or semi-public environment and were wide-ranging in their setting, function and purpose. For example, many were located within various public toilets, car parks, pedestrian thoroughfares, public amenities (such as telephone boxes), disused/abandoned buildings, doorways of retail units, rooftop locations and areas of waste ground. Injecting drug use was also a widely-reported aspect of living in high rise tower blocks, in which communal areas of shared space (stairwells, electric intake rooms and shared areas for depositing refuse) were regularly reported as drug using environments. Similarly, injecting environments were identified within premises that were managed within the private and public sectors. Examples of the former include business premises and retail units (parking lots, toilet facilities, shopping centres, travel centres); whereas facilities and properties managed by the relevant statutory authorities comprised the latter (examples as above, in addition to parkland and other council-owned property). Other injecting environments were visited in areas associated with street-based sex work. These particular settings were typically referred to as a 'red light district', in which residential areas historically-associated with street-based (female) sex workers also provided settings for injecting drug use. Injecting spaces in these areas were typically located in alleyways, but also included parkland, doorways and recesses of residential/business properties within the immediate vicinity.

All street-based drug using environments identified were categorised by their *authentic* function, environmental design and public purpose. This classification is summarised below in Table 5.1. It should be noted that these data have not been categorised by geographic location in order to maintain some confidentiality regarding the specific environmental settings of injecting episodes.[1] From these data, it may be noted that almost 37 per cent (150/409) of all drug using environments were located in some form of public convenience. These included male and female facilities; those providing disabled access, those located in business premises (such as fast food restaurants, retail units) and those that were 'unsupervised' and 'supervised' (by the relevant frontline service personnel within public/private sectors).

---

1   In some circumstances it would be possible to easily identify the relevant public injecting sites by naming the location of the categories concerned. It is not the intention of this book to specifically name and identify public injecting sites visited during the course of this research. This lack of disclosure maintains some anonymity and avoids any on-going sensitivity possibly associated with injecting drug use within the various geographic settings of research.

Drug Using Environments as a 'Continuum of Descending Safety'

Table 5.1   Frequency and Type of Injecting Environment

Public Injecting Site Type	Frequency
Disabled Access Toilets (Unisex)	16
Supervised Toilets (Male)	20
Supervised Toilets (Female)	20
Business District Toilets (Male)	15
Business District Toilets (Female)	15
Unsupervised Toilets (Male)	12
Unsupervised Toilets (Female)	12
Isolated Toilets (Male)	5
Isolated Toilets (Female)	5
Blue Light Toilets (Male)	15
Blue Light Toilets (Female)	15
Supervised Car Parks	12
Unsupervised Car Parks	5
Derelict Outdoor Sites	7
Stairwells (shopping centres)	10
Doorways/Recesses/Rooftops	9
Parkland/Bushes/Green Areas	27
Alleyways (shopping centres)	20+
Alleyways (residential centres)	c.20+
Tower Block (stairwell)	c.30
Tower Block (refuse room)	c.60+
Tower Block (electric unit)	c.30+
Tower Block (basement refuse)	5
'Red Light Areas'	c.20+
Private Land (business sector)	4
Total	c.409

A further 41 per cent (167/409) of drug using environments were found in a range of street-based public settings that included supervised/unsupervised car parks, stairwells, and green areas such as parkland and/or urban greenery. A number of injecting environments were also identified within various alleyways, doorways and other recesses and were often associated with rough sleeping sites. In contrast to these more 'individualised' settings were those associated with more frequent, regular outdoor injecting. A total of seven large-scale, public injecting environments were identified throughout the study in which these settings were frequented almost exclusively by drug users for the purposes of injecting heroin/crack cocaine. These particular sites were usually located within derelict buildings (x 3), overgrown green areas (x 2) and businesses that had been abandoned by the relevant owners (x 2).

A further category of injecting environment was associated with communal areas situated within and around high rise tower blocks in all four locations. Approximately 31 per cent (125/409) of all drug using environments identified were within this category and consisted of settings within stairwells, communal waste areas (known as 'bin chute rooms' – see Figure 5.1), electric intake rooms (containing electric meters) and/or basement areas where refuse is collected in industrial-sized 'skips'. In summary, 20^2 different categories of drug using environments were identified during the course of all fieldwork and associated analysis.

Environmental Features of Public Injecting Sites

Having established 20 *physical* categories of drug using environment located throughout four different geographic settings, it is possible to further refine this classification by the *environmental* characteristics that constitute individual settings. For example, as evident in Table 5.1, some car-parks and public toilets were supervised by frontline service personnel in order to maintain cleanliness, safety and security as a specific aspect of their employment. Similarly, other comparable locations were only partly-supervised or completely unsupervised. Still others operated a system of semi-formal 'policing' in which employees monitored facilities whist engaged in other primary duties (such as those employed in fast-food restaurants). Those drug using environments that had little or no formal supervision by frontline service personnel were more likely to be characterised by varying degrees of dirt and discarded drug-related litter (including injecting paraphernalia).

Accessing drug using environments during all fieldwork was, on occasion, an overwhelming sensory experience involving pungent, overpowering odours coupled with a lack of adequate lighting within enclosed environments in which the slightest sound echoed all around. The following fieldnotes provide an insight into these sensory encounters:

> Throughout the ascent to the top floor of the car park, the stairwells stunk of urine. Participant explained that this didn't matter if you were ill and desperate for a hit as you knew it wouldn't be long before 'feeling well' again. (The actual injecting site) was covered in pigeon excrement and there was various drug-related litter scattered around. Overall (the site) was an unpleasant place to see and smell. (*Fieldnotes, Car Park*)

Similarly:

> The bin chute room was approximately 8 feet by 8 feet by 6 feet, no windows, lit with a dim fluorescent light bulb and accessed by a heavy steel door. The right

---

2   This figure relates to the assumption that all male and female toilet sub-categories (such as 'supervised toilets') are regarded as single entities and not as separate typologies.

Drug Using Environments as a 'Continuum of Descending Safety' 109

side of the wall had some kind of shelf built into the wall and spaces either side of the chute formed alcoves within the room. The left alcove was probably long enough to accommodate a person sitting down with their legs fully stretched, whereas the right alcove would do the same, but would be struck if/when the door opened. From this position it was easy to visualise how drug users would secure the door by sitting with their backs against the chute and their feet pressed against the door. In this particular room there were no items of litter other than household items on the floor (tin cans and cardboard boxes). The floor appeared to have been recently washed as it appeared wet with some small puddles on the concrete surfaces. Although it was not a 'dirty place' – it wasn't exactly clean. I could understand the attraction/utility from an interruption/secrecy/privacy point of view – but from a hygiene perspective, there were limited surfaces, poor lighting, dark, dusty environment, no running water and nowhere to safely prepare solutes. (*Fieldnotes, High Rise Tower Block*)

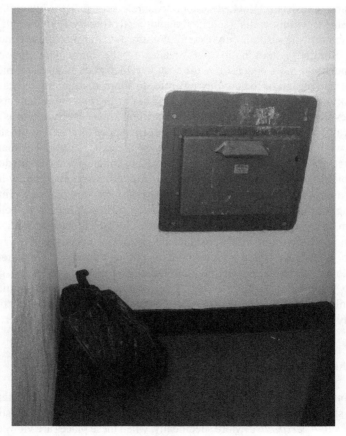

Figure 5.1   Bin Chute Room

Concealment and Marginality

An environmental constant noted throughout each research location were the related, shared, characteristics of concealment and marginality attached to almost all injecting environments visited. These inter-related features became evident during successive visits to the relevant sites and were observed as characteristics that served to completely screen injecting environments from the view of (non-injecting) others. Indeed, these features of concealment and marginality provide naturally-occurring urban camouflage so that those *not* involved in drug use would not necessarily be aware that such places of injecting drug use even exist. In purposely selecting environments containing these features, it became apparent during environmental visual assessments (EVA) that injecting drug users were deliberately attempting to make their presence *invisible* within highly *visible* locations.

For the purpose of this text, concealment relates to the immediate *material* environment that provides primary screening for drug using practice. Typically, concealment consists of 'locked doors', 'concrete screens' (for example, walls), flora (bushes), 'within walls' (stairwells) and/or 'temporary shelters'. Of all drug using environments visited, only three did not provide any of these concealment features. Similarly, marginality here relates to the immediate *physio-spatial* environment and more specifically the way in which such places are interwoven into the urban design of the city/town centre. In short, marginality exists on three levels: 'sky-level', 'eye-level' and 'subterranean'. Injecting environments located in 'sky-level' sites involve a physical *ascent* from street-level settings as a means to physically conceal drug use (for example, the upper floors of multi-storey car parks, or within the upper stairwells of buildings' fire exits). 'Eye-level' marginality relates to street-level 'nooks and crannies' used for similar appropriation (doorways, toilet cubicles and behind street furnishing). 'Subterranean' marginality however, involves a physical *descent* from street-level walkways, into places of diminished natural lighting and/or semi-darkness (examples being stairwells to cellars, fire exits from basements and/or public conveniences located in underground settings).

When these environmental constants are categorised accordingly, a hierarchy begins to emerge in which concealment in public settings is characterised by locked doors, concrete screens, within walls and screens of urban greenery. Similarly, marginality is more likely to be located at 'eye-level' (within alleys, public toilets), but also incorporates 'subterranean' and 'sky-level' settings that physically remove injectors from the immediate *street-level* public sphere.

Establishing a 'Continuum of Descending Safety'

In addition to the above typology, that prioritises shared environmental features of injecting sites, it is possible to further categorise the same venues from a distinctively *harm reduction perspective*. More specifically, when these places are viewed *only as drug using environments* (and not in terms of criminality, morality or other sanction) they may be further characterised in terms of how compatible they are (or not) with the practice and principles of (injecting-related) harm reduction. For the purposes of this research these harm reduction ideals were available in two formats from which all relevant comparative analyses could occur (see Chapter 4). In using these as the relevant benchmarks for 'safer injecting practice', it was possible to further organise all drug using environments in terms of how they are able to reduce, produce and/or reproduce established harms associated with injecting drug use.

As an *aide memoir* to these harm reduction comparisons, all initial assessments of drug using environments relate to how similar or distant each setting is (or is not) to those contained within formalised 'safer injecting facilities'. This form of state-sanctioned intervention typically provides controlled, hygienic and medically supervised settings for the explicit purpose of injecting illicit substances. An example of such a setting is noted in Figure 4.1 and depicts the injecting cubicles found within the Medically Supervised Injecting Centre in Sydney, Australia. Accordingly, *all* injecting environments visited (and photographed) throughout this research were compared to images similar to Figure 4.1 as part of a harm reduction-focused comparative analysis, in which similarities and differences relating to street-based 'environmental control', 'injecting hygiene' and 'levels of supervision' (including presence of others) were noted and recorded.

The second comparative benchmark used throughout this study is a harm reduction manual known as *The Safer Injecting Briefing* (Derricott, Preston and Hunt 1999). This document provides a pedagogical approach to safer injecting technique and practice. As such, the chapters within this guide relating to the preparation of drug solute, injecting technique, routes of administration, overdose management and vein care provided a similar, (although textual), foundation upon which to compare drug user accounts of their injecting experiences in all street-based settings.

From such an analytical and epistemological stance, all street-based injecting sites could be situated within a three-tier schema that prioritises the practice and principles of harm reduction. Furthermore, this visual and text based representation of injecting environments prioritises notions of *control*. It should be noted that 'control' here relates to the content of manufactured environments and how these settings may have been shaped and constructed by *human* intervention for *human* application (that is, built, made: 'control' in this context does not in any way relate to sociological constructions of structural power and/or dominance). Accordingly, 'control' within this hierarchical and classificatory model equates to the co-presence of amenity made available to facilitate safer injecting and harm reduction practices (such as access to water, adequate lighting, injecting space, sterile surfaces).

As such, when drug using environments are viewed from such a perspective, *a continuum of descending safety* (Parkin 2009a) may be noted within the environmental spectrum of street-based settings used for injecting drug use (visually-presented in full below). The continuum of descending safety aims to classify individual street-based injecting sites into one of three environmental categories from the applied standpoints of harm reduction intervention and safer injecting practice. For simplicity each of the classes within this hierarchical model are termed Category

A, B and C respectively. Category A settings are regarded as the most 'controlled' places for injecting purposes as they typically afford greater opportunities to conduct safer injecting episodes; Category B as 'semi-controlled' and Category C as the least controlled ('uncontrolled') of all environments identified. In addition, 'upper-level', Category A sites (disabled-access toilets, see Figure 5.2) typically contain some similarities that are consistent with safer injecting facilities as well as provide *some* environmentally-based opportunities for conducting safer injecting techniques (larger spaces, cleaner surfaces, emergency alarms/ripcords, running water, sharps bins). However, at the lower-levels of the continuum, (within Category C environments such as those within Figures 5.11–5.16), are places identified as those most inconsistent (visually and environmentally) with safer injecting facilities, where injecting episodes become more problematized (due to an overall lack of any *facilitative* amenity). Between these two categories lies the range of semi-controlled (Category B) sites, which provide positive and negative opportunities for conducting safer injecting episodes. However semi-controlled environments are typically spatially, visually and environmentally disconnected from formal, medically-supervised safer injecting facilities.

In order to further clarify this typology of street-based injecting settings, the physical, environmental, and social attributes of each category are explicated below in greater detail.

Category A (Controlled) Public Injecting Sites

These locations are considered as the most 'controlled' injecting environments in street-based settings due to their location in places frequented by the general public and are normally occupied on a regular (or semi-regular) basis by the relevant frontline service personnel. All Category A sites are public toilets and may be provided by businesses within the private or public sectors, in which the latter may be managed by local, statutory authority. Consequently, these 'controlled' sites are typically an aspect of a formal 'working environment' where evidence of drug-related behaviour (for example, discarded paraphernalia) is generally addressed in an immediate manner by those employed in such settings (cleansing operatives, janitors etc.). Examples of such controlled environments include the range of public toilets listed in Table 5.1 and are predominantly located in shopping precincts, supermarkets, bars and fast food restaurants. Figures 5.2–5.6 [below] visualise a range of toilet environments that typify this particular category of within the continuum of street-based injecting environments.

From a harm reduction perspective, Category A injecting environments are further interpreted as providing places more conducive (but not the most ideal) to the safer preparation and injecting of drugs. This is because public toilets typically provide a range of essential requirements to practise safer injecting. These include sanitised surfaces within semi-private settings that are generally well-illuminated (whether by natural or artificial lighting), provide access to clean, running water, tissue paper and informal discarding facilities (litter bins). Street-based toilets are also typically *cleaner* public environments in general due to the various hygiene regimes adopted by the frontline services/local authorities managing and operating such premises. Although frontline personnel within such facilities are more likely to discourage and prevent drug use from taking place, the presence of these people (and the general public) also inadvertently provides an unofficial 'safety-net' in the event of drug-related harm. Injecting safety (relating to overdose management) is therefore further consolidated by the 'natural' presence of non-drug using others, in which people may intervene and/or assist in the event of drug-related overdose.

However, despite this commonality in amenity, environmental and hygienic parity within public toilets is by no means a universal feature of these particular street-based settings. Indeed, multiple visits to the range of public toilets listed in Table 5.1 during fieldwork identified descending levels of hygiene. For example, disabled-access toilets were often the cleanest in contrast to unsupervised, 'stand-alone', street-based facilities that were often characterised by more visible levels of excrement, urine, vomit, soiled paper tissue, blood-stained material and alcohol-related detritus. Indeed, if only Figures 5.2 and 5.6 are compared to one another, one may immediately recognise falling standards of hygiene towards less sanitised settings of injecting drug use that essentially characterises the wider typology of descending safety. Similarly, regardless of any harm reduction amenity provided within public toilets, the presence of locks on cubicle doors to secure privacy (associated with intimacy) has the effect of negating all attempts at safer injecting procedures in the event of drug-related hazard (especially overdose).

Furthermore, the intra-categorical variation associated with public toilets descends even further, from a harm reduction ideal, if one considers conveniences illuminated by fluorescent, ultra-violet lighting ('blue lights'). These installations are purposely designed to prevent injecting drug use from occurring in the relevant settings as they aim to make the task more arduous by means of visual distortion. In such settings, sensory experiences of injecting drug use shift from 'sight' towards 'touch' and injectors are unable to completely 'see' what they are doing with needles and syringes (Parkin 2013, Parkin and Coomber 2010). From a wider public health perspective, blue lights also contribute to physical and visual disorientation that may be problematic for those who are elderly, infirm or experience epilepsy, seizures and/or certain forms of light sensitive visual impairment (Parkin and Coomber 2010).

Due to the monochrome printing within this text, it is not possible to incorporate images of these environments within the visual representation of the continuum model (below). Nevertheless, public toilets equipped with 'blue lights' would be situated between Categories A and B. This positioning (between Controlled and Semi-Controlled categories) relates to the availability of harm reduction amenity typically contained within toilets (hygiene, water, privacy, space) but are made impotent by the presence of lighting purposely designed to problematise injecting episodes.

Injecting Drug User Motivations

Respondent motivations for accessing public toilets typically referred explicitly to the environmental conditions that facilitated drug preparation and injection described above. This is evident in the following multi-site illustrations:

> (I go to) ... the disabled toilets in (fast food restaurant) at the *bottom* of town – the disabled toilets in (fast food restaurant) at the *top* of town. The disabled toilets ... in the mall and basically anywhere you can get into a disabled toilet. Cos it's basically a toilet on its own. There's no one else, you can lock the door and it's just you there and no one else can hear what you're doing. ... It's a bigger space, you can sit on the floor and do it, you're not cramped up in a little tiny cubicle worried that if a policeman come into the toilet he can see your feet hanging out underneath the cubicle door, 'cos your kneeling down on top of the toilet trying to sort your stuff out.[3] (*Respondent 058*)[4]

> See for me I always go in a public toilet cos I'm always behind a locked door. So they (police) never get through the door if they know I'm in there. They'd never get through that locked door, I would of got rid of everything (drugs) by the time they did. (*R042*)

> I went to a ward up in the hospital. Went into the toilet there and I thought 'well if anything happens, I'm in a hospital innit'. If anything drastic happens or something, a nurse is gonna be there, know what I mean? So it is outside and totally illegal to fuck but I was in a cancer ward, sitting there in the staff toilet having a dig. (*R055*)

> ... most of the time ... they're (toilet attendants) that busy if they see you coming in, their minds are occupied and they ain't gonna look at ya and think 'oh he's a bit dodgy' like, you know. They're always busy so there's less attention on you. (*R068*)

---

3 Throughout this book all interview responses have been presented verbatim. Whilst no attempt has been made to recreate the local dialect with appropriate phonetic representation, all utterances have remained unchanged in terms of grammar and informal speech (for example, 'ya' for 'your'). Similarly, the use of ellipses (that is, '...') has been used as in conventional academic citations; to present clarity in syntax whilst retaining the *original meaning* of the words spoken. Ellipses have *not* been used as means of censure or to indicate problems in finding the correct phrase by the speaker. This convention follows that adopted by Bourgois and Schonberg (2009, 12–13).

4 For all further *injecting drug user responses* (R), the following convention applies: *R001-R071* = the collapsed cohort.

Harm Associated with Injecting Drug Use within Category A (Controlled) Sites

Despite the range of amenity within public toilets that may facilitate harm reduction, experience of drug-related hazard within such settings was reported by injecting drug users throughout each geographic setting of the study. Listed below is a summary of key harms associated with injecting episodes conducted in public conveniences (Parkin 2009a, 2013). Each of these harms should be regarded as a manifestation of the various environmental influences (social, spatial, physical and legal) associated with 'toilet' settings. Furthermore, all harms below were reported with varying degrees of experience throughout the 71-strong cohort across all four geographic settings.[5]

- death of peers (due to drug overdose occurring behind *locked* cubicle doors).
- overdose (fatal and non-fatal).
- cerebral hypoxia (following rushed/slammed injecting to avoid detection/ interruption in a public place).
- groin injecting (considered rapid practice to ensure drug intake and hasty departure from public places).
- opportunities for viral and bacterial infection to emerge from the recycling of discarded (used and unused) paraphernalia (including water and cookers).
- rushed preparation of drugs (to avoid interruption by public, frontline service personnel) involving shared use of paraphernalia.
- rushed injection technique (to avoid interruption public, frontline service personnel) that causes or extends injecting-related injury.
- sharing paraphernalia (especially cookers) to minimise time in setting, creating opportunities for viral/bacterial infection.
- minor burns resulting from using swabs as improvised 'lighters' whilst holding uncapped cookers.
- engaging in tactile-oriented injecting (in groin, neck or peer injecting) to counter the effect of 'blue lights' in areas.

Category B (Semi-Controlled) Public Injecting Sites

Figures 5.7–5.11 (below) provide generalisations of injecting environments within this category. Category B sites are typically frequented and attended mainly by drug users and for the specific purpose of drug injecting. These locations are regularly situated within areas associated with other street-based activities (such as drug markets, street-based sex work) that typically exclude full-access by the

---

5 The precise details of how these harms are made manifest are documented at length in *Habitus and Drug Using Environments* (Parkin 2013).

wider-public due to their hidden (and 'invisible') nature. Semi-controlled sites are known throughout drug user networks as places where substances may be injected with minimal contact with other people (non-drug users, police, security guards, neighbours) and are generally more marginal, clandestine locations when compared to those of Category A. The most recurring feature within semi-controlled settings is the limited access to water and other sanitary conditions (if existing at all), in which drugs are prepared for injection in settings characterised by dirt and detritus (of human and organic origin). This environmental descent may be noted in the relevant images below, in which the 'communal' and shared nature of semi-controlled environments of injecting drug use may also be apparent (evidenced by the volume of drug/alcohol-related litter below in Figures 5.7–5.11). Category B sites may also be regarded as locations defined by pre-arranged, pre-planned injecting behaviour as well as being secluded environments that often require a specific 'insider' knowledge of their actual whereabouts. These locations also offer less of the protective features afforded in more controlled environments (such as hygienic surfaces, running water, with adequate injecting space). Indeed, contact with other people (specifically non-drug users) in these settings is typically limited and social encounters in such sites are more through happenstance than design. Further 'semi-controlling' characteristics of these sites relates to the absence of regular 'opening hours', a lack of security patrols and/or the frequent cleansing programmes by frontline service personnel within such settings. Instead, these locations are generally defined by their exact opposites; namely *the lack of* safety, *lack of* cleanliness and *lack of* restricted access.

From a harm reduction perspective, injecting environments in this category are defined as 'semi-controlled' sites on the basis of shared sociality *by other injecting drug users*. Although lacking the fundamental hygienic locations needed for safer injecting episodes, they do provide opportunities for contact with other people due to the fluctuating and frequent attendances by other injecting drug users. This element of social and physical contact with others (regardless of how hostile or unfamiliar these encounters may be) provides a potential safeguard in the event of drug-related harm (for example, providing access to paraphernalia, providing assistance with resuscitation, reporting overdose, calling emergency services prior to fleeing injecting site[6]).

Numerous injecting sites of this variety were identified within various alleyways and stairwells surrounding areas of street-based sex work, within derelict buildings and untended green areas across all four urban centres of the study. Other examples within this category include the wide range of car-parks (multi-storey, underground, supervised and unsupervised) and the various settings associated with high rise tower blocks (see Table 5.1).

---

6   Assuming that these forms of assistance *would* be provided.

Injecting Drug User Motivations

Respondent motivations for attending Category B injecting environments purposely prioritises the limited access they provide to the wider (non-drug using) public. For example:

> Someone just showed it to us one day. Up at the top there's little (fox)holes you can get into. Someone just showed us, get in there, out the way, nice and quiet, no one is ever going to come along there and disturb you. So you can take as much time as you want; relax. Before you could sit in the undergrowth and watch people walking past along the park – but they couldn't see you. Unless you knew where these holes were, you wouldn't look at 'em. I didn't even know they were there till someone showed me! It's a nice little place to go if you've got nowhere to sleep and you could sleep there, there's no wind and it's ideal actually. The only dis … . down thing about it, is all the junk you've got to climb through to get to it. An' there's a lot of horrible stuff lying around up there! (Including drug related litter and human faeces). (*R065*)

> … so you're down in the corner, behind bushes, and you can see out and see the whole park. But you know, people just walking past wouldn't know you were there. Nice and quiet, they wouldn't know you were there. … unless they were actually looking for ya. But you can see them, you know what I mean? And people won't wander in because, you know, why would you jump over a fence of a bowling green? You just wouldn't would ya? The average man, woman, kid, just wouldn't! (*R059*)

> I look for a secluded place. Anywhere, where I know no one can come in or if they did come in I could hear them coming in. A safe place … I've never done it in crack houses or places like that cos when you're gouching you don't know what people could do to ya. That's why we go in the bin chute rooms, cos you can sit down on the floor and lay your stuff out in a safe kind of environment. But in (toilets) I could never do that. Cos someone would be thinking I've been in there too long. The bin chutes are like a homely environment. (*R039*)

> (Security guards are) usually in their little hut. They don't usually venture out, so long as you don't act suspicious or there's a big group of you, any you're quick an' that, then there is pretty good. (It's) well-down there, it's out of the wind basically and it's pretty dry and out of the way. The best concealed place if you are in a hurry, or you are ill an' it's pretty good just to get out of the way. The threat of people coming and going is pretty low as most people that use this car park are either here at nine or ten o'clock in the morning, or four or five when they're leaving work. (*R006*)

Category C (Uncontrolled) Public Injecting Sites

Category C injecting sites are the most concealed/less obvious injecting environment of all three categories within the continuum of descending safety (see Figures 5.12 –5.16). They are typically more-related to individual and opportunistic injecting episodes instead of the more environmentally-focused, socially-organised settings of drug use associated with Category A and B respectively. Uncontrolled sites are spatially more random, more transient and more difficult to trace due to the often spontaneous nature of their organisation. This is due to Category C sites having greater associations with homeless/roofless individuals that may have temporarily appropriated specific places for the dual purpose of 'pitching' (sleeping) and injecting. In contrast, such locations may also be settings of opportunistic injecting due to the nearby presence of drug sellers, needle and syringe programmes and/or spontaneous street-based contact with other drug users. Unlike Category A and B environments, these sites are not static in time and place and may be used less frequently by fewer drug users (perhaps only known to one or two individuals at any given time).

Uncontrolled environments are often characterised by small, dark, recessed areas that are, paradoxically, both public and private locations. This is because such places are usually more public oriented during working, daylight hours when compared to the relative privacy they provide between dusk and dawn (for example, a loading-bay at the rear of a shopping centre). These locations are usually within the scope of CCTV cameras or are subject to other security arrangements (such as security guards, locked gates, perimeter walls and/or fencing). No amenities to facilitate drug preparation are associated with such settings and it is for these reasons that they are classified as 'uncontrolled' injecting environments. Similarly, the almost spontaneous emergence of these injecting environments (in locations more deeply concealed, more deeply marginalised) provides greater opportunities for drug related harm and hazard to occur.

Injecting Drug User Motivations

The more spontaneous and opportunistic nature of injecting within this more marginal injecting category may be observed in the following responses:

> My favourite spot is a telephone box. And I call it my 'Superman turnout' because I'm usually ill when I go in the phone box and it's normally not because ... well, yeah, it is convenience. You know, you travel a certain distance to go get your bit of gear; you're sweating, you're sneezing, you're puking, and you don't want to have to walk all the way back to the estate to do your thing. And it's hard to get into the flats that are nearby ... because of drug using, you know, so I go in a phone box. (*R037*)

It depends as well where you score and you know the areas well 'cos you know whereabouts your dealer lives. So you know then if there's cemeteries nearby. They're quite good place to inject 'cos usually they're quiet and safe as well because you can hide behind tombstones and graves. (*R046*)

If you go into any of the back alleys in the city centre … they've got bins there. So you can crouch down next to a bin in a back alleyway … and nobody sees you till they are right on top of you. And if it's a long alley it'll take them a minute to get there, so you'll see them coming (and can leave quickly). (*R070*)

No, it's the other way around (for me). Having more people there makes it more difficult for me. … It's easier for it to be peaceful not hectic, (but) quiet, quieter – for me, personally, I find that's better for me. … Heroin is not a social drug, you know, *it's just not*. I mean I've got a few problems at the moment. … and I don't wanna sit there with anyone. The whole thing about heroin is the nothingness of it. You know, the obliteration so that I haven't got any problems … so you don't really want anyone chatting in your ear in that time. You just wanna be asleep basically. I suppose it's the closest to being dead you can get (without actually being dead) … (*R055*)

Harm associated with injecting drug use within Category B (Semi-Controlled) and Category C (Uncontrolled) Sites

As with public toilets, environmental settings within the continuum of descending safety defined as semi-controlled and uncontrolled injecting environments also produce and reproduce drug-related harm. Listed below is a further summary of key harms associated with these less controlled environments (Parkin 2009a, 2013). It may be noted that these environments house a more comprehensive spectrum of drug-related harm. This is turn may be correlated to the situated nature of injecting drug use in more social and more marginal environments. As such, and as with public toilets, each of the harms presented below represents the manifestation of the harmful effects of place upon agency in the context of injecting drug use. (Similarly, all harms below were reported with varying degrees of experience throughout the 71-strong cohort across all four geographic settings).

- death (due to overdose in isolated, *concealed* settings).
- overdose (fatal and non-fatal).
- cerebral hypoxia (due to rushed/slammed injecting practice following to avoid police detection whilst in a public place).
- groin injecting (considered rapid practice to ensure drug intake and hasty departure from public places).
- opportunities for viral and bacterial infection to emerge from the recycling of discarded (used and unused) paraphernalia (including water and cookers).

- needlestick injury caused by greater volume of discarded sharps (used and unused).
- peer-injecting (including inappropriate hygiene and injecting technique by injector).
- peer-mediated injection injury (especially in neck and legs of the injected).
- 'dirty hits' due to unsanitary environments (and increased opiate use as self-medication to reduce associated pains), also increased opportunities of bacterial infection.
- rushed preparation of drugs (to avoid interruption by public, frontline service personnel) involving shared use of paraphernalia.
- rushed injection technique (to avoid interruption public, frontline service personnel) that causes or extends injecting-related injury.
- sharing paraphernalia (especially cookers) to minimise time in setting, creating opportunities for viral/bacterial infection.
- diminished injecting technique due to inadequate lighting – especially in outdoor settings during the hours of darkness.
- minor burns resulting from using swabs as improvised 'lighters' whilst holding uncapped cookers.
- violent confrontation with other drug users seeking drugs/money.
- swallowing drugs to avoid arrest (police) or assault (by other drug users).

Environmental Liminality

Although the continuum model summarised above provides an account of three specific injecting categories, it should be equally noted that all drug using environments are not mutually bound within a particular, single category. Indeed, in some instances there may be an overlap in the variation of harm reduction control and it is possible that some locations may overlie two categories within the proposed model.

As an illustration, the previously mentioned toilets that contain 'blue light' installations may be jointly-considered as an example of a 'controlled environment' (due to the cleaner environment, co-presence of others and the privacy afforded by cubicles) and an 'uncontrolled environment' (due to way in which blue lights aim to make injecting more difficult).

When viewed from a harm reduction perspective some places may therefore exist in an environmental liminality between two different categories (for example, Categories A and B) affording both safety (hygiene and security) and danger (poor lighting and locked doors). Similar liminality may be observed in settings where injecting-related practice is diminished in facilities that are completely unsupervised, occasionally supervised or monitored on a regular basis (for example, toilets and car parks). Nevertheless, this model of a *continuum of descending safety* aims to provide a categorical and sociological condensation of environmental features, spatial and social settings associated with public injecting drug use in an attempt to correlate harm with 'place'.

Visualising the Continuum

Whereas the above sections sought to *describe* the typology of street-based injecting environments encountered during all fieldwork, the remainder of this chapter aims to *visualise* the same model. The following visual dataset is intended to be viewed as a complement to the above text-based summary of over 400 environments affected by injecting drug use.

The 15 injecting environments portrayed below therefore re-present the three hierarchical categories of street-based environments contained within the continuum of descending safety. These images demonstrate the way in which each

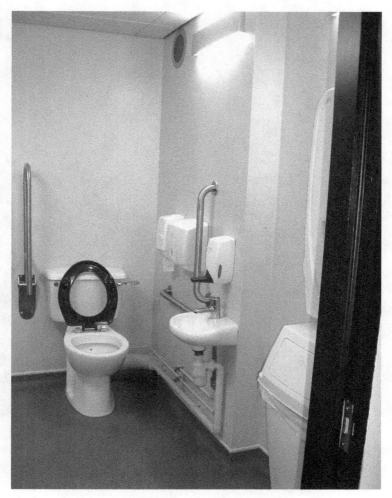

Figure 5.2   Category A (Controlled) Injecting Environment (1)

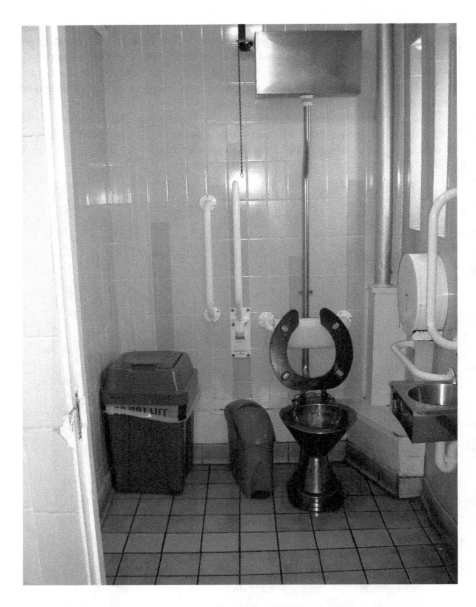

Figure 5.3   Category A (Controlled) Injecting Environment (2)

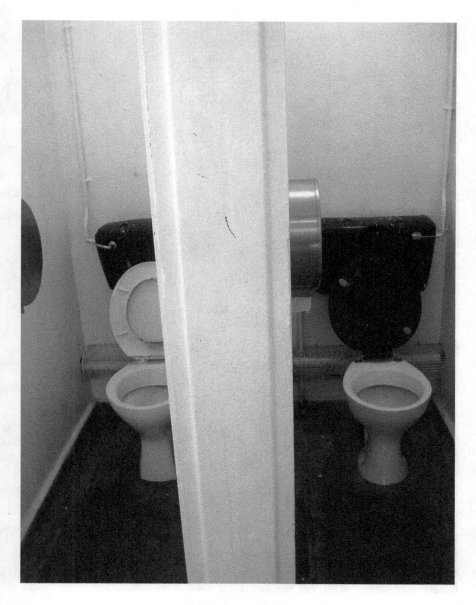

Figure 5.4   Category A (Controlled) Injecting Environment (3)

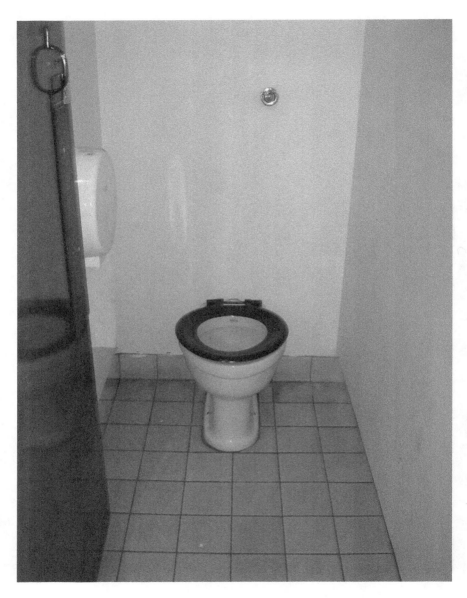

Figure 5.5   Category A (Controlled) Injecting Environment (4)

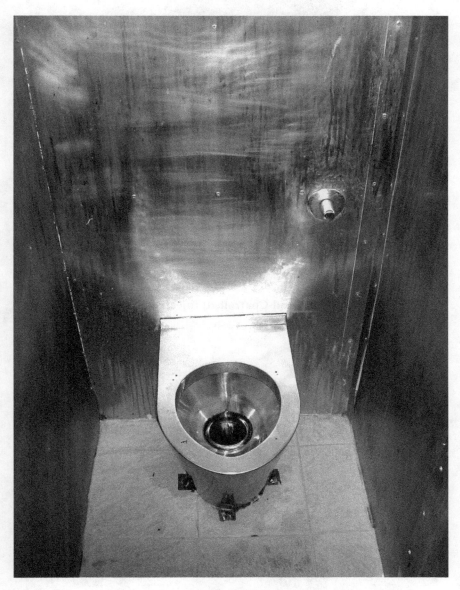

Figure 5.6   Category A (Controlled) Injecting Environment (5)

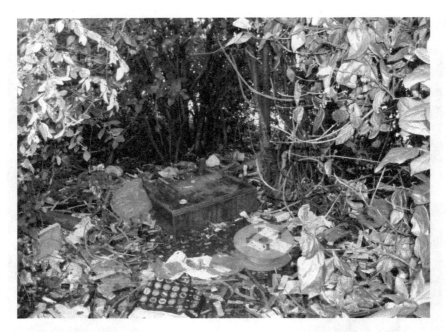

Figure 5.7   Category B (Semi-Controlled) Injecting Environments (1)

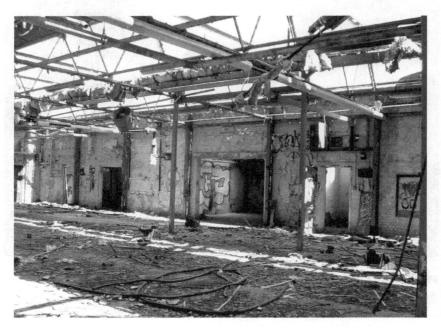

Figure 5.8   Category B (Semi-Controlled) Injecting Environments (2)

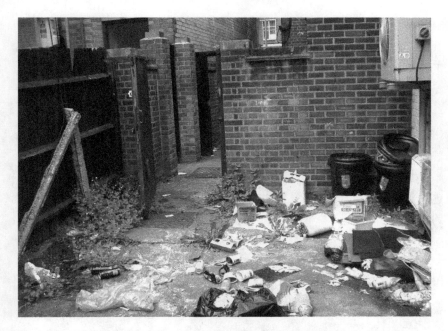

Figure 5.9   Category B (Semi-Controlled) Injecting Environments (3)

categorical and environmental setting problematises the harm reduction-focused safer injecting procedures outlined in Chapter 2. As such, the 15 photographs have been organised in a vertical manner (top-down) to best portray the hierarchical model associated with 'descending safety'. In considering the environmental conditions portrayed throughout Figures 5.2–5.16, one may appreciate the spatial diversity in which street-based injecting occurs and simultaneously visualise the physical and environmental descent from hygiene and safety (Figure 5.2) towards dirt and danger (Figure 5.16).

Harm Reduction Implications

When viewed alone as single artefacts, the various photographic images included in this chapter may be considered rather 'meaningless' and bereft of any 'applied value'. Indeed, if viewed in such a manner, it may be argued that each individual photograph merely contains a representation of everyday, mundane settings found in almost every urban environment in the developed world. However, when a series of seemingly unexciting images become connected by a particular theme (injecting drug use) and linked by a variety of analytical foci (harm reduction, injecting environments and associated practice), the wider visual dataset becomes significantly more evocative and meaningful. More specifically, when viewed as a complementary component of a mixed dataset comprising of text and photography (that incorporates reflexive

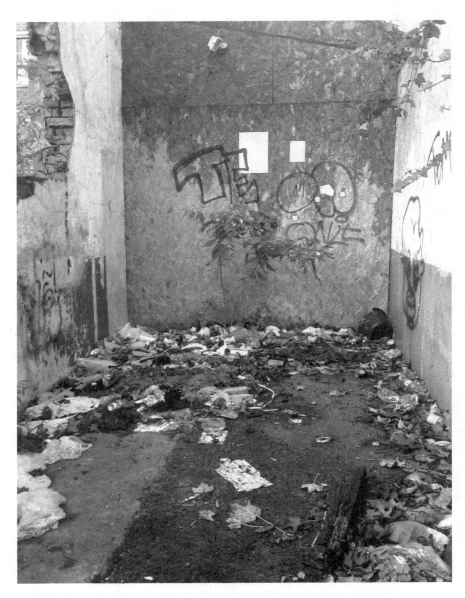

Figure 5.10 Category B (Semi-Controlled) Injecting Environments (4)

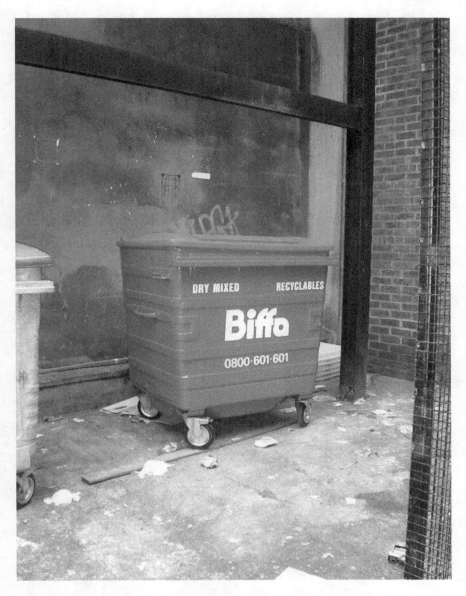

Figure 5.11   Category B (Semi-Controlled) Injecting Environments (5)

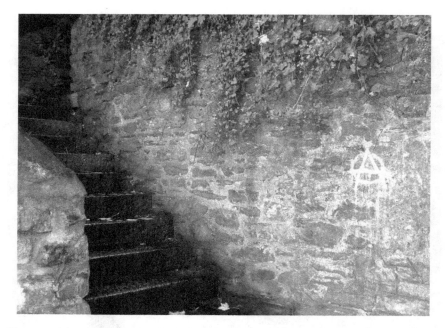

Figure 5.12   Category C (Uncontrolled) Injecting Environments (1)

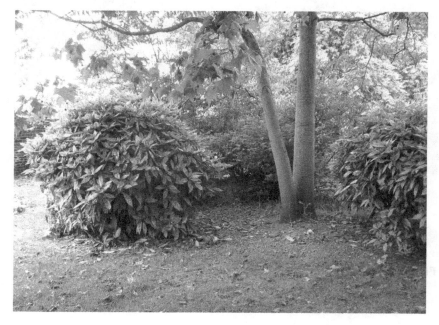

Figure 5.13   Category C (Uncontrolled) Injecting Environments (2)

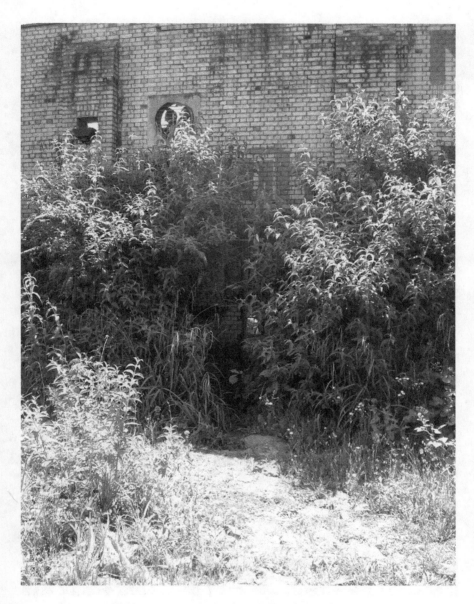

Figure 5.14 Category C (Uncontrolled) Injecting Environments (3)

132   An Applied Visual Sociology: Picturing Harm Reduction

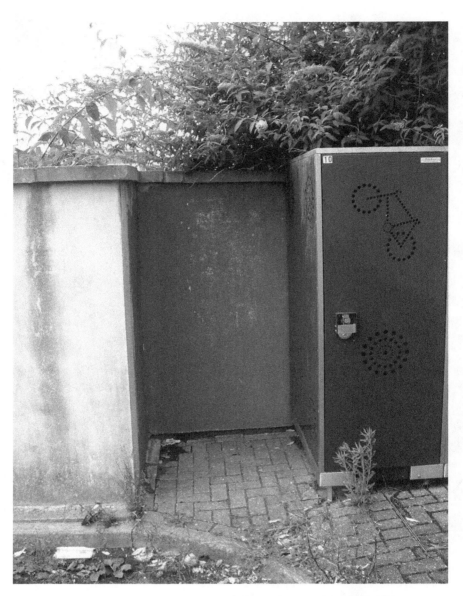

Figure 5.15   Category C (Uncontrolled) Injecting Environments (4)

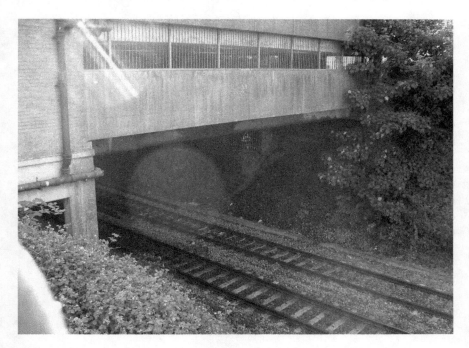

Figure 5.16   Category C (Uncontrolled) Injecting Environments (5)

fieldnotes, interview transcripts, ethnographic observation and visual materials) an amalgamated unit of qualitative material emerges for analysis. Accordingly, when these data are viewed through the analytical lens of an applied harm reduction, the relationship between 'health' and 'place' in the context of injecting drug use is characterised by associated harm and hazard.

This negative health-place nexus becomes further evident if one considers the photographs of environments alongside accounts of injecting episodes reported by drug users in such places. For example, the principles of safer injecting practice outlined in Chapter 2 are consistently made difficult by the environmental characteristics that typify street-based locations. This consistency relates to injecting practice that is made more problematic from sensory perceptions (sight, sound, touch and smell) and the perspectives of safety (locked doors, poor lighting, insecure settings), comfort (unsanitary, makeshift conditions, frenetic environments), hygiene (dirt, excreta, drug-related litter, lack of water, lighting), ambience (noise, stress, rushed), drug preparation (frantic and anxious) and ultimately injection itself (hasty, assisted, rapid, distracted and frenetic). All of which are settings and behaviours that better characterise the *antithesis* of harm reduction practice. Instead, accounts of injecting in these environments typically reflect a conscious and unconscious participation in the practice of harm production. Indeed, the contributory environmental qualities of harm production may be noted in the images attached to the continuum of descending safety portrayed throughout this Chapter (Figures

5.2–5.16). Indeed, if the relevant images within this 15 image dataset were permitted to 'narrate' the principles of harm reduction and safer injecting, then the over-riding message from this non-fiction account would be that these settings amplify harm production and contribute towards the re-production of established hazard in street-based injecting environments (Parkin 2009a, 2013).[7]

To conclude this chapter, the *methods* involved in data generation (Chapter 3) coupled the associated *analytical* processes (Chapter 4) attached to this study provide a genuine attempt at synthesising academic research towards applied, service-relevant, value (this chapter). In Chapter 9, the findings described in this Chapter (relating to the 'continuum of descending safety') and the collected conclusions described in Chapters 6–7, are totalised in the context of 'picturing harm reduction' within a framework of 'applied visual sociology'. The intention of consolidating individual chapter conclusions in this way is to purposely accentuate the potential of research (with more applied visual sociology) for informing intervention.

---

7   To further validate this point, each photograph in this chapter should be further compared to the suggested social, physical and hygienic settings recommended for safer injecting outlined in Chapter 2.

Chapter 6
Drug Related Litter as Visual Data

For the purposes of this book, 'drug related litter' and 'discarded equipment' are terms that are used interchangeably to refer to paraphernalia that facilitates injecting episodes and are items that have been deposited in settings associated with episodes of street-based injecting. Such items principally relate to needles that are attached to syringe barrels; as well as interchangeable needle attachments, syringes with no needle attachment and syringes with fixed needle attachments. In addition, drug related litter includes items such as filters, steri-cups®, improvised cookers, water ampoules/bottles, swabs, tissue, needle caps, portable sharps boxes and various wrappings and seals associated with all of the above. Furthermore, the term drug related litter and discarded equipment refers to both *used* and *unused* items that may have been deposited in public settings. All of the aforementioned items may be noted in Figures 2.1–2.3.

The issue of drug related litter is arguably more contentious and more emotive than the physical act of public injecting drug use itself – especially when viewed from the perspective of community safety. This paradox in public health possibly relates to the potential for wider social contact with discarded paraphernalia, particularly when such litter may have been used (directly or indirectly) for the purposes of administering injections of illicit drugs. In a previous article (Parkin and Coomber 2011) the author suggested that this situation was associated with sociological constructions of 'fear' in which non-drug user perceptions of injecting equipment is synonymous with infection, disease and contamination of health. Similarly, when such 'pollution taboos' (Douglas 1966) are extended and associated with people who inject illicit drugs, the latter are subsequently perceived as 'threats' within a particular social setting. In turn, morally-founded constructions of 'social threat' (relating to 'dangerous infections' emanating from 'dangerous bodies') become the bases of stigma and prejudice. This view may be substantiated in the following news items that report upon drug related litter throughout the British Isles (England, Scotland, Wales, Northern Ireland and the Republic of Ireland) and simultaneously contextualise the issue in community settings. As these articles are contemporaneous with the research period (2006–2011) described in this text they further reflect a view of drug related litter (and injecting drug users) that is representative of the time in question.

We want the junkies out

Angry residents who say they are sick of finding used hypodermic needles in their gardens have rounded on a housing association they blame for placing suspected heroin addicts in their street. (*Plymouth Herald*, 15 December 2006)

Jamie, 5, pricked by dirty needle

The mother of a five-year-old boy has described her anxious wait for tests results after her son was pricked by a hypodermic syringe while playing in a children's park. (*Plymouth Herald*, 22 February 2007)

Five-year-old boy who sucked on discarded hypodermic needle faces tests for HIV and hepatitis

A boy of five must have an HIV test after sucking a hypodermic needle he picked up near a playground. (*The Mail Online*, 18 April 2008[1])

Used needles found in post boxes

Postal workers in Derby are being warned to take care after a rise in the number of used syringes being found in post boxes. (*BBC News Online*, 17 October 2008[2])

Police set sights on fly tippers and litter bug drug addicts in Blackheath

The police have pinpointed St Paul's Church Hall as a trouble spot after complaints of wanton fly tipping and drug addicts littering the area with needles. (*Halesowen News*, 14 December 2009)

Shock as tot, 3 finds dirty needle in West Howe

A mother was horrified when her three-year old daughter found a used hypodermic syringe near their home in Bournemouth.(*Bournemouth Daily Echo*, 7 September 2010)

Addicts get special bins for needles

Soaring drug use at the St Paul's protest camp has forced council bosses to install special containers for used needles. The City of London said 'sharps bins'

---

1 http://www.dailymail.co.uk/news/article-560505/Five-year-old-boy-sucked-discarded-hypodermic-needle-faces-tests-HIV-hepatitis.html (accessed: 29 March 2013).

2 http://news.bbc.co.uk/1/hi/england/derbyshire/7675689.stm (accessed: 29 March 2013).

were needed after police found addicts' syringes around activists' tents (*The Daily Star*, 24 November 2011)

Used needles found on route to Maesycoed Primary School

Mothers in Graig have lifted the lid on a potentially serious drug problem after finding needles in bushes near their local school. (*Pontypridd Observer*, 5 April 2012 (*Wales*))

Junkies terrorising pensioners in town centre

Battling junkies are terrorising pensioners and traders in Airdrie town centre. One shopkeeper described a fight between two female drug addicts at Airdrie Cross as "like the OK Corral". Several traders told the Advertiser that their customers are being frightened and intimidated by a large crowd of addicts congregating outside Farmfoods each day. And we also discovered a drug den behind one shop which is littered with used needles and drug paraphernalia where addicts are shooting up to get high. (*Airdrie and Coatbridge Advertiser*, 1 August 2012 (*Scotland*))

Children at risk from discarded needles

Children have been exposed to deadly diseases after picking up needles discarded by heroin users who inject themselves on Cork streets. (*Irish Examiner*, 13 September 2012 (*Republic of Ireland*))

Media Reportage of Drug Related Litter

The various media reports of drug related litter presented above typify the way in which the issue is reported in printed and online publications throughout England, Scotland, Wales and the Republic of Ireland. Although each of the above reports originates from numerous sources, from four different countries, the underlying moral and political message is resoundingly similar throughout. Namely, 'drug related litter is a danger to public health and those who deposit such items are an unwanted menace to society'.

To elaborate upon this view, a basic 'content analysis' of each media item above would identify noticeable common ground between the relevant provincial and national reports. For example, the dominant theme to emerge from these stories is one of 'conflict', in which outraged members of the public allocate blame and voice moral indignation on the issue of drug related litter and injecting drug use/rs. This conflict is made further evident in the chosen vocabulary within many of the reports above. For example, accounts of 'refusing' to comply with taxation, 'mothers lifting the lid' on social problems, in addition to 'blaming' and 'rounding-on' authorities, who in turn 'pinpoint' people and places in a 'battle' to protect public space are all clear expressions of social and community unease. Similarly, a language of 'psychological warfare' underlies several reports in which accounts of 'horror', 'terror', 'intimidation', 'shock' and 'anxiety' are used in conjunction with drug related litter, drugs and/or drug users. This stance is further perpetuated in the pejorative use of terms such as 'junkie' and 'addict', in which the provision of legitimate facilities to drug users (such as 'sharps bins') is somehow misrepresented as extraordinary and undeserving intervention ('special bins').

Whereas the above interpretations may be regarded as more 'politically-oriented' responses to drug related litter and injecting drug users, a more 'moral' imperative is also inferred throughout each of the reports. For example, reports of discarded injecting equipment are typically juxtaposed alongside accounts of childhood innocence, in which designated social space (typically 'playgrounds') have been made corrupt by dirt and danger. These accounts of contaminated childhood are made more explicit when the report(er)s attempt to personalise particular events in the 'naming' and 'aging' of children involved in accidental injury. Strategically and emotively constructed sentiments such as this present a quintessential illustration of the global social uncertainty, unease and anxiety documented within theses of risk society and reflexive modernity (Beck 1992, Giddens 1990, 1991).

A further constant that may be observed throughout each of the reports is the underlying threat of illness and infection inferred – or explicated – in each account of drug related litter. This typically relates to an 'exposure' to 'HIV', 'hepatitis', and/or 'deadly disease' as a result of injury from 'dirty needles' and is made yet more sensational when it involves younger members of a given community. Finally, the importance of 'place' in the context of injecting drug use is also apparent throughout many of the sample stories presented above. This is perhaps only evident when reports of drug related litter such as these are presented *en masse* in which the locations of street-based injecting environments may otherwise go unreported. For example, listed above is an indication of many of the 'hidden' settings that appear consistent with Category B and Category C injecting environments described in the previous chapter. Concealed locations described above that are compatible with the continuum of descending safety comprise churchyards (including 'protest encampments'), undergrowth ('bushes') and areas associated with and/or adjacent children's playparks (that are more typically public and/or 'green areas'). However, whereas the continuum of descending safety prioritises the relationship of health and place, the accounts of public space in the above media reports is more aligned to moral constructions of place and social (im)purity.

It is perhaps necessary to emphasise that a societal role of the mass media is, essentially, to report upon *extraordinary* and *remarkable* events that occur in provincial, national and international settings. For example, at a macro level, this may include commentary and analysis of world affairs, current events, political concerns and celebrity 'news'. At more micro-levels of society this may involve accounts of individual success and achievement, local business developments, government investment/cutbacks and other important community/public events. In the context of these wider social and political affairs, reports of isolated and individual events of needlestick injury (regardless of age, identity and place) that occur in local and provincial settings are hardly remarkable or extraordinary events.

In reality, it is debateable whether reports of needlestick injury are actually newsworthy in *any* capacity; otherwise the national news would be dominated by reports of mundane accidents occurred in community settings on a daily basis. Accordingly, news items regarding needlestick injury rarely make national headlines and will more likely feature in provincial newspapers due to their relevance to specific communities and, perhaps, to highlight drug-related issues in those specific locales. However 'the mass media tend to represent the world as predominantly uncivil, violent and threatening' (Lupton and Tulloch 1999, 509) in which 'lay knowledge, in local dialogic exchange with a variety of circuits of communication (… local papers, television …) constructs specific causal chains in relation to 'unemployment', 'drugs', 'crime' … ' (ibid., 521).

In considering these interpretations of the mass media, reportage of drug related litter (such as those presented above) in community settings possibly contribute to a limited understanding of social problems experienced at a local level of society. Similarly, such distorted reporting may initiate and justify social responses considered appropriate *from the perspective of a 'moral' majority*. Whilst such reporting may reflect a particular agenda for those directly concerned, a further possible inference is the general discrediting and destabilisation of harm reduction approaches to drug use. More specifically, negative constructions of needles/syringes in community settings imply a de-legitimisation of valid public health intervention and the problematisation of international policy that has a demonstrable record of efficacy (O'Hare et al. 1992, Pates and Riley 2012, Rhodes and Hedrich 2010, Strang and Gossop 2005a,b).

The Politics of Drug Related Litter

It is important to further emphasise that the issue of drug related litter has been included in this text as the topic was often *politically* synonymous with the wider study that prioritised the health effects of injecting episodes conducted in public places (Parkin 2009a, 2013). Similarly, discarded, drug-related paraphernalia was *– without question –* always regarded as a controversial, emotive and political issue by the majority of frontline service personnel and community-based participants throughout all four geographic areas of fieldwork. Furthermore, the various concerns voiced by the latter were equally articulated by the 71 injecting drug users that participated in the study, who themselves had engaged in episodes of street-based injecting. However, whereas the latter sought to distance themselves from acts of other drug users perceived as 'anti-social' and 'irresponsible' (Parkin 2013) the views of non-drug users were typically less rationalised. Instead, the various responses offered by those directly and indirectly affected by discarded injecting equipment were often vehement criticisms that reflected antithetical opinions of harm reduction, injecting drug use and/or users. In short, the views, emotions and moral stance of non-injecting drug users involved this study were not dissimilar to the pejorative politics outlined and contained within the above media reports.

There can be no dispute that on an *individual* level, needlestick injuries in community settings are tragic and unfortunate accidents. Such events will inevitably cause immense distress and anguish for those directly and indirectly affected by such incidents. Nevertheless, media interpretations and misrepresentations of this issue serve to inflame irrational responses towards an important public health issue, in which prejudice and stigma directed at particular members of society typically prevails (see Box 6.1; Appendix I). This chapter therefore attempts to re-contextualise the politics of drug-related litter within a harm reduction approach to community safety and public health management. This chapter *does not* seek to provide an 'apologist's viewpoint' of drug related litter within community and street-based settings and the author is cognisant of, and overtly familiar with, the psychological distress contact with such paraphernalia (and associated injury) may initiate (Blenkharn 2008, Parkin and Coomber 2011, Sohn et al. 2006). Nevertheless, the aim of this chapter is to summarise qualitative data obtained from the processes of serial triangulation (Chapter 3) and to re-consider the relevant findings obtained from varied analyses (Chapter 4) in an attempt to further debate on this controversial subject in a manner that prioritises a harm reduction approach to drug related issues.

> In an attempt to reflect the applied agenda of this book and in support of harm reduction intervention in particular, a proactive and responsive resource may be found in Appendix I. This item may be used as a template (copied and adapted as required) by relevant agencies and individuals who may wish to respond to any inaccurate accounts of drug related litter contained in local media reports.

Box 6.1 A Harm Reduction Response to Negative Media Accounts of Drug Related Litter in Community Settings

Rationalising Harm Associated with Drug Related Litter in Public Settings

As noted above, a recurring theme within accounts of drug related litter in community settings is a 'symbolic' association between potential transmission of infectious disease and discarded injecting equipment. Whilst it is well-established that needle and syringe programmes were introduced throughout the UK as a harm reduction response to various HIV epidemics during the 1980s, it would be erroneous to associate all injecting paraphernalia with viral infection. This view relates specifically to HIV and assorted 'strains' of the hepatitis virus (primarily hepatitis B, and hepatitis C) and may be substantiated with a sizeable body of research literature that critically evaluates the viability of needlestick injury, discarded needles and syringes within community settings as potential sources of viral transmission.

For example, Philipp's (1993) study of individuals given treatment for hepatitis B (following needlestick injury) found that, of the 958 relevant cases throughout the UK, there were no reports of seroconversion amongst those affected. Similarly, Wyatt et al's (1994) examination of the medical records of 67 children presenting needlestick injury to a Scottish hospital concluded that viral transmission associated with such accidents remained speculative. In a later study (Nourse et al. 1997) of 52 children treated for similar needlestick injury, only two incidents were categorised as 'high risk' of infection. However, none of the children concerned developed hepatitis (B or C) or HIV. Research conducted in Australia, also confirms these conclusions and suggests that viral infection from needlestick injury in community settings remains low (Russell and Nash 2002).

Other studies have focused more upon the longevity of blood borne viruses outside of the body and within hypodermic equipment. For example, Nyiri et al. (2004) collected 106 *used* needles from four separate public locations and tested all for viral presence. Of these, 4.7 per cent (5 items) returned positive for hepatitis B and hepatitis C. HIV could not be detected in any of the items due to inadequacies in the analytical procedures attached to the study. Nevertheless, Nyiri et al. (2004) conclude that discarded needles possibly raise some public health concerns relating more to hepatitis than HIV. Similarly, Thompson et al. (2003) studied the survival rates of hepatitis and HIV in syringes stored at room temperature and found that all viruses could survive outside of the body for several weeks if kept in optimal (manufactured) environments. More specifically, they found that hepatitis B is able survive up to 8 months and does not decline in its sensitivity (that is, its ability to infect); hepatitis C may survive a similar period but its sensitivity decreases nine-fold during a similar time scale, whereas HIV is able to survive up to 30 days – but is generally limited to 1–2 days. Each survival rate is largely determined by the level of the virus titre (amount of antibodies within the solution), the volume of blood contained within the needle and syringe, room temperature and levels of exposure to sunlight. From these analyses, the researchers conclude that the 'risk of blood borne virus from syringes discarded in community settings appears to be very low' (Thompson et al. 2003, 602). However, as with most other studies, the researchers also concede that this potential is 'unlikely to be zero' (ibid.), particularly with regard to hepatitis B (due to its ability to survive longest) and hepatitis C (due to its higher prevalence amongst injecting populations). As such, Thompson et al. (2003) argue the most likely scenario for potential viral infection is to experience needlestick injury from a recently discarded needle by an injecting drug user who is hepatitis C positive. (However, the researchers fail to give any indication or definition of 'recent' in this 'worst-case scenario').

Despite the absence of a completely conclusive statement that wholly confirms or refutes the potential for infection from needlestick injury, there is sufficient evidence to state that viral seroconversion and life-threatening infection is *not* a commonly reported consequence of such events (Blenkharn 2008, Gomez et al. 1998, Nourse et al. 1997, Philipp 1993, Russell and Nash 2002, Wyatt et al. 1994). Nevertheless, it is perhaps important to reiterate that whereas viral infection from needlestick injury may be considered a form of 'low risk' exposure, such injury should not be dismissed as 'no risk' (Nyiri et al. 2004, Thompson et al. 2003). More precisely, (and perhaps the most conclusive statement on the issue to date), the chances of seroconversion following community acquired needlestick injury 'where the source is unknown but assumed to be an (injecting drug user), is 12–31% for hepatitis B, 1.62% for hepatitis C and 0.003–0.05 per cent for HIV' (Blenkharn 2008, 727). In lay terms, this translates to: of every 100 episodes of needlestick injury less than one will transmit HIV infection; approximately two of every 100 episodes of needlestick injury will transmit hepatitis C and for every 100 injuries there is variable potential for infection from hepatitis B.

To conclude the politics of drug related litter, from an *epidemiological* perspective, there is perhaps only limited rationality in the aforementioned symbolic associations between viral infection and drug related litter (and especially needles and syringes) in community settings. Similarly, from a *sociological* perspective, there is equally sufficient evidence from the studies cited above to counter-balance the provincial hysteria inferred within the various news items presented at the onset of this chapter. In the following section, an empirical account of drug related litter is presented in an attempt to further challenge fear and stigma associated with all discarded paraphernalia found in street-based settings. In addition, these collective accounts of experiences connected to drug related litter aim to advance and promote the continued need for applying harm reduction approaches to community-based issues.

Categorising Harm Associated with Drug Related Litter in Public Settings

As noted in Chapter 3 this multi-site, longitudinal, research involved field visits to over 400 street-based environments affected by injecting drug use. Each of these environments were classified within a continuum of descending safety (Chapter 5) in which one aspect of this categorisation process relates to the presence and volume of drug related litter associated with particular places. Accordingly, throughout all visits to individual street-based injecting sites, the amount of drug related litter was variable in amount and frequency at all stages of fieldwork. As such, some sites (such as public toilets, communal areas in high-rise tower blocks) that were frequently attended by injecting drug users, somewhat paradoxically, rarely contained any drug related litter. This absence typically related to various cleansing routines employed by frontline service personnel and/or the presence of refuse bins in which persons unknown may have deposited the relevant discarded litter. Other sites however (such as stairwells, alleyways, and areas associated with sex work) were regularly littered with single or multiple sharps (used and unused) in addition to paraphernalia such as cookers, spoons, filters and/or swabs. However, within some Category B settings, (especially those frequented almost exclusively by injecting drug users), the amount of discarded items (all paraphernalia) was often so severe that it was impossible to provide any accurate assessment of the actual volume involved.

Despite the variation in public injecting sites noted in Chapter 5, wherever and whenever drug related litter was noted during all environmental assessments, a visual record (photograph/s) was made of the volume, location and position of all items concerned. Whereas the applied value of such photography was not immediately apparent whilst in the field, the actual significance of these data became increasingly evident during the various coding procedures attached to analyses of all visual images (see in Chapter 4). For example, focused analysis of photographs *per se* provided opportunities to revisit and reflect upon environments affected by injecting drug use in a manner whereby the author was not pressured by time spent within, (or the policing of), the relevant locations. Similarly, software associated with digital photography permits opportunities to magnify (or 'zoom') particular features within pixel-based images. The post-fieldwork process of 'zooming' into previously visited settings of injecting drug use permits the visual analyst to get 'physically closer' to the places and objects within the images without actually crawling on hands in knees in the actual environments concerned. Indeed, the latter aspect of visual analysis essentially provided opportunities to revisit injecting environments and to 'forensically observe' (Parkin and Coomber 2009b) items that may have gone unnoticed or unobserved during the actual field visit.

The coding processes attached specifically to images of drug related litter produced outcome similar to the analysis of injecting 'places' (described in Chapter 5). More specifically, when considered from the perspective of harm reduction, drug related litter found within street-based settings may be similarly ordered within a schema that reflects notions of 'descending safety' associated with injecting environments. In the context of drug related litter however, this categorisation of harm involves discarded equipment that may be regarded as 'harmless', 'harmful', or be present as 'a hidden harm' or a 'massed harm'. Each of these categories of drug related litter is summarised below in which visual and text based data is used to substantiate and evidence this (controversial) classificatory system.

Harmless Drug Related Litter

A recurring observation of drug related litter noted in street-based settings was the frequency of items that may be considered as 'harmless'. Although classified as 'drug related' litter, the reality of discarded items such as seals, wrappers, empty sharps bins, in addition to *unused* items (such as steri-cups®, filters, swabs) is that they are simply 'waste' that has been discarded in an inappropriate manner. Similarly, when viewed from a harm reduction perspective discarded and unused paraphernalia pose no immediate hazard to public or individual health. Such littering may be compared to the equally inappropriate practice of discarding food and drink containers, cigarette butts and chewing gum in public places.

This absence of harm equally relates to those *unused* sharps (including items such as 1ml insulin syringes, with needle attachment and protective cap, still contained within the protective seal) that may have been discarded in public settings (such as public toilets, or 'stashed' in hiding places). This is perhaps a contentious, if not controversial, claim. However, as these items have not been used for *injecting* purposes, they are still considered sterile and 'fit for purpose'. They almost certainly do not raise concerns about 'infectious, deadly disease' suggested in the media reports included above. To suggest that injury from such items may require stressful blood-testing and/or may lead to viral infection would be grossly inaccurate and epidemiologically impossible. Similarly, as such items are categorised as 'sharps' (as with broken bottles in public places), then they will inevitably cause injury if handled inappropriately by persons unfamiliar with such equipment (as with broken bottles in public places). Instead, such items are perhaps aesthetically offensive to the wider population, in which their presence may only *symbolise* threat and danger from an unknown – but assumed as attributable – source.

Throughout fieldwork, there were numerous occasions when packs of unused equipment (including sharps) were found discarded in street-based settings (especially in toilets). In Figures 6.1 and 6.2 (taken in two different public conveniences), one may note that a plastic bag, containing all essential paraphernalia required to facilitate ten individual injections, has been torn open. From each package, only a strip of 10 insulin syringes (contained within individual 'seals') has been removed. As the latter items were not evident within each relevant toilet cubicle, there is no physical harm presented by the package, other than alerting others of a previous presence of at least one *probable* injecting drug user within the same setting. The following fieldnotes seek to explain this form of drug related littering from a variety of perspectives.

> Inside the toilet cubicle was a ripped drinks can that had been used as a cooker and there was an opened pack of kit on the floor. (Outreach worker) believed somebody was going to go back to the cubicle as all the equipment was still inside. Participant countered this and explained that such discarding was typical, as users will not necessarily keep the whole 10-pack and use only one set for a single hit. (Outreach worker) seemed quite disheartened by this and it led to a discussion regarding the availability and distribution of needles and syringes in packs. Participant felt local pharmacies should be able to distribute steri-cups® with water amps and reduced amounts of needles (suggesting packs of 5, or even as a single item) in preference to the current multi-packs available from local outlets (containing 10 insulin syringes, swabs, filters but no cup and no water). (Outreach worker) felt that this would be a financial difficulty for services. Participant argued against this adding that the costs saved in reducing needle content (in packs) could be used to include water and cups. ... Regarding

the unused, discarded content in the toilet, participant was also disheartened by such littering and was angry about it. He went to pick it up to dispose of it but (outreach worker) asked him not to touch it 'just in case'. (Outreach worker) was concerned about leaving such litter and wanted to report it for immediate collection by the local authority. Participant was not concerned about picking-up the drug related litter as he said he knew how to handle it safely. He understood (outreach worker's) concern about not wanting to touch it, but I got the impression he thought (outreach worker) was overreacting due to the *unused* nature of the items. (*Fieldnotes, Category A Site*)

Similarly:

'This looks quite recent', he said and showed me the inside of the pack as we stood next to a tree, looking into a plastic bag of approximately 8 unused syringes, as the rain came down upon us. (Outreach worker) stumbled into the bush at this point and made a comment that participant shouldn't be handling litter as he was. He brushed off the comment and said he didn't want to leave it where it was. As we stood around the base of the tree it became very apparent that this was a very claustrophobic place in which there was 'standing room only' due to the extensive low branch cover. Respondent explained that this was a place used only by a select few people, and was an injecting site that had emerged partly a consequence of dispersal/clearance procedures associated with a larger site nearby. We pushed back out the bushes and headed over to that site and respondent carried the bag of unused works for disposal in a sharps bin contained within the boot of the car. (*Fieldnotes, Category C Site*)

Finally:

When asked why injectors may be going to local green areas, the Park Manager was of the opinion that it was connected to the free availability of easily-accessed needles from local drug services. He felt that agencies were *over-providing* injecting drug users with equipment to the extent that *unused* needles had been left in park areas alongside those that have been used. Although he agrees with the harm reduction ethos of needle distribution he felt that prior to these conditions users had to reuse their needles and would keep them for longer. Now that they are able to use them once, discard and get new ones, the Park Manager believes users deposit them irresponsibly in public areas. He was more in favour of a '1-for-1 exchange policy' and he stressed that this was *his* view and not the council's opinion (although I have a feeling this opinion was shared by many others I met too). (*Fieldnotes, Category C Site*)

146   *An Applied Visual Sociology: Picturing Harm Reduction*

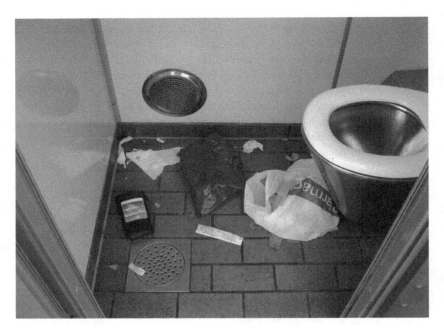

Figure 6.1   Harmless Drug Related Litter (1)

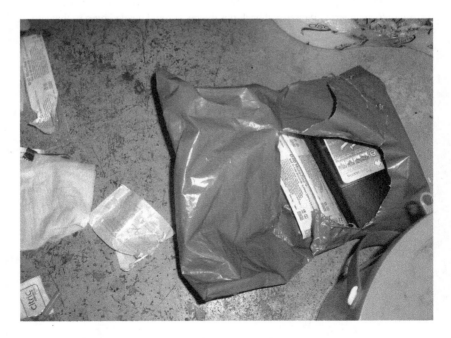

Figure 6.2   Harmless Drug Related Litter (2)

Harmful Drug Related Litter

Visits to street-based injecting environments included frequent observations of injecting paraphernalia that may be classed as examples of 'harmful' discarding. In this category, needles attached to syringes are fully exposed and may inflict needlestick injury if inadvertent contact is made with such items (see Figures 6.3–6.6). Other items in this category include used/unused needles/syringes that are discarded with the protective cap attached to the needle-point (see Figure 6.7). Although the presence of the protective cap may prevent accidental contact with the relevant sharps, this does not completely neutralise harm in the event of inappropriate handling by those unfamiliar with injecting paraphernalia. Used condoms containing seminal (or other) fluid that has been deposited alongside or adjacent injecting paraphernalia (see Figure 6.8) is a further addition to this category of drug/sex-related litter considered harmful.

'Harmful' drug related litter was typically identified with greatest frequency in settings regarded as Category B and Category C injecting sites. As noted earlier in this book, Category B sites are those associated with semi-public settings such as concealed stairwells, multi-storey car parks, alleyways as well as abandoned/disused buildings that are attended almost exclusively by injecting drug users. Similarly, Category C settings are those that exist within more marginal, more secluded spaces and have greater associations with individual injectors, rooflessness and/or homelessness. Category B and Category C sites may also be noted within environs associated with street-based alcohol use and/or street-based sex work. Such locations may also provide additional 'drug using niches' for those individuals also participant in either street-drinking and/or sex work. Due to the largely concealed nature of Category B and Category C settings, evidence of 'harmful' discarding was noted more frequently in locations that are not widely accessed, or commonly attended, by members of the public (or by those with without 'legitimate' reason for being within the immediate vicinity). People that are most likely to frequent Category B/C settings are specialised cleansing teams, frontline service personnel (employed in the vicinity of the area affected), street-based outreach workers and those who own premises affected by public injecting drug use (for example, abandoned buildings). For these reasons, one would not expect to encounter casual observers from the general public within places of environmental seclusion, geographic marginality and public exclusion. Instead, one would more likely expect to observe individuals from those services listed above, in addition to street-based alcohol users, drug users, sex workers (and their clients), and users of local services/charities (relating to homelessness) within the immediate vicinity.

Throughout all research, accounts and experiences of 'harmful' discarding were widespread during semi-structured interviews held with frontline service personnel *and* injecting drug users. There was consensus throughout both interview cohorts that such discarding practices were unacceptable, anti-social and irresponsible. The following interview extracts reflect this unanimity between figures of authority *and* injecting drug users.

> (Business Manager) believes that there are two types of injecting drug user in (the area). These being, 'younger users who have no regard for others and who will discard randomly as soon as they have had a hit', compared to the 'hardened users who will carry (used) works with them and dispose of them safely at needle and syringe programmes or in litter bins'. (Business Manager) believed that the 'hardened users' were probably more likely to be homeless. (*Fieldnotes*)

Views similar to the above, regarding drug related litter, were widely shared amongst the injecting drug user cohort. For example:

> ... there's two type of heroin addicts right. There's what I call 'a user' and then you get 'the smackhead' ... You've heard the term 'smackhead'? A user is someone like me who do their drugs, take everything with 'em, make sure everything's clean. A smackhead is a person who will do their injection and chuck their needle down and not give a fuck. They're disrespectful and they don't care about anything but themselves. (*R058*)

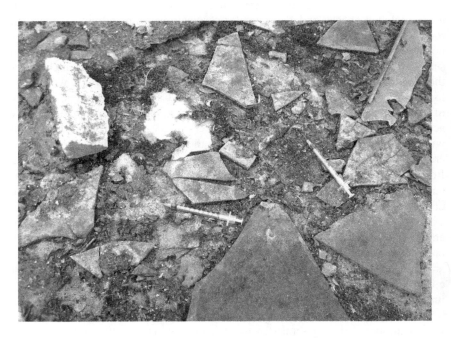

Figure 6.3   Harmful Drug Related Litter (3)

Drug Related Litter as Visual Data 149

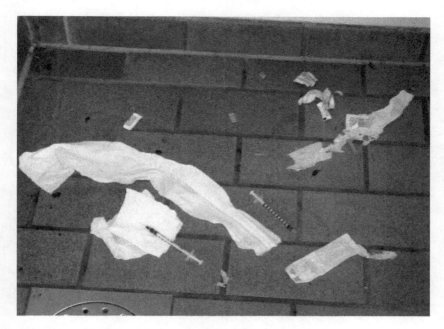

Figure 6.4   Harmful Drug Related Litter (4)

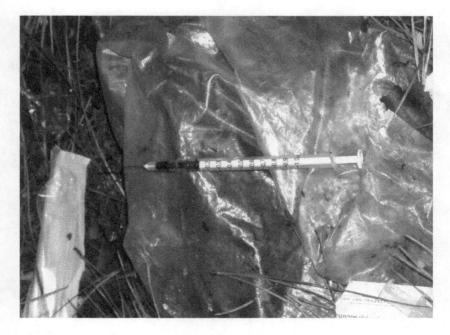

Figure 6.5   Harmful Drug Related Litter (5)

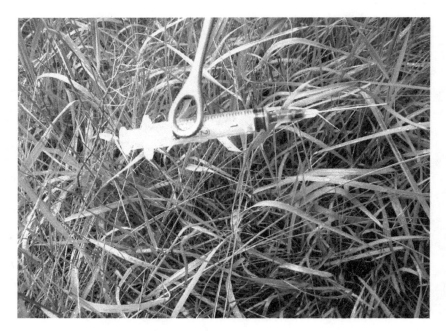

Figure 6.6   Harmful Drug Related Litter (6)

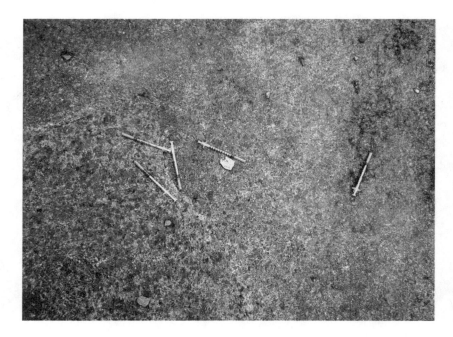

Figure 6.7   Harmful Drug Related Litter (7)

Drug Related Litter as Visual Data 151

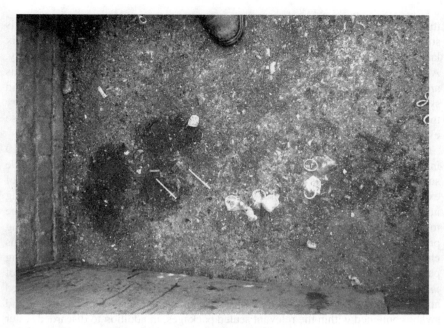

Figure 6.8   Harmful Drug Related Litter (8)

Massed Harm

A further form of drug related littering noted across all geographic locations of this study is here categorised as a 'massed harm'. This aspect of littering is limited only within those Category B sites that are accessed almost exclusively by injecting drug users for the purposes of preparation and injection of illicit substances. Such settings may be termed pejoratively in mass media reports as street-based 'shooting galleries' and are usually located in abandoned, makeshift and outdoor settings. A total of seven environments formed this sub-category of Semi-Controlled settings that were identified throughout all research. All seven sites were concealed within abandoned or derelict buildings, or within marginalised 'green' areas on the outskirts of central business districts associated with each town/city of the study. All injecting environments of this nature were typically near to drug markets and accessed at all times of the day by drug users who were alone, in pairs or as part of a larger group. These settings were typically well known amongst injecting cohorts within a particular area and were attended by those known to one another in addition to those regarded as 'socially distant' (that is, unknown). These settings were also known to local emergency services (particularly police patrols and ambulance crews).

Figures 6.9 and 6.10 depict the environmental characteristics of these particular injecting environments. From these images, one may note that such concealed locations are typified by the presence of larger volumes of drug related litter that spreads across a wider surface area. In one particular location during this study, a Category B site of this nature (located within a wooded area between six lanes of vehicular traffic) was physically uprooted by the relevant local authority. According to the relevant Environmental Health Manager, the clearance of this area included the removal of an 'estimated 3,000 used and unused needles and syringes'. This information perhaps demonstrates the frequency and regularity that the site was accessed by local drug users (and does not intend to sensationalise events in disclosing the volume of litter involved).

Injecting drugs within social spaces such as those in Figures 6.9 and 6.10 involves the negotiation of discarded equipment that has been strewn across a wide surface area in which it is almost impossible to note (during daylight) the presence of exposed sharps. Indeed, accessing such areas often involves inadvertently walking upon paraphernalia that has spread across all available 'floorspace'. Similarly, due to the absence of appropriate surfaces and seating areas within such settings, drug preparation and injection typically involves sitting/squatting in makeshift conditions characterised by dirt and yet more discarded equipment. In addition to used injecting paraphernalia (whether capped or not), these sites also contain larger volumes of *unused* equipment that has been discarded in a manner similar to that described above. This typically includes a variety of syringes, needles, cookers, filters and swabs contained within the relevant sealed packages, in addition to discarded water (in bottles), blood-stained materials (tissue, cloth, swabs), makeshift tourniquets and sharps boxes (of unknown content). Other non-drug related items also located within the area may increase wider hazards associated with drug related litter. For example, one may note in Figure 5.7 an unusual amount of wire cable (that has been stripped of its copper content to be sold for cash at a local scrap metal merchant) surrounding the injecting environment that may cause trips and falls upon exit/entry to the site in question. Similarly, Figure 5.8 depicts an area characterised by all of the above, in addition to broken glass, uneven concrete surfaces, scrap metal and rusting tools; all of which make access/exit to the injecting areas more arduous and dangerous.

Due to the increased volume and extraordinary spread of discarded items (whether used or not) within such confined and concealed settings, drug related litter of this nature is here categorised as representing a 'massed harm'. Injecting drug users accessing environments such as this appeared to be cognisant of the harm associated with drug related litter massed in such a manner. Similarly, such settings were often described with abhorrence and repulsion in which injecting drug users described their attendance within such environments with regret, shame and self-loathing (Parkin 2009a, 2013). However, such environments were also regarded as providing acceptable spaces for addressing drug dependency (cravings, withdrawal symptoms) whilst simultaneously offering limited privacy outwith the gaze of the public and law enforcement. The subsequent acceptance of environments characterised by dirt, danger and environmental hazard may be noted in the following experiences reported by injecting drug users.

I hate going there actually 'cos the place is full of needles and that. You don't know where you are treading and that ... I mean, I'm one of these people who cleans up after myself. I can't abide people who throw their needles on the floor and everything. It's disgusting, there's no need for it and it's so dodgy at the end of the day. And for them reasons I hate going in there. It's just skanky, dirty, horrible. (*R054*)

Similarly:

But I think (drug related litter is) disgusting, 'cos I wouldn't leave my pins about, 'cos there's children about. But when I went in these bushes, the amount of needles that were there, I thought it was disgusting how anyone could leave it there. *I know I'm bad for doing it there* but I wouldn't leave anything lying around for anyone to hurt themself. (*R059*, emphasis of shame added)

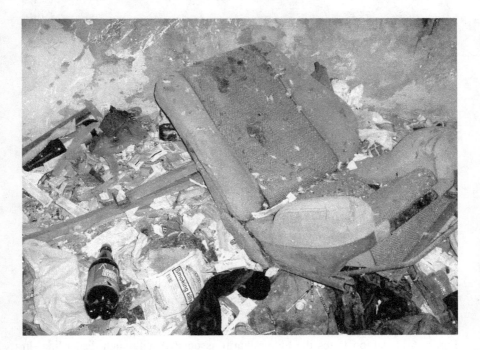

Figures 6.9   Massed Harm (1)

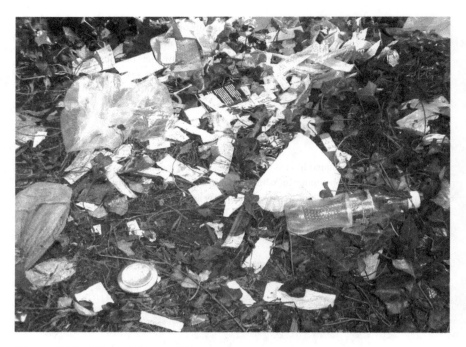

Figure 6.10   Massed Harm (2)

Hidden Harm

A final category of drug related litter relates to items that may have been discarded in locations considered 'safe' by injecting drug users, but may have been deposited in locations associated with particular working environments. Examples here include paraphernalia that has been deposited in conventional litter bins (in toilets, shopping centres, high streets, residential settings), dropped into toilet cisterns or drainage systems, buried in flower beds and/or concealed amongst other naturally-occurring materials. When such items relate to used and/or exposed needles, this form of litter may be described as representing a more 'hidden harm' as individuals within the associated 'working environment' may not necessarily be aware of (or expect) any presence of injecting-related sharps. Figure 6.11 demonstrates the hidden harm associated with such discarding, in which sharps partially buried in a 'planter' (a portable flower/plant container used for decorative purposes) have been made 'safe' to some degree (presumably by an injecting drug user) and are items that have been physically removed from *public* view. However, such items also remain out of view from those who may attend to such items as part of their employment, in which the harm presented from sharps also remains hidden. Similarly, Figure 6.12 depicts various used sharps and a clear blood presence (on tissue paper). From one perspective, these items have been appropriately deposited in a street-based litter bin and have been appropriately removed from any *public* contact. Whereas this may appear at first sight to be a commendable disposal strategy, frontline service personnel typically remark that the content of these particular litter bins often has to be transferred, by manual labour, into larger plastic sacks and transported to other locations for further disposal. This final destination may involve the manual sifting and sorting through refuse as it is emptied onto various conveyor belts. As such from another perspective, the discarding strategies of drug users reflect wider contestations relating to space and place are perhaps made more evident.

In practical terms, there is the possibility that 'hidden harms' may also be present sharps puncture/tear the plastic sacks and cause injury to those handling such equipment during all processes attached to waste disposal (Figure 6.13). This aspect of litter management and associated hidden harm was reported exclusively throughout the study by frontline service personnel (such as car park/toilet/garden attendants, refuse collectors, street cleansing operatives and incineration staff). Similarly, many of those describing such 'hidden harm' also reported wider experiences associated with needlestick injury as a result of the concealed nature of sharps in this manner. This may be noted in the following accounts:

> (Refuse operative) was the more experienced of the team and told me about various needlestick injuries he has received during his cleaning duties. To date, he has been stuck twice, both times during house-clearances involving needles contained within a refuse sack. He explained the process he went through involving hospital attendances, a course of vaccinations and a 12-month wait for various test results to be confirmed as negative. He was of the opinion that he wouldn't get HIV ('as it can't live very long outside of the body') but added that he was nervous/anxious for about 2 months after the injuries about Hep B/C. He also spoke of the tension these blood tests put upon his relationship with his wife, the enforced celibacy to 'protect' her and the embarrassment of calling in his wife to hospital for her to be tested too ('just cos I'm doing my job'). He also described the suspicions that this can cause when this happens a second time as his wife began to question if he was actually 'playing around' (being 'unfaithful'). (*Fieldnotes*)

Drug Related Litter as Malicious Intent?

Overall, those with experience of 'harm' associated with drug related litter hidden in concealed settings (*sic*) were of the opinion that such discarding was done with malicious intent. That is, frontline service personnel believed that purposely depositing used injecting equipment in potentially dangerous positions was the equivalent of setting 'booby-traps' designed to inflict deliberate harm upon those most likely to make contact with such items. This may be noted in the following comment:

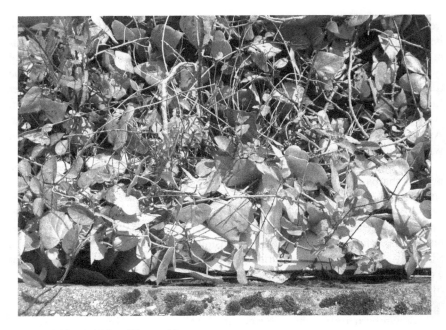

Figure 6.11 Hidden Harm (1)

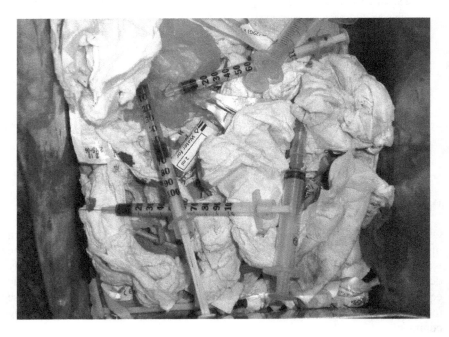

Figure 6.12 Hidden Harm (2)

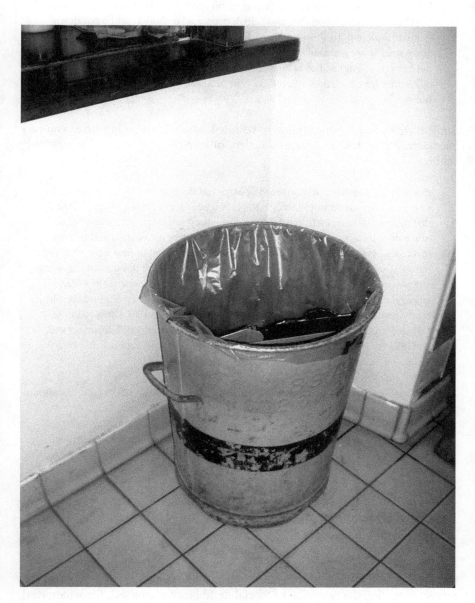

Figure 6.13 Hidden Harm (3)

> I wasn't surprised to hear (the cleansing team) speak bitterly about drug users as 'sick' (minded), irresponsible and selfish people who should 'all be put down' (similar to dogs)! To illustrate these feelings (driver) actually stopped the van and turned to me and said – 'you tell me, people that tape needles (i.e. the pin – not barrel) to door handles of houses, light switches and sockets, abandoned cars or on door frames so they can fall on your head and inside toilet rolls – are they not sick people?' (*Fieldnotes*)

Similar views and experiences were reported by a Security Operative who had encountered drug related litter in a variety of employment roles and recreational settings.

> (Security) pointed out where blood splatter has been cleaned and showed me where needles put down toilets caused blockages in the S-bend. (Security) stated that needles had been left in places to cause injury to others, such as on the top of the door frames, wrapped in paper towels and was of the opinion that this was malicious, done by 'people who don't care' and 'who want to pass on a virus to others'. (Security) felt that this was not only in the toilets but throughout the city and provided a number of 'needle stories' from his previous experience as a 'Parks' employee. For example, he recalled a sandpit that had been used a disposal site for used paraphernalia, with needles pinned point-down into the sand. Other examples included needles in planters, needles on shelves and ridges of park furnishings and on top of roofs; all of which were used to support his claims that drug users were acting 'maliciously' in their disposal strategies. (*Fieldnotes*)

Similar sentiments were expressed by a manager within a high street cafe/restaurant.

> (Manager) explained that drug users had also secreted needles within the lining of the seats we were sitting on, under metal rims of the seating frame and ledges found under the table tops. She felt that these were deliberate attempts to hurt other people rather than attempts to secretively discard or stash needles for re-use. (*Fieldnotes*)

Indigenous Discarding Procedures

In contrast to the above views regarding drug related litter were those offered by drug users to explain various discarding strategies employed whilst engaged in episodes of street-based injections. Although some caution may be noted in this respect regarding the provision of 'social desirability responses', the widespread condemnation of reckless drug related littering expressed by all 71 drug users in the study was unanimous and undisputed. More simply, almost all participants with experience of public injecting were critical of other drug users who discarded used equipment in public places. Such actions were repeatedly regarded as 'irresponsible', 'immoral' and 'disrespectful' actions that could lead to accidental injury amongst non-drug users (especially children). Discarding paraphernalia in public places was also condemned on the basis that it may reveal concealed injecting sites to authorities and identify particular 'injecting hotspots' for increased surveillance (and result in the displacement of temporary safety from settings appropriated for injecting purposes). Those with experience of rooflessness also believed that discarding near a 'sleeping pitch' was equally offensive and was regarded as an intrusion of their 'personal space'.

Indeed, many of the criticisms directed at other drug users who deposited used equipment in a reckless and irresponsible manner were supported by counter claims that highlighted practice considered 'safer discarding'. For the purposes of this text, these strategies are termed collectively as 'indigenous discarding procedures' in an attempt to situate street-based practice that emerges from street-based experience.

'Snapping and Dropping'

Throughout the study, the most frequently cited indigenous discarding strategy involved removing/destroying used needle attachments from syringe barrels or depositing used items into drainage systems (via street guttering). These disposal strategies were considered appropriate by injecting drug users as they removed 'sharps' from public contact. These swiftly applied strategies were also regarded as compatible, and consistent, with the 'rapid' process of accessing/exiting street-based settings where 'rushed' technique characterised injecting episodes. The rapid discarding of injecting equipment in this way therefore facilitates successful 'movement' through social and physical environments that generally seek to penalise and criminalise illicit drug use/rs. These discarding strategies (of rapid 'snapping and dropping') may be noted in the following remarks:

> I put (used needles) in tin cans, put them inside the can and crush them over. So a bin man can't put his hand in and spike himself, 'cos that's fucking horrible. You know, if I was a bin man I'd be pissed off with that, so just out of respect for anyone else, put it in there, it doesn't take 2 minutes. I mean coming up here (to needle syringe programme) with a bin full of needles is a big pain in the arse. I mean, walking around with a bag of needles, getting asked 'what's in the bag' or whatever (by police) .... (is not going to happen) (*R070*)

> ... so like it's just commonsense, you shouldn't even have to throw them on the floor, know what I mean, they shouldn't touch the floor. Shove it in your arm, put the lid back on, snap it off, in a can or something and in a bin. (Even) not putting the can in a proper bin, but then it's in a can isn't it, (so) ... if someone changes the bin bag, it's not gonna go in them. But it is gonna go to a landfill and be disposed of in a landfill. (*R046*)

I'd put it in a drain. I'd just snap it. I used to use 1 mils with the orange tops, I used to snap the orange tops with the pins in the top and put em in a drain. Yeah, wherever I was, yeah. Down the nearest drain. Which is probably not, you know, ideal, but at least it's better than leaving them on the street. (*R058*)

As intimated in the above extracts, relevant respondents appeared cognisant that 'snapping and dropping' strategies were not ideal and inferred that they were not entirely appropriate from a community safety perspective. However, from a public health and harm reduction perspective, those concerned were equally convinced that such practice minimised chances of needlestick injury in various settings and stressed the reduced potential for viral infection from street-based, indigenous discarding strategies.

Post-interview analyses of photographs containing items of drug related litter (taken across all four geographic locations of the study) appears to confirm many of these claims regarding 'snapping and dropping' discarding strategies. For example, Figures 6.14 and 6.15 depict drug related litter in two different Category B settings. The syringe in Figure 6.14 has had its needle attachment removed and has been discarded alongside various alcohol-related items (in which the glass

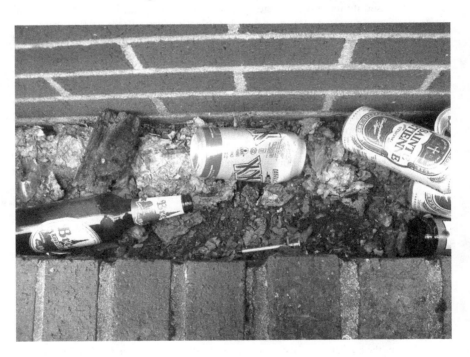

Figure 6.14 'Snapping and Dropping' (1)

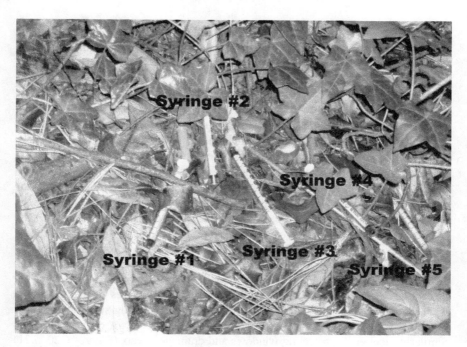

Figure 6.15 'Snapping and Dropping' (2)

bottles are arguably the most 'harmful' items in this image). Figure 6.15 however shows five syringes discarded in a large-scale outdoor site that was used on a daily basis by injecting drug users. However, what is perhaps most notable about this image is the almost regimental manner in which the five items have been placed onto and into the earth. From this image one may assume at least five injecting episodes have taken place at this particular spot, and each episode would almost certainly *have not* involved the same individual due to the frequency with which the site was used on a daily basis. As such, it is feasible to infer that multiple persons had injected at this spot and the equipment had been 'positioned' (rather than thrown aside in a random, haphazard manner) in an attempt to apply some degree of 'safety' and harm reduction management within this particular drug using environment (whether applied consciously or unconsciously).

In addition to the above, further analysis of the photograph reflects specific interview responses and associated experiences regarding the removal of needle attachments following injection. Of the five insulin syringes pictured, those numbered 1–4 have had the *fixed* needle attachment removed from the syringe barrel, whereas Syringe 5 is partially submerged into the soil. This image (and many others like it within the overall visual dataset) would appear to provide a forensically-based visual resource (Parkin and Coomber 2009b) that is consistent with reports of injecting behaviour provided by (drug user) interview respondents.

Furthermore, verbal accounts of drug users' attempts to reduce harm associated with used, discarded equipment have been substantiated by images of this nature.

Facilitative space

A further form of indigenous discarding has a direct correlation with the immediate environmental setting that contains individual or multiple injecting episodes. The term 'facilitative space' is used here to describe the way in which injecting drug users may appropriate street-based furnishings (present in the injecting environment) as a means of rapidly disposing (or storing) equipment to facilitate more hasty injecting practice. Various examples of these facilitative spaces are presented in Figures 6.16–6.21, in which the presence of fixed bins provide a convenient disposal whilst *in situ* (Figure 6.16); where door ledges and damaged light fittings on the upper levels of multi-storey car parks floors provide 'shelving' and storage/waste space respectively for particular items (Figure 6.17: equipment is concealed within the damaged 'down arrow' above the escalator door located on the right). Other facilitative space for discarding and/or storing equipment may be noted in Figures 6.18 and 6.19 in which the presence of street-based furniture adjacent injecting sites further assist rapid practice associated with injecting episodes (as a point of disposal/storage). Similarly, steel grills protecting windows and drainage covers (Figures 6.20–6.21) may provide naturally occurring barriers to inadvertent or accidental contact with used/unused items. Steel grills also partially conceal discarded items and one may not observe items located behind such screens without scrutiny.

Colliding Perspectives of Drug Related Litter

Each of the above may/would be regarded as examples of 'malicious discarding' from the perspective of those affected by drug related litter in work-related environments. However, when viewed from the perspective of lifestyles shaped by transience, drug dependency, urgency and limited social, economic and physical resources (especially with regard to housing), 'facilitative discarding strategies' appears as a culturally relevant response to structural constraints that seek to impose sanction and penalty upon injecting drug use/rs. This may further apply to those living in temporary hostels (where penalties/eviction for paraphernalia possession may apply) as well as those who are of no fixed abode or considered 'roofless'.

Accordingly, from perspectives that prioritise the lived-experience of street-based injecting, 'facilitative discarding' may also be interpreted as a response shaped by need (of 'place' in which one has to be quick, in order to maintain liberty, avoid arrest, detection and interruption). The perceived benefits of facilitative discarding may be noted in the following extract in which the respondent provides an account of concealing and storing equipment as a result of homelessness:

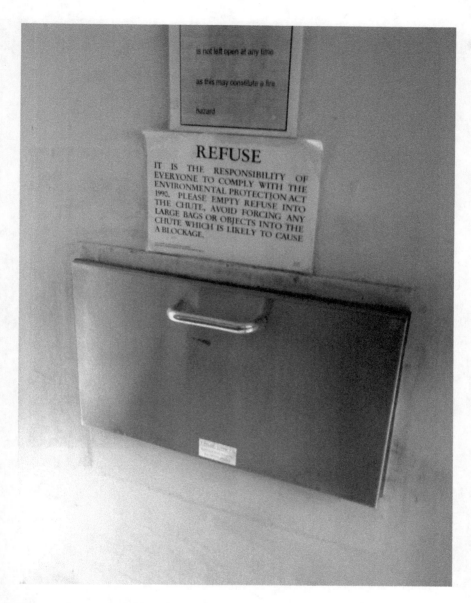

Figure 6.16 Facilitative Space (1)

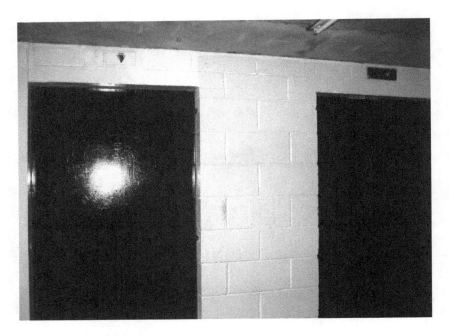

Figure 6.17 Facilitative Space (2)

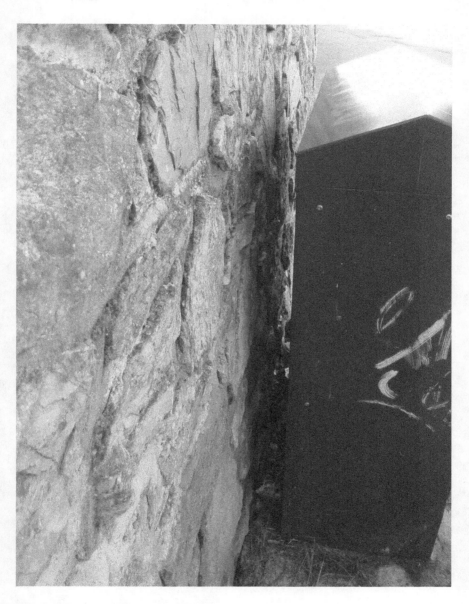

Figure 6.18 Facilitative Space (3)

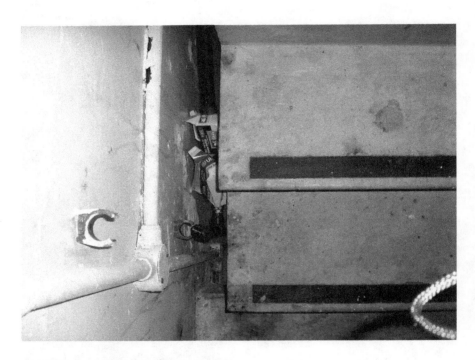

Figure 6.19   Facilitative Space (4)

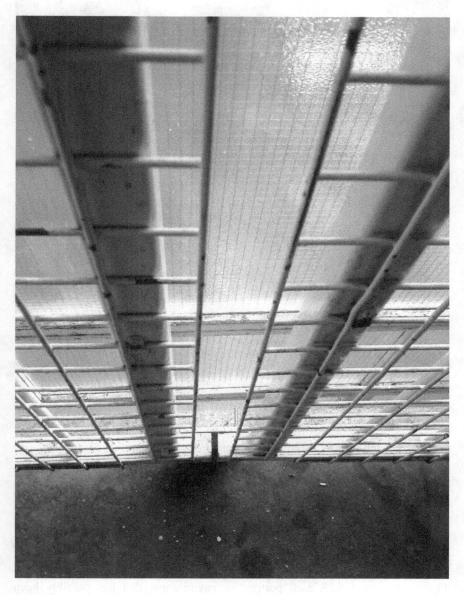

Figure 6.20 Facilitative Space (5)

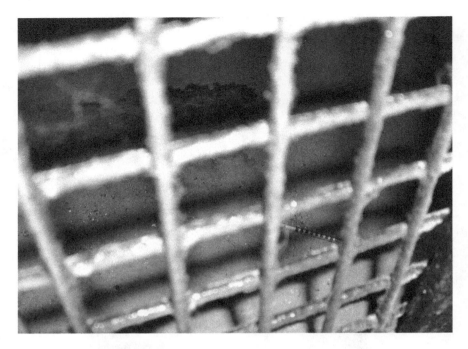

Figure 6.21   Facilitative Space (6)

There's a park near the dealer's house, and I know it is a secluded area with a small brick wall to (conceal) me. So I parked my bike and it just took me 5 minutes and I left everything behind as well. Stashed it in the wall, in case I have to go back there. I have some citric, and some clean water stashed, 'cos that's another thing as well when you find a place like that – you tend to leave something just in case you have to go back again and then you're prepared. Because this is one of the problems as well when you are homeless, occasionally you don't have the needles all the time, or citric or a spoon. So if you can you wrap it up and stash in a safe place and then you tend to go back and use there again. Or if – for an emergency – if you're in the area, you can go and pick it up and use it indoors or outdoors again. (*R026*)

Shaping Space

Figures 6.22 and 6.23 each portray an environment that has possibly been purposely *shaped* to introduce safer injecting guidelines within an area of absolute dereliction. This deliberate shaping and altering of an abandoned setting was noted in only two environments throughout the entire study (in which over 400 injecting settings were visited). As such, this particular indigenous discarding strategy may not be regarded as fully representative of the wider study. Instead, the visual data pertaining to this particular location provides a useful resource (and under-reported insight) regarding injecting procedures attached to street-based settings. Nevertheless, the 'exclusivity' of this practice and the somewhat unique visual data do not disqualify such matter from inclusion in this text.

In Figures 6.22 and 6.23, one may note attempts to establish control upon a derelict environment characterised by dirt, disorder and disarray. Furthermore, the environmental management observed and recorded in the following fieldnote suggests concerted efforts at spatial manipulation and/or environmental adaptation in which the fundaments of applied harm reduction (relating to injecting drug use) may also be noted:

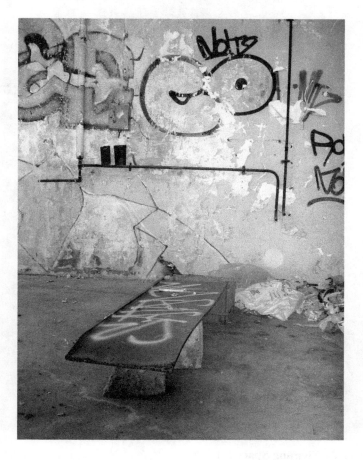

Figure 6.22 Shaping Space (7)

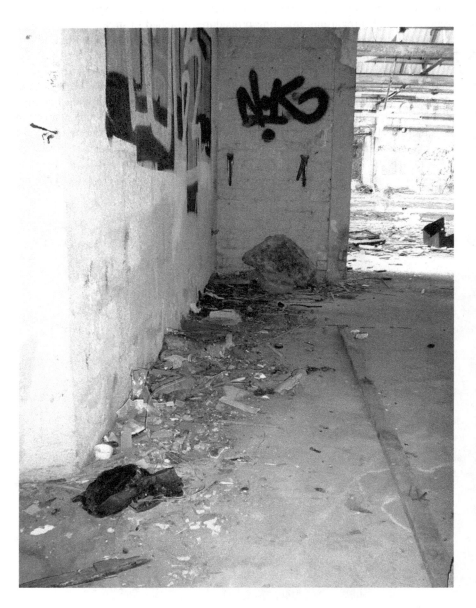

Figure 6.23 Shaping Space (8)

On the left side (from the point of entry) of the foundry room were two adjunct rooms that were clearly used by drug users for the purposes of injecting (due to high levels of discarded paraphernalia noted within the rooms). 'Room 1' was the most active and seemingly current (2 injecting drug users were arrested during a similar police-accompanied inspection by council workers earlier in the week). This small room measured approximately 15x12x12 feet; had an artificial sun roof (that provided an ambient tone to the setting during the midday sunshine) and provided shelter, security and privacy within the main complex. It would be possible to reside in this room without being seen by others who may also be in the premises at the same time.

In two corners of this room, obvious attempts had been made to physically clean and brush all drug-related litter into contained piles, most likely by those with reason to visit the 'injecting' room (i.e. injecting drug users). The floor was relatively clean in contrast to the other spaces throughout the building and genuine attempts had been made to create a cleaner/safer injecting environment. This was confirmed by the positioning of 2 small black hazardous material bins (for sharps disposal) onto a surface adjacent a makeshift seating/injecting/ preparation area (made of rocks and boards: see Figure 6.22). Persons unknown had apparently made attempts to make this particular room a communal resource, that was 'cleaner' and 'safer' than the wider setting of the complex. Indeed, the relative 'cleanliness' and 'orderliness' of this room made it, ironically, more conspicuous within the site of wider dereliction (see Figure 6.23 – note the brushing of debris towards the wall).

It was simply not possible to estimate the large volume of drug-related litter and needles/syringes that had been swept into piles in this room due to the way in which the site had been managed by those using it. Consequently, in order to estimate the levels of discarded equipment in this room, it would perhaps be more practical to collect all waste into a single container for the purposes of weighing rather than counting. (*Fieldnotes*)

Despite the large volume of discarded injecting material described above, the suggestions and inferences of environmental 'ownership' should not be overlooked nor understated. That is, there appeared to be evidence of responsible/ organised decision-making in attempts to establish cleaner, safer and more hygienic injecting spaces *within* a centre of total dilapidation. However, as these reflexive and analytical interpretations are premised only upon environmental visual assessments and associated visual data, the claims of indigenous discarding strategies in this setting cannot be fully confirmed (or denied) with interview data from injecting drug users. This was because no opportunity was made available for arranging contact with those attending the location for injecting purposes and consequently did not participate in the wider study.

Nonetheless, injecting drug users that had attended a similar setting (a squat), described practice that appeared consistent with the shaping of 'safer' environments depicted in Figures 6.22 and 6.23 All settings were located in the same geographical area of the study and were separated by a distance of approximately 1.5 km (1 mile). In the following interview extract, the respondent describes a process of clearing large amounts of discarded equipment as a strategy to avoid police detection and identification of the relevant derelict building appropriated for injecting purposes.

> ... a couple of the lads got together and we all cleaned it all up, the whole place up and that, but ... .you know, then left it there so someone could pick it up and it all did get removed (when the squat was closed by the council). ... It just makes you think because, other people like give you a bad name kind of thing. Because like not everybody just leaves their stuff, you know, we try and keep the stuff with us, even the used ones, you put them back in your bag like, then you can dispose of your whole bag, so you've got used ones with clean ones, so you know, you don't go back to using your used ones. But you just don't leave them where you use basically, because then what it means is it's gonna 'get hot' (attract police attention) if you use the same place again, isn't it? ... So, you're not gonna leave stuff there so you can't go back there again. (*R055*)

Although contextualised within a legal framework (to avoid police interest), the account above describes a process of making a squatted environment more 'safe' for injecting purposes. Similarly, inferred in the practices of avoiding arrest, the respondent above also (perhaps inadvertently) describes a form of grassroots, harm reduction-focused, activism that is made manifest in the resistance strategies of the relevant cohort of injecting drug users (Parkin 2013). Although such conclusions can only be speculative in the absence of focused interview data regarding these particular settings, the overall implication of such practice may be noted in the following observation made by a Public Health Specialist in the relevant setting. In viewing further images of the environment contained in Figures 6.22 and 6.23, this individual was encouraged to remark that 'it's not all injecting chaos out there'.

Deconstructing the Debate

This chapter has focused upon the contentious issue of drug related litter in community settings. More specifically, it has attempted to provide a more empirically-grounded perspective that seeks to avoid demonisation of drug use/rs and similarly circumvent health related hysteria regarding discarded injecting paraphernalia. Throughout this chapter, visual data has played a significant part in formulating this alternative perspective of a thoroughly modern concern and in concretising the various findings described above. Indeed, the various analytical processes attached to the visual dataset of drug related litter has assisted in confirming/refuting drug user views of discarding procedures, consolidated a negative health-place nexus associated with injecting environments and also provided a 'forensic' resource for conducting visually-based analysis of street-based, drug-related harms. Accordingly, the central aim of this chapter has been to 'deconstruct' more dominant representations of drug related litter that may prove to be less helpful in generating pragmatic, harm reduction responses to a politically sensitive, public health issue. Similarly, the visual data attached to this chapter should also be interpreted as a further attempt to demonstrate the 'picturing of harm reduction' (and the disciplinary move towards an applied visual sociology) due to the overall emphasis placed upon applied interpretations.

As an indication of the magnitude attached to the political and structural interest in drug related litter, the following chapter further addresses this sensitive and emotive topic. However, in Chapter 7, the issue is viewed almost exclusively and uniquely (perhaps for the first time) from the perspectives of those frontline service personnel who are required to handle and manage drug related litter in public settings as part of their employment.

Chapter 7
The Management of Drug Related Litter in UK Settings

In the previous chapter, various perspectives of drug related litter were presented in order to illustrate conflicting interpretations of what is undoubtedly a politically and emotionally sensitive issue in UK settings. Whereas Chapter 6 prioritised the views of injecting drug users, the following chapter seeks to summarise the lived experiences of *frontline service personnel* who have been directly affected by discarded injecting paraphernalia during the course of their work. These particular perspectives of street-based injecting drug use have been greatly understated in the literature to date, although some notable exceptions do apply (for example, Parkin 2013, Parkin and Coomber 2009a).

In order to contextualise these particular lived experiences of drug related litter, the following chapter commences with a summary of an advisory document (and its recommendations) issued by the UK's Central Government for consideration by authorities at a local level. This is followed by a series of ethnographic insights on how drug related litter is managed at street level, with particular reference to various experiences of frontline service personnel regarding their applied (and observed) cleansing procedures. A further section focuses upon the advantages and disadvantages of installing dedicated sharps bins within public conveniences (namely, toilets) from the perspectives of frontline service personnel and injecting drug users. As with previous chapters, each of these various accounts is supported with reference to image- and language-based data that were generated throughout the entire research period (2006–2011) as previously described in Chapter 3.

Tackling Drug Related Litter

In October 2005 the UK government's Department for Environment, Food, and Rural Affairs (Defra) published a report titled *Tackling Drug Related Litter*. This document is dedicated to the issue of drug related paraphernalia found discarded in community settings and the document attempts to provide guidance on 'tackling' many of the issues raised and discussed in the previous chapter. *Tackling Drug Related Litter* was produced in recognition that discarded injecting paraphernalia may 'create a very real fear of infection and disease, (and) acts as a stark reminder of the wider harm caused by the misuse of drugs' (Defra 2005, ii), whilst equally acknowledging that:

the *health* risk to the general public of litter from drugs is actually very small, but the *perceived* risk is considerable, making individuals feel unsafe and negative about where they live and work ... (ibid., iii, emphases added)

Tackling Drug Related Litter aims to provide a series of recommendations for managing and reducing the 'growing problem' (Defra 2005, 1) of discarded paraphernalia in various locations, the concomitant 'fear, anger, disgust and frustration' (ibid.) this may generate, in addition to the perceived and actual harms attached to discarded injecting equipment in community/public settings. Similarly, throughout the report, Defra continuously advocates the formation of local partnerships and joint-working initiatives as a means of implementing co-ordinated and effective responses to the management of discarded drug related paraphernalia. This latter point perhaps infers that drug related litter management is a *community*-level issue rather than an individual-level issue.

Defra Recommendations

In essence, Defra's (2005) vision of a joined-up approach to community development prioritises on-going liaison and intervention between local authorities, community organisations, police, drug/alcohol services and all employees that may be affected by drug related litter (whether in the public or private business sectors). Of further import is that whilst the report and its various recommendations seek to promote community safety and public health, there is also an underlying support for the practice and principles of harm reduction made evident throughout the document. For example, the benefits of harm reduction intervention as part of the UK National Drug Strategy is made explicit throughout the text, particularly with regard to needle and syringe distribution, HIV prevalence and the relationship between drug use and sex work (Defra 2005, 3–4). Similarly, many of Defra's recommendations for 'tackling' drug related litter in community settings are premised upon pre-existing examples of 'good practice' noted throughout the UK, in which public health, community safety and *harm reduction* are often central tenets of the interventions cited.

A total of 14 recommendations regarding the management of drug related litter are made by Defra. Of these, almost all emphasise the importance of co-ordinated responses to the surveillance, management, collection and disposal of drug related litter. Similarly, at least 11 of these 14 recommendations endorse some form of harm reduction intervention. For example, Defra suggests that local authorities and community organisations may be more proactive in formalising agreements regarding positive policing of *used* needle possession, the siting of sharps bins in public toilets, avoiding the installation of blue lights in public settings and providing training for all people who may encounter discarded equipment during the course of their employment. However, throughout the various recommendations, Defra also cautions that any person coming into contact with discarded sharps 'should take the view' that such items 'could be infected' (Defra 2005, 48). Furthermore, any information disseminated to the general public 'should not include any suggestion that needles can be moved or touched' or provide any guidance on how community members may handle discarded sharps (ibid.).

Other significant health, safety and harm reduction guidance contained within Defra's report relates to the most effective tools required for drug related litter collection by frontline service personnel. Although Defra states that all relevant organisations should provide appropriate personal protective equipment (PPE) to all affected employees, consideration should also be given to the suitability of some equipment for particular working environments. Amongst the key Defra-recommended utensils required for the collection and disposal of drug related litter are portable sharps boxes, tongs, brushes, dustpans and protective gloves that afford a suitable level of safety against potential needle puncture.

It should be noted however, that Defra is *not* responsible for any government policy regarding illicit drug use. Nevertheless, it is a body that works in conjunction with other central government departments (namely the Home Office and Department for Health) in promoting the current National Drug Strategy (Defra 2005, i). As such, *Tackling Drug Related Litter* may be regarded, at best, as only an advisory document that provides good practice guidance, for consideration by local authorities throughout the UK. Accordingly, Defra's (2005) recommendations provide *options* for local government application and they – regrettably – should not necessarily be interpreted as a template of mandatory expectation.

Guidelines for Clearing Drug Related Litter: An Illustration

Perhaps due to the proliferation of drug related litter in community settings noted by Defra (2005), in conjunction with the latter's recommendations regarding drug related litter management (especially for those in contact with discarded sharps), there are currently many organisations and individuals operating throughout the UK that provide bespoke services for clearing injecting paraphernalia and/or specialised training in drug issues. An illustration of the latter may be noted in the 13-step guide to managing drug related litter (Blacklock 2010) presented below in Box 7.1. These guidelines are designed specifically for street-level operatives involved in the removal of drug related litter from affected environments.

Rigorous cleansing processes such as those summarised in Box 7.1 essentially aim to ensure that safer disposal of discarded sharps takes place within community settings and/or workplaces. Each aspect of the meticulous cleansing regimes described above also aims to avoid needlestick injury amongst those collecting the items as well as reduce potential sharps-contact with members of the public in the affected setting. Similarly, the pragmatic procedures outlined above comply absolutely with Defra's (2005) recommendation regarding the

> 1. Risk assesses the whole area
> 2. Always wear gloves from the start of the procedure to the end
> 3. Never place your hands into an area you cannot see
> 4. Always take the sharps box to the needle/syringe. (The shorter the distance the syringe travels the smaller the risk)
> 5. Place the open sharps box on the ground
> 6. Use tongs to pick up the syringe and place into the sharps box. (Needle facing down)
> 7. Close the sharps box ensuring the lid is locked
> 8. When removing contaminated non-sharps, place them into clinical waste bag using tongs and seal the bag
> 9. Clean up the area where needles have been collected, to ensure no bio-hazard (blood, vomit etc.) is left for subsequent visitors
> 10. Decontaminate all equipment used
> 11. Place collected items into a secure drugs cabinet
> 12. Place gloves into clinical waste bag
> 13. Log the items found (to establish a database of drug related litter)

Box 7.1 A 13-step Guide to Managing Drug Related Litter

constant need to err on the side of caution when handling potentially hazardous equipment. Indeed, these specific guidelines are entirely commensurate with the relevant recommendations contained within *Tackling Drug Related Litter*.

However, the reality of street-based, drug related litter management may not fully reflect the thoroughness and diligence suggested in the above protocol. As such, the remainder of this chapter seeks to juxtaposition the lived experiences of drug related litter management with the various recommendations regarding good practice guidelines cited above. This account is based upon interviews, ethnographic attachment and street-based observations with those frontline service personnel whose employment is directly affected by street-based injecting drug use (such as café staff, car park attendants, refuse operatives, street cleansing teams, toilet attendants and each of their various line managers). Similarly, this account has been informed by data generated from each of the four geographic settings involved in this research (see Chapter 3). As such, this account is therefore *not* exclusive to one particular location and aims to provide conclusions that are representative of all four locations involved in the study. However, for reasons relating to confidentiality and anonymity, the actual organisations, employees and locations described throughout this Chapter (as with drug users and the various environments housing street-based injecting) cannot be revealed or identified.

Summarising Drug Related Litter Management Across All Field Sites

It is perhaps necessary to acknowledge from the onset that all local authorities (and numerous businesses within the private sector) involved in this study had implemented some form of drug related litter management in community settings prior to any research taking place. Furthermore, many of these measures were in accordance with the various good practice guidelines advocated by Defra and all authorities sought to provide a co-ordinated response to drug related litter. Examples of shared intervention noted throughout all four field sites included the availability of rapid response cleansing teams, designated freephone 'hotlines' (for members of the public to report drug related litter) and the availability of training/ equipment for personnel handling discarded sharps and paraphernalia in street-based locations. Similarly, established *cleansing* protocols were reported in almost every setting that had been affected by street-based injecting episodes (involved in the study) whether they were located in the public or private business sector. This included settings such as car parks, public toilets, high street shopping centres, entertainment venues and travel termini.

However, some differences were also noted. For example, some locations openly supported and provided sharps bins in public locations (whereas others did not) and some supported blue lights in public toilets as a strategy to prevent drug injecting (others did not). Some private businesses formalised training in drug related litter management – others did not. Similarly, not all statutory authorities meticulously recorded the volume of drug related litter collected on a *daily* basis (and only one was able to provide a wealth of quantitative data relating to public injecting drug use that covered a period of several years). Other variances related to the way in which street-based injecting was managed by different police forces. For example, in one setting, possession of un/used injecting equipment was considered legitimate grounds for temporary detention and questioning in local police stations. Despite these similarities (and variations) regarding Defra-related good practice guidelines, there was also a *shared unawareness* (across all four geographic areas) of the relevant document concerned with *Tackling Drug Related Litter* in community settings. In conclusion, one may assume that regional policies regarding the management of drug related litter in four different urban areas throughout the south of England were consistent in aims and objectives but, paradoxically, *inconsistent* in design and delivery. The *qualitative significance* of this observation is discussed below.

The Lived Experience of Drug Related Litter Management

The following section seeks to provide an insight of the way in which drug related litter management is experienced from the perspective of those personnel responsible for the implementation of such tasks. In this account, no attempt has been made to differentiate the experiences of local authority employees from those who work within private business sector settings. This deliberate absence of data segregation aims to portray a collective, lived experience of drug related litter management, from a particularly 'street-level' outlook. More importantly, this more generically-focused account simultaneously and conveniently avoids the identification of particular working procedures noted within specific organisations involved in the study.

Training, Equipment and Assorted Responses

Almost all of the *street-based*, frontline service personnel that participated in this study were each familiar with a range of 'in-house' procedures designed to manage drug related litter in affected settings. In most cases, these individuals were directly responsible for the actual removal of discarded sharps (and related injecting paraphernalia) as well as the cleansing of environments found to contain 'litter' in general. As such, most operatives interviewed had received varying degrees of formal training by their respective employers regarding hazardous materials, appropriate cleansing procedures and the use of suitable equipment. Similarly, many individuals described a cleansing routine that they were *expected* to follow whilst engaged in drug related litter cleansing procedures. Indeed, these accounts typically paralleled the procedures outlined above (in Box 7.1) by Blacklock (2010). Figures 7.1 and 7.2 portray the typical range of PPE (sharps boxes, tongs and protective gloves) issued by employers to facilitate safer collection and discarding procedures. However, when individuals were observed (or asked to describe) how they actually performed these guidelines, a variety of responses were noted during all fieldwork. Indeed, the various working *practices* noted by frontline service personnel may be categorised as 'formal', 'semi-formal' or 'informal' responses to drug related litter management. Furthermore, the relevant responses often reflected the formal working environment and wider duties of the operatives concerned, *in which both were consistent with the relevant category of injecting environment* (see Chapter 5). Each of these work-related responses is described in further detail below.

Formal Responses

The cleansing procedures that were identified as those most 'operationally' close to those suggested by Blacklock (2010) are here defined as the most 'formal' responses to drug related litter management. These procedures were typically described by frontline service personnel by individuals employed within static, fixed locations in which sites of discarded injecting paraphernalia were typically enclosed within a wider public sphere. Illustrative examples of such locations housing these formal responses include shopping centres, disabled-access toilets and public conveniences located within private sector businesses. Accordingly, there is perhaps little coincidence that more duteous cleansing protocols were reported within environments that contain greater numbers of the general public, as the former attempt to maintain appropriate standards of 'customer care' (especially in relation to sanitation and hygiene). In Chapter 5, these settings of injecting drug

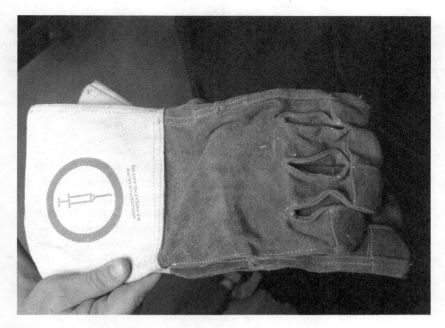

Figure 7.1   Protective Equipment (1)

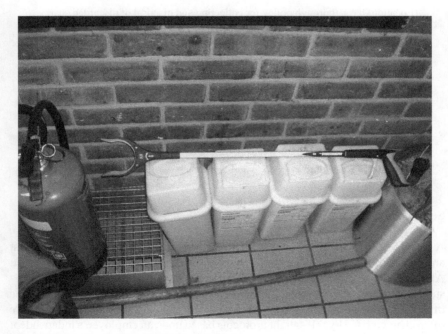

Figure 7.2   Protective Equipment (1)

use are categorised as 'controlled' (Category A) environments and, from a harm reduction perspective, typically contain the most hygienic, street-based, location for episodes of drug injecting. The following fieldnotes summarise examples of 'formal' cleansing routines noted in two settings affected by drug related litter and injecting drug use.

> Certain individuals within the workplace are designated as drug related litter cleaners. These individuals have been given training in collecting all sharps (needles, bottles, glass) and (respondent) reamed off the entire procedure from a safety training sheet she had brought with her. This provided instructions on the type of gloves to wear; how to clean the area and disinfect the needle before picking-up, how to place items correctly in a sharps box, how to clean the immediate vicinity (that would be 'guarded' by another member of staff in order to prevent others contacting the needle/syringe before the designated cleaner arrives) and how to handle the sharps box for disposal. A similar procedure was in place for cleaning any bodily fluids present and involves the use of a solidifying foam/gel for removing blood, excrement, urine and vomit. In 7 years there have been no incidents of needlestick injury amongst all staff. (*Fieldnotes, Shopping Centre*)

Similarly:

> (Location) has a thorough policy for collecting and disposal of discarded sharps. Staff are given training by external contractors in how to collect and dispose of sharps safely. (Location) is fully-equipped with various sharps boxes, *steel-lined gloves*, tongs and various cleaning fluids. All discarded items collected on site are subsequently given to a sub-contracted cleansing unit. The latter will exchange any used 5 litre sharps bins for a new set of unused bins. The used bins are then sent to an unknown location for incineration along with other hazardous waste. As well as this (staff) may also use a local telephone hotline to the local council. Respondent spoke positively of the rapid response they receive from local services whenever they report drug related litter found on the premises in this regard. (*Fieldnotes, Public/Civic Amenity*)

Semi-formal Responses

A second set of responses noted across all geographic locations were those that are here defined as 'semi-formal' responses to drug related litter management. Although the relevant respondents attempted to emulate Blacklock's (2010) 13-step guide to sharps retrieval, these procedures usually occurred *in the absence* of any formal training provided by the relevant employers. Such procedures were often characterised by self-taught protocols based upon an employee's independent review of the relevant 'health and safety' literature. Furthermore, decisions to adopt these *ad hoc* procedures typically reflected the relevant workers' level of independence (or responsibility) in the workplace when compared to those who were monitored and regulated by supervisors and/or line managers. That is, those who made the relevant decisions to implement improvised strategies of drug related litter management in their work environment were more likely to hold positions of limited responsibility and decision-making. Similarly, the enthusiasm with which they articulated this volitional (and unexpected) responsibility was also perceived by those respondents as a reflection of their own personal dedication to providing 'quality customer-care'.

The semi-formal, improvised and self-taught protocols noted in the following Fieldnotes occurred within fixed settings that provided semi-public access to all members of the community. Examples of such locations include supervised settings contained within multi-storey car parks, as well as 'unsupervised' amenities and conveniences in similar locations (and cleansed as part of a rolling-rota system). Semi-formal responses may therefore be noted to occur within injecting environments previously defined (in Chapter 5) as Semi-Controlled (Category B) settings. As such, the environmental consistencies relating to place-based hygiene (from a harm reduction perspective) should once more not go under-stated. For example:

> (Respondent) explained that sharps collection involves wearing thick rubber gloves, a plastic apron and placing sharps into 'a yellow box'. This is collected by a local pharmacy for appropriate disposal when respondent decides it is full (possibly with a 'collection fee' attached). Training appears to have been self-taught, as all information was gathered from manuals and training sites accessed online. There has never been an incidence of needlestick injury reported at in this setting. (*Fieldnotes, Unsupervised Convenience in Basement Car Park*)

Similarly:

> As a means of illustrating the extent of injecting in the car park, (respondent) showed me a 10 litre sharps box that was stored in the cabin. Respondent removed the *insecure* lid and showed me the contents (Figure 7.3). Inside was approximately '330 needles' that had been collected in the last '2–3 months'. Inside I could see thicker barrelled syringes and many of the standard 1ml insulin syringes. There were long pins in there too and lots of cookers, foils and improvised cookers. (Respondent) explained that staff are not actually required to pick up this litter – as instructed by the management – and they are supposed to report this to the local authority who will then arrange collection and disposal. However, such assistance costs the company £60–70 per call out. Because of the amount of drug related litter and because respondent (and colleagues) appeared to be concerned about the safety of children and customers using the car park they arranged to collect themselves as and when necessary. As such, they personally obtained a sharps bin from (a local needle and syringe programme)

and bought (at their own expense) a pair of tongs for collecting drug related litter. Once the bin is full they take it to the source for disposal and exchange. They each stated that they have received no training in collecting drug related litter (and throughout our walkabout tour I noticed one respondent using unprotected fingers to poke around in the dirt looking for foils and other paraphernalia). Respondent was of the opinion that you 'need some kind of special licence to pick-up needles'. However, I was most surprised at the presence of the open sharps bin (with detachable secure lid) left open and exposed in the car park cabin. There were no reports of needlestick injury at this location. (*Fieldnotes, Multi-Storey Car Park*)

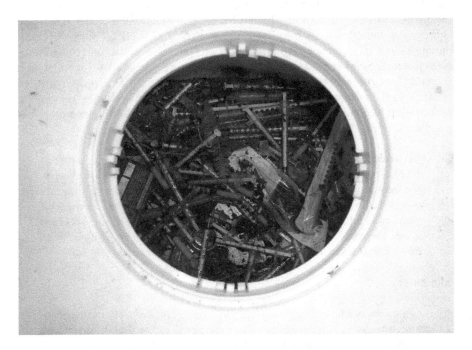

Figure 7.3   Semi-Formal Drug Related Litter Collection

Informal Responses

A third variation of drug related litter management noted throughout all research is here termed as an 'informal' response to collecting discarding equipment. In more simplistic terms, this relates to adopting a reported 'common sense' approach to handling potentially hazardous materials. In these circumstances, operatives had more often than not received formal drugs training within their workplace and were often aware of various harms and hazards associated with discarded injecting equipment. Similarly, almost all these individuals had been issued with PPE from their various line managers and were issued for the specific purpose of collecting discarded needles and syringes. Furthermore, there was a managerial expectation that this equipment (typically heavy duty gloves, tongs and various sharps containers) would be used whilst collecting drug related litter. Many individuals within this body of frontline service personnel had also been given a course of 'hepatitis vaccinations' as part of 'health and safety at work' procedures. As such, these employees may be regarded as the most drug-aware, best equipped and most 'hepatitis-alert' cohort within the entire frontline service personnel sample throughout all research.

For many of these individuals, the presence of drug related litter in street-based settings was typically regarded as mundane and commonplace items that they frequently encountered during their working hours. As one operative nonchalantly commented, the collection of drug related litter 'is a job for life innit'. This work-related statement perhaps demonstrates the normalisation of the extraordinary in daily routines, in which the collection of drug related paraphernalia is regarded with indifference and as a task to be completed as a matter of course. Similarly, many of these individuals worked routine shift systems, based on 8-hour time periods, that varied on a weekly basis. Others were organised as mobile units and were expected to cover a wide geographic area within a given time period (relating to shifts/rotas). In addition to collecting drug related litter, a further requirement involved the sanitising of public conveniences *per se* (of vomit, urine, excrement, general litter etc.) in addition to cleansing areas affected by chewing gum, graffiti, glue, paint, fly tipping/posting and the collection of sex related litter. In some locations there was also the added expectation that each individual task was 'logged' within a record book that was maintained by the relevant crews responsible for geographic zones within a given area. Ethnographic attachment to these units involved visits to numerous locations within a given time period in which cleansing had to performed competently, efficiently and rapidly whilst simultaneously restore hygiene standards considered satisfactory by the relevant management/supervisory teams (who often followed mobile cleansing teams, checking work completed for final approval). Indeed, many observations of this form of employment noted that frontline service personnel were under constant pressure to complete tasks and targets. For example:

> Respondent explained wider problems relating to anti-social behaviour within the toilet setting; such as 'winos and drunks sleeping in toilets, refusing to move as so inebriated', 'kids causing havoc at weekends when pissed up', (and taunting him as they know he 'can't touch them'); others waiting until he has mopped the floor and deliberately dropping/smashing bottles on the floor for him to clean again and taunting him with the comment that 'he's just a cleaner'. Respondent explained that sometimes he gets so angry he wants to 'lash out', (verbally and physically) as he gets so frustrated by the abuse. ... Respondent said that 'if the public knew

the shit (he had) to deal with everyday', he wondered if they would be 'so forward in condemning (toilet attendants) as they do'. (*Fieldnotes, Public Convenience*)

This pressure was further intensified – and made more stressful – when members of the public openly challenged and confronted street cleansing operatives bemoaning the unacceptable condition of particular environments (typically accessed by members of the public). For example:

(As we sat outside the toilets discussing the cleaning rotas) a middle-aged woman approached (respondent) after visiting the toilets and gave him a torrent of abuse about the state of the toilets. She remarked how 'unclean they were' and felt they 'were not fit for public use'. She stated she was going to raise this issue at a meeting with a local MP and would be writing to the authorities to complain. Respondent stood silently as she complained for about 5–7 minutes, during which time she even told him 'not to say anything' as she 'wasn't interested in his answers'! Ironically, I had left the women's toilet only minutes before her and had taken photos of some of the cubicles (of places where needles have previously been found) and have to say that I found them clean and of an acceptable standard. I told (respondent) this and he said he might need my photos to respond to the letter he was expecting from the complainant! Two frontline staff, also present, stated 'we get this all the time'. One of which chortled and added, 'she should be around when the drunks and druggies are using the toilets!' (*Fieldnotes, Public Convenience*)

It was perhaps due to these work-related and wider social pressures that many frontline service personnel adopted what was frequently termed 'a common sense approach' to drug related litter collection. The application of this informal response aimed to gather discarded items by the most rapid and most safe method, in a manner that removed items from public harm and facilitated progress in their own daily duties and related tasks. Furthermore, this more informal response was especially noticeable amongst those who were comparatively mobile and independent in carrying out work-related tasks across a range of settings and locations. As such, these informal strategies were employed in all environmental categories relating to injecting drug use (that is, Category A, B and C) as the former reflected the rapid and mobile nature of the work expected. However, in adopting this informal, 'common sense' approach, employees were often noted as 'cutting corners' in order to facilitate more positive progress in their daily routines and associated duties. This is made evident in the following fieldnotes.

As we walked up the length of (street name) I estimated about 20 condoms were collected and between 6–10 needles/syringes. All needles and syringes were hidden under empty beer cans, in long grass, under other rubbish and retrieved from a gated alleyway. There was a lot of other drug related litter, including foil (a whole tube of it), needle caps, wrappers, swabs and other seals. I noticed that (the cleansing team) only collected needles/syringes and condoms and did not bother with this other paraphernalia as we had to move onto the next site before premises began to open for business. (*Fieldnotes, Street Cleaning, 6am-shift*)

Similarly:

Staff stated they tended to apply a 'common sense' approach to drug related litter. They will treat materials cautiously and will collect sharps using rubber gloves and a sharps collection box (using tongs). They added that if the sharps box was not nearby, they would deposit needles in 'normal' bins whose contents are taken to landfill sites. Those items that are collected in sharps boxes are disposed of in hazardous waste bins along with paints, chemicals and other toxins to be dealt with by the designated hazardous waste contractors. The manager had considered issuing heavy duty rubber gloves to his staff for the purpose of collecting sharps. But when asked if they would wear them, his patrol team said they wouldn't. So he never bought any and the team opted not to wear them (as they are considered too cumbersome) ... (*Fieldnotes, 'Park Patrol' Focus Group*)

Similar experiences were reported by a unit dedicated to the regular cleansing of all public conveniences located throughout one particular setting. Namely:

A discussion with all 3 operatives in the toilet area noted that each were prepared to apply improvised cleansing procedures that involved putting needles/syringes into drinks-cans and avoiding the use of the designated gloves issued to them because they were 'too awkward'. Each described a 'common sense' approach to avoiding injury when handling sharps. (*Fieldnotes, Public Convenience*)

Of all PPE issued to frontline service personnel, it was the heavy duty 'anti-syringe' gloves (Figure 7.1) that were the most unpopular and most under-used of protective items issued by various employers. The rationale provided for not wearing these items typically related to the bulky, rigid design that made gathering pencil-like objects (such as syringes) almost impossible. A further justification for not wearing protective gloves equally related to the rapid and mobile nature of the work conducted by the relevant operatives. For example, several caretakers and concierges reported that carrying bulky equipment on their person unnecessarily hindered an already 'busy' (frantic) daily work routine. As such, excess equipment (that may or may not be needed during a specific task) was often deliberately left, surplus to requirements, in the relevant utility/rest rooms or canteen areas. In the event of subsequently encountering sharp items (especially needles) within a community setting, a shared response reported by those concerned was to further apply 'a common sense' approach to the matter. In short, without the assistance of protective gloves, respondents reported that they would 'fling' discarded sharps into a nearby litter bin without actually touching the needle or making contact with any obvious blood presence (that is, replicating discarding procedures considered inappropriate when conducted by injecting drug users). For these reasons, many operatives believed that 'anti-syringe gloves' did not provide value for money, especially when estimated at '£160 a pair'. These views/actions are perhaps encapsulated in the following focus group response with an assembly of caretakers (CT1-CT4) in a residential setting:

> CT3: Yeah, we do get trained (in how to dispose of needles and syringes). But I mean, basically, if you find a syringe and that, I mean, you used to get (a box for it). But the proper way now is, is to come back here (canteen) and get the yellow sharps box put these 'super gloves' on, go back and dispose of it.
>
> CT2: Do you know, with those 'super gloves' though, you can't bend your fingers ... ((incredulous laughter)).
>
> CT4: You can't bend your fingers can you? ((more laughter)).
>
> CT2: They're about a hundred quid a pair aren't they?
>
> SP: So if you do find one, do you generally do that procedure where you go back and get your bin, get your gloves, get your sharps box and tongs?
>
> CT3: No.
>
> CT1 You just put them in the nearest bin ...
>
> CT4: Common sense. You don't get hold of the sharp end and just dispose of it. My sharps box is in my little room down there (so I) just put it in (the nearest bin).

Comparing Lived Experience

When the work routines of frontline service personnel are *qualitatively* compared to the drug using routines of street-based injectors (Parkin 2013), one may note some similarities in the lived experience of social environments. More specifically, both lifestyles are characterised by movement and motion across a wide geographic area within city environs; both involve a degree of transience and operating independently to complete necessary 'chores' and, most importantly, both parties aim to perform their respective 'tasks' (cleaning/injecting) in a manner that is rapid and hasty in order to 'save time'.

Whereas these similarities clearly relate to opposing roles that may be defined as licit (employment) and illicit (drug use), the commonalities of mobility, transience and rapidity serve to facilitate competent performance (completing jobs *vs.* administering drugs), in a satisfactory manner that avoids challenges from authority (line managers/supervisors *vs.* police/public); all of which need to occur within a specific time-frame (that is, as quickly as possible). Moreover, as noted in Chapter 5, environments characterised by rushed and rapid injecting practice contribute towards injecting-related harm amongst drug users. Accordingly, it is perhaps of little coincidence that rushed and rapid cleansing practice conducted by frontline service personnel within similar environments may produce 'drug related harm' in the form of needlestick injury.

Indeed, throughout all geographic areas of the study, those frontline service personnel who reported greater incidents of needlestick injury were typically those that utilised more 'informal' cleaning responses and, ironically, were those that had received greater levels of formalised drug training from their employers. Accounts of (single and multiple) needlestick injury were myriad amongst those with cleaning responsibilities within this sector of frontline service personnel. Similarly, those affected often recounted the events surrounding their needlestick injury with anger and loathing directed specifically at injecting drug users *per se*. In addition, these recollections of drug related harm were often characterised by accounts of anxiety and stress as respondents described lengthy time-periods awaiting blood-test results regarding viral infection. The following accounts typify this experience:

> (Respondent) recalled an event involving the collection of a needle from a sink basin that resulted in needlestick injury for the attendant concerned. The latter had been unaware of anything wrapped inside a paper towel that had been discarded in the basin, and as he picked it up he was 'jabbed' by the needle concealed within. He was taken to hospital and 'tested for viruses'. He was distraught for a few weeks after this event, worrying about what may happen, but had recently been given the 'all-clear' as his tests came back negative. (*Fieldnotes, Public Convenience*)

Similarly:

> In the ten years (respondent) has worked the 'toilet-rota' she has had one needlestick injury – which happened only recently. About 6 months ago she was removing a sanitary bag from a cubicle. As the bag swung it caught her hand and she felt a prick in her finger. She opened and emptied the bag, found a needle and then immediately bled her finger over a sink basin. She went to hospital and had blood tests. She is still waiting for the 'all-clear' but is confident they will return negative. She based this opinion on the fact that there was no 'wet' blood present in the needle ... (*Fieldnotes, Public Convenience*)

Whereas the latter example perhaps demonstrates the value of drug training and how to respond to needlestick injury, it should also be noted that many frontline service personnel articulated the potential of viral infection (such as hepatitis and HIV) from discarded needles. Similarly, several caretakers and cleansing operatives each reported completion of various courses of hepatitis vaccinations and/or reported previous histories of hepatitis B infection. However, there was also a concomitant belief that the relevant course of vaccinations would provide *complete* immunity from the hepatitis virus and there appeared to be a shared lack of clarity regarding the various 'strains' of the virus. In short, many frontline service staff were of the mistaken belief that their hepatitis vaccinations/previous hepatitis B infections provided total immunity from hepatitis C (for which there is no current immunisation program and is the most chronic and persistent form of the hepatitis virus).

From this qualitative account, one may conclude that those frontline service personnel whose work routines emulate the transient nature of public injecting drug use; whose cleansing routines adopt a 'common sense' approach to drug related litter management (despite having received training in drug issues and viral infection) and whose working practices are most characterised by rushed and rapid performance are those possibly most *susceptible* to drug related harm (needlestick injury).

Drug Related Litter Bins in Public Conveniences

One possible response to issue of discarded sharps in community settings, as recommended by Defra (2005), may be the introduction of dedicated sharps bins in public conveniences. These containers aim to minimise contact with sharps in public environments and appear as appropriate intervention for promoting safer disposal strategies to reduce drug related harm that emerges from needlestick injury (whether by members of the public, frontline service personnel or injecting drug users). A summary of the advantages brought about by such intervention is summarised in the following section. Furthermore, all findings relate to research located across all four sites involved in this multi-site study of drug-related litter/ street-based injecting drug use.

The Politics of Drug Related Litter Bins

Decisions to introduce drug related litter bins into public places may be surrounded by controversy, condemnation and even public outrage. For example, research conducted by Environmental Campaigns (ENCAMS), notes community-wide suspicion and scepticism of sharps bins situated in public settings. More specifically, ENCAMS (2004, 39) reports that members of the public *assume* drug users lack the required lucidity and social responsibility to actually utilise the bins for depositing injecting equipment. The organisation also reports that perceptions of drug related litter bins in community settings typically signal wider social unease (relating to a particular 'drugs problem') and/or make an area appear unattractive to tourists and other visitors. Similarly, ENCAMS further identify valid community concerns relating to children that may encounter sharps bins, as well as consequences relating to vandalism (or other damage). As a result of these sensitivities, ENCAMS conclude that 'the public do not want services that seem to condone drug usage or bring more users into their neighbourhoods' (ibid.).

However, for each and every one of these concerns, there is an equal and opposite harm reduction response that would counter the relevant contention. Namely, *empirical* research (Parkin and Coomber 2011) has shown that injecting drug users will engage with appropriately placed (and environmentally-relevant) drug related litter bins in a manner that is responsible and is behaviour that may occur immediately after injecting drugs. Furthermore, the same article (ibid.) did not note any 'honey-pot effect' associated with drug related litter bins (and this is more likely to occur with the presence of drug markets rather than waste receptacles). A counter-argument relating to the perceived anti-aesthetic value of drug related litter bins is that such initiatives would signal *positive* messages (to all community members, tourists and visitors alike) that the relevant authorities have chosen to adopt a proactive public health policy aimed at reducing drug related harm (whilst simultaneously addressing public health and community safety issues). Similarly, concerns relating to children/vandalism may be reduced when sharps containers are securely located in fixed settings and raised off the ground at appropriate heights to avoid mishandling by young people/children.

Due to the range of potentially negative public responses identified by ENCAMS (2004), Defra's (2005) report to Central Government clearly acknowledges the contentious nature of drug related sharps bins positioned in public settings. However, Defra equally suggests that subsequent public outcry may be diminished by a process of public consultation in which partnerships (consisting of statutory bodies and community organisations) seek public advice and assistance prior to any actual installation of the bins. Similarly, in an attempt to minimise concerns relating to children accessing used injecting equipment, avoiding vandalism and making containers fully secure, Defra makes a number of suggestions regarding the appropriate design and location of drug related litter bins when installed in public settings. More accurately, Defra recommendations in this regard state that drug related litter bins in public sites should:

- be secure.
- be designed to either allow for single items or personnel sharps containers.
- be able to receive other drug related paraphernalia (cookers, filters, swabs) without causing blockages.
- be weatherproof, vandal-proof, graffiti-proof and fireproof.
- be designed for regular maintenance.
- not cause injury by their design.
- be out of sight from CCTV (in order to maximise service uptake by drug users).

- be positioned in discreet locations (to avoid unnecessary provocation).
- be attached to locations to minimise opportunities for vandalism and break-ins.

As a consequence of the cumulative desirable features listed above, Defra further recommend the most appropriate environments for considering the installation of drug related litter bins should be public conveniences. This conclusion relates to the 'privacy' that cubicles afford in addition to the varying degrees of security (cleaning, shelter, supervision, public access, restricted hours of access) associated with settings of public toiletry and hygiene. The three key recommendations that specify a positive correlation between public conveniences and the installation of sharps bins are reproduced (verbatim) below in Box 7.2.

Tackling Drug Related Litter: Guidance and Good Practice
Recommendations relating to public conveniences
Plans for managing drug related litter *should* include close liaison with those responsible for the design, maintenance and management of public toilets
Due to the increased risks to users and lack of evidence as to its efficiency, blue lighting *should not* be used in public toilets to deter drug use
Partnerships *should* fully explore the potential for sharps bins, liaising closely with drug users and services to ensure the siting and promotion of bins is as effective as possible
Department for Environment, Food and Rural Affairs (2005, 48 emphases added)

Box 7.2   Key Recommendations Relating to Public Conveniences and Drug Related Litter Bins

Examples of Drug Related Litter Bins in Public Places

Figures 7.4–7.8 show an assortment of sharps bins that the author has noted in numerous public settings throughout the UK during 2006–2011 (some of which were not necessarily in the geographic areas of fieldwork described in Chapter 3). As may be noted from this particular montage, the range of drug related litter bins fixed into community settings may vary in their design, installation and environmental setting. Furthermore, each image is of a static sharps box that represents a form of 'real world' intervention and each were actively used for collecting/disposing injecting paraphernalia in public settings at the time each image was recorded.[1]

---

[1] Due to the variation noted within these particular images, readers are directed to Chapter 10, (Assignment #6) in order to further consider these photographs from the perspective of an applied visual sociology.

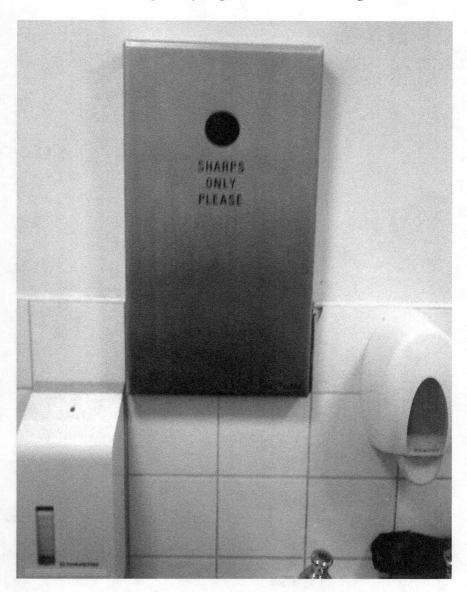

Figure 7.4   Drug Related Litter Bins in Public Place (1)

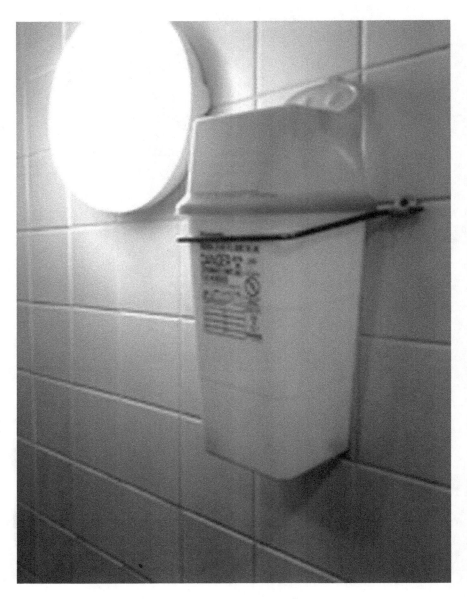

Figure 7.5   Drug Related Litter Bins in Public Place (2)

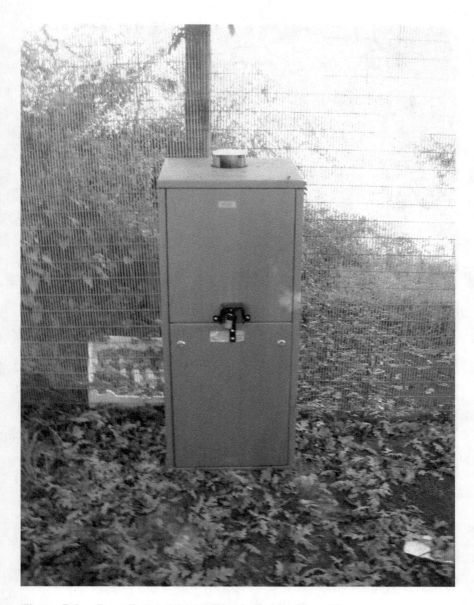

Figure 7.6   Drug Related Litter Bins in Public Place (3)

196   *An Applied Visual Sociology: Picturing Harm Reduction*

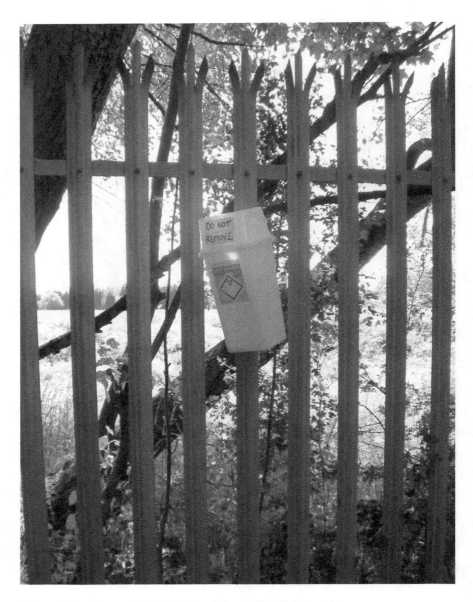

Figure 7.7   Drug Related Litter Bins in Public Place (4)

The Management of Drug Related Litter in UK Settings 197

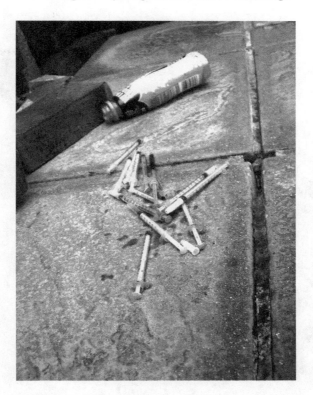

Figure 7.8   Drug Related Litter Bins in Public Place (5)

Although each of the bins displayed in Figures 7.4–7.8 may be commended and criticised from a variety of conflicting viewpoints,[2] it is the design featured in Figures 7.9–7.17 that has been met with the most approval by Defra. Throughout *Tackling Drug Related Litter*, Defra provide exemplars of developing community safety by means of improving facilities within public toilets. An explicit illustration of good practice guidelines in this regard relates to an initiative identified by Defra in the city of Cambridge (UK) and operated by the local authority of that location. In this example, the provision of public conveniences, such as those contained within the aforementioned images, is applauded and commended as an appropriate method to 'tackle' drug related litter in community settings. More accurately, the relevant toilet design aims to minimise incidents of needlestick injury (via spatial planning and spatial management) and simultaneously provide opportunities for the disposal of sharp items in public places. It is for these latter reasons that the overall design is regarded as a model of good practice in the management of public health and community safety.

---

2   For example from the perspectives of harm reduction, community safety, public health and enforcement.

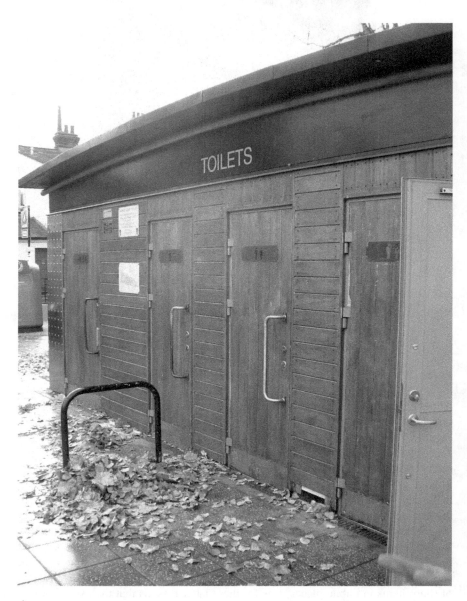

Figure 7.9 'Gold Standard' Public Toilet/Drug Related Litter Bin Design (1)

Figures 7.9–7.17, therefore represent a series of images that visualise and demonstrate a 'gold standard' design for drug related litter bins in public settings as suggested by Defra (2005). However, it should be stressed that these images are *not* of the public toilets in Cambridge described in the Defra (2005) report. Instead, they depict a form of public toilet provision noted during fieldwork that may be regarded as 'almost identical' to the 'Cambridge model' advocated by Defra.

In the first image of this particular dataset (Figure 7.9), the design of several stand-alone, unisex, toilet cubicles grouped together as a single unit is perhaps most noteworthy. This design feature essentially aims to provide private spaces of public convenience in community-based settings. However, the overtly public location and eye-catching 'chalet' design of the unit (less noticeably) aims to maximise naturally-occurring surveillance of any suspect behaviour associated within or around the immediate vicinity of the unit. These design features are applauded by Defra, as they facilitate the provision of public amenity where formalised supervision (by local authority employees or other frontline service personnel) can/may not necessarily be able to occur.

The commendable design of the chalet-unit continues within each individual cubicle and may be noted throughout Figures 7.10–7.14. In these five images (of three different units), one may note discrete signage notifying patrons of the location of sharps bins adjacent and above the respective sink basins. Furthermore, these notices feature visual icons of objects deemed suitable for disposal within the 'birdhouse' opening located upon the internal fascia unit. As may be evident in Figure 7.10, appropriate items for disposal include needles and syringes in addition to other objects associated with washroom attendance (such as razor blades and safety pins). In some settings, Braille notification also accompanied these icons in order to alert those experiencing visually-impaired difficulties of the relevant disposal facilities. Overall, the symbolic, textual, tactile and visual ambiguity of the signage is a further demonstration of creditable design. This is because the non-specific notice advises the public of facilities designed for the discarding of sharp items *per se* rather than identify specific objects relating explicitly to injecting drug use. As such, this more neutral and impartial notification possibly minimises concerns relating to any community unease associated with the immediate social and physical setting (pertaining specifically to drug issues).

In Figures 7.11–7.14, it is further possible to appreciate an overall 'safer toilet design' when compared to other 'Category A' environments described throughout Chapter 5. For example, one may note the self-contained hand-washing facility (providing access to hot, running water, soap and drying facilities); comparatively more comfortable and more hygienic space in private settings and the provision of alarms in the event of emergency (Figure 7.12 only). Moreover, the absence of flat surfaces, ledges and shelves further minimise the amount of littering spaces available for the discarding of injecting paraphernalia (whether 'stashed', or as part of any so-called 'malicious intent', by injecting drug users) should also be noted within these images. Indeed, the

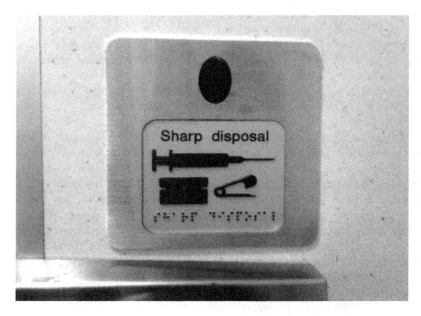

Figure 7.10   'Gold Standard' Public Toilet/Drug Related Litter Bin Design (2)

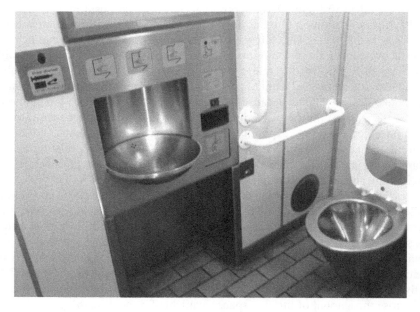

Figure 7.11   'Gold Standard' Public Toilet/Drug Related Litter Bin Design (3)

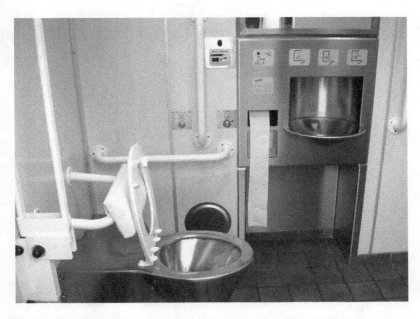

Figure 7.12 'Gold Standard' Public Toilet/Drug Related Litter Bin Design (4)

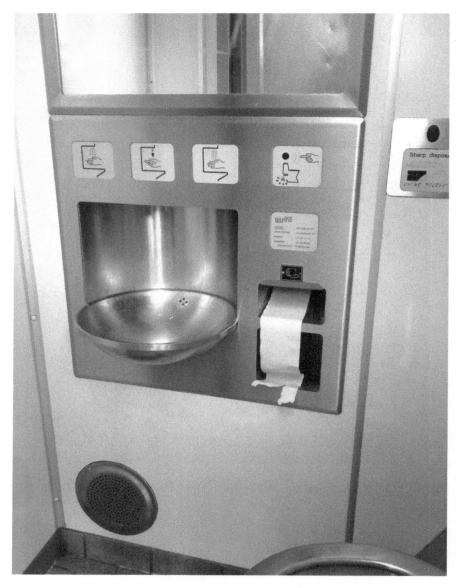

Figure 7.13 'Gold Standard' Public Toilet/Drug Related Litter Bin Design (5)

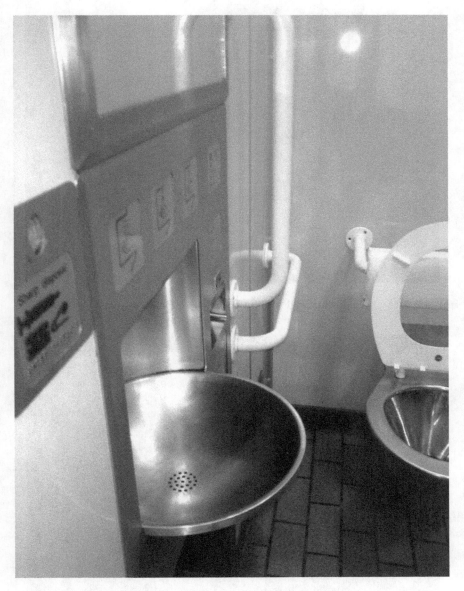

Figure 7.14 'Gold Standard' Public Toilet/Drug Related Litter Bin Design (6)

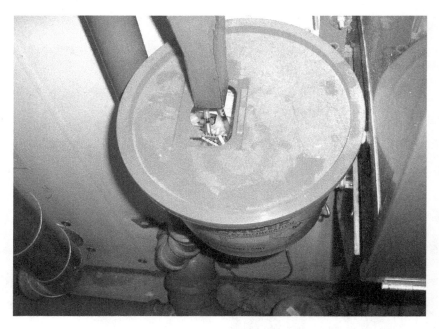

Figure 7.15 'Gold Standard' Public Toilet/Drug Related Litter Bin Design (7)

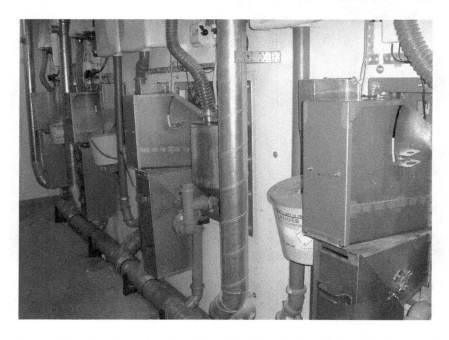

Figure 7.16 'Gold Standard' Public Toilet/Drug Related Litter Bin Design (8)

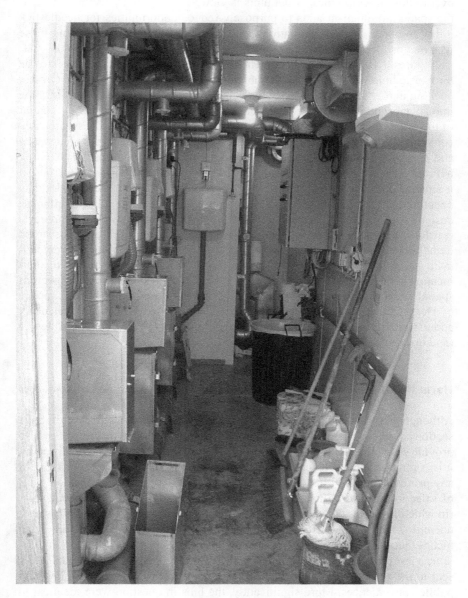

Figure 7.17 'Gold Standard' Public Toilet/Drug Related Litter Bin Design (9)

overall design *within* these toilet units is viewed positively by Defra (2005), as the spatial minimalism aims to purposely reduce opportunities for needlestick injury to occur amongst all patrons who attend public toilets (including those who may work there).

Figures 7.10, 7.15–7.17 document the journey of items deposited into the birdhouse hole within each toilet cubicle. As items are placed into the circular opening in the 'functional area' of the cubicle, they fall through a metallic chute into an appropriately placed container located within a 'service area' at the rear of the toilet unit (Figure 7.17). The latter space is a 'restricted-access' area that contains all necessary items and equipment required for general maintenance and operation (relating to cleaning, plumbing, repair, storage) within the entire unit. As such, for each toilet within the unit, a dedicated hazardous material bin is situated directly behind each cubicle. Accordingly, individual receptacles may be monitored, removed and replaced as required. Similarly, the raised birdhouse design, that screens a chute positioned in a downward trajectory, prevents restricted access to children (or others) who may attempt to retrieve discarded items placed into the bins. This has the effect of making the bins *environmentally-detached* from the public 'functional area' of the toilet cubicle due to their location in the private 'service area' at the rear of unit. These particular aspects of spatial management are correspondingly regarded as examples of good practice by Defra (2005), as the units provide public convenience, whilst simultaneously address public health and community safety by means of environmental design (and manipulation).

Harm Reduction Impact of Drug Related Litter Bins in Public Conveniences

Although bespoke public conveniences such as that portrayed in the above section have been designed specifically with community safety in mind, they also provide environments for housing opportunities of harm reduction. At this point, it is perhaps crucial to emphasise that it would be reckless and irresponsible for any professional body to advocate toilet environments as 'recommended' sites of safer injecting drug use. However, in the context of street-based injecting, (in which lifestyles are characterised by transience, homelessness, rooflessness, unemployment and poverty), public conveniences *per se* do provide injecting niches that facilitate attempts at reducing drug related harm (Parkin 2013). This latter view may be further supported in the following personnel communication sent to the author regarding the impact of drug related litter bins installed into public conveniences. More significantly, the bins in question were identical in design to those portrayed above (Figures 7.9–7.17) and concern a city-wide, public toilet, initiative in a location outwith the geographic areas of this research and associated fieldwork.[3] Nevertheless, in the following extract, the relevant individual outlines the perceived value brought about by the introduction of bespoke public conveniences that contain dedicated drug related litter bins (identical to those described above).

> We have 60 toilet cubicles with this type of disposal. I can say these disposal facilities are heavily used. We use 7 litre sharps containers and in some high use toilets we can change a bin once a week. We have never counted the number of syringes but know that the majority of syringes seem to be 1 or 2 mil (barrels) but there are also a significant number of 5 mil (barrels). What (the bins have) done is greatly reduce the number of needles found in the area around the toilets. In one case, where the toilets are in a multi-storey car park, prior to the toilets being modernised, used needles were regularly found in the car park. Since the toilets now have needle disposal, it is rare for a used needle to be found in the car park.
>
> The approach taken (by the relevant local authority) in providing needle disposal in public toilets was quite controversial. However, our legal advice and risk assessment at the time put public- and staff-safety first and therefore needle disposal was introduced in the toilets. It was also recognised that the legitimate users of needles (diabetics) may want to dispose of used equipment. (*Project Manager, Street Services, personnel communication via email*)

In short, the inferences made throughout this missive are that injecting episodes previously located in street-based environments (such as multi-storey car parks) occur less frequently following the modernisation and introduction of public conveniences equipped with sharps bins. Similarly, the presence of sharps bins is similarly correlated with a reduction in the volume of discarded drug related litter found in the aforementioned street-based settings. Although the Project Manager explains these outcomes specifically within a framework of public health and community safety, they may also be interpreted from the perspective of harm reduction. More accurately, reduced opportunities for harm production may be noted in the reported decrease of street-based injecting within Semi-Controlled (Category B) settings in addition to the (presumed) concomitant shift towards more hygienic and Controlled (Category A) environments of public convenience. This may be interpreted, (in somewhat Orwellian terms), as a form of 'positive displacement' in which drug users relocate to a less harmful setting for injecting purposes. Similarly, the reduction of drug related litter in public settings reduces potential needlestick injury to occur amongst community members and also minimises opportunities for the recycling of previously-used

---

3   The relevant information was obtained following a written request by the author and was made in connection with a literature review regarding the wider research agenda pertaining to public injecting drug use *per se*.

injecting equipment by other drug users. Indeed, the harm reduction value of such initiatives may be further shown in the following accounts of this particular toilet design from the lived experiences of injecting drug users that participated in this study.

Drug Users' Views of Defra-recommended Drug Related Litter Bins in Public Conveniences

In a previous article (Parkin and Coomber 2011), the author provides a comparative analysis of injecting drug users' views (and service uptake) of drug related litter bins. This earlier work focused upon responses to differing designs that were observed in public settings throughout all geographic settings visited during fieldwork. Presented below, however, is a summary of injecting drug users' views, opinions and experiences that relate exclusively to the sharps bins portrayed in Figures 7.10–7.17.

All of the relevant injecting drug user cohort, (that is, resident in the location that provided facilities for discarding sharps within public toilets), were familiar with the intervention and believed that the drug related litter bins were a positive attempt by local authorities to address street-based injecting in the town/city concerned. Of these respondents, several individuals recognised the public health and community safety agenda that typically underlies such initiatives. For example:

> I've noticed in some places they are putting sharps boxes and I think, "well, that's not encouraging (street-based injecting)". I think it's realistic. They know (street-based injecting) is happening. And, it's better than people leaving (injecting paraphernalia) on the floor, because, like, Hep C virus can stay alive for 90 days (outside of the body) ...(*R008*)

Likewise:

> I think it's a great idea. I thought it was very well thought out because obviously there are people that are injecting and they don't want (to keep) needles on them ... and not everyone is of the state of mind just to put the lid back on. So you don't want people coming across (discarded sharps) and getting it in the foot or whatever. I think it's a great idea that there is a place where they can be disposed of safely ... (*R014*)

However, the presence of public toilets equipped with facilities for depositing injecting paraphernalia was also viewed with some confusion relating to 'operational ambiguity'. For example, some respondents were of the belief that the local council were explicitly 'catering for' street-based drug users in providing informal, locally-sanctioned, settings of injecting drug use. In these particular responses, the term 'safety' is not used in the context of public health. Instead, 'safety' is used as an indigenous expression to describe the absence of police intervention, in settings (toilets with sharps bins) which appear to offer a temporary sanctuary from possible arrest. For example:

> I don't know if it's because they've (injecting drug users) been told it's a safer place, but what I've noticed in them toilets is you've got a hole for sharps and stuff like that. So I don't know if they've like ... they probably like seen that in the past and thought, "Yeah you can go there (to inject) ... it's a *safe* place to come and go" because of that. (*R018*, emphasis added)

Similarly:

> Well it's *safe* I suppose because if you didn't have a 'cin bin (portable sharps container) on you, you can at least discard your needle safely (in there). (And) because you can lock the (toilet door) and if people are sort of like 'pee-ing' in there when they (inject), they'd be able to discard everything anyway. So nobody would know that they had been (injecting) there anyway. (*R005*, emphasis added)

Indeed, this spatial ambiguity is further supported in the following extract in which the respondent perceives toilet facilities as semi-formal injecting settings that are simultaneously centres of increased police surveillance of drug users (and their arrest).

> I've been arrested in a few toilets as well, when I've been standing (injecting) in the toilets (cubicles). I've used them a lot of the time (for injecting heroin). And there's also toilets which are the same (design at a nearby location). And they've got the ... on the wall they've got the needle bin ... where you put needle disposals and all sorts like that. So really, they like sort of ... (street-based injecting) is sort of, like, being catered for, isn't it? It is, isn't it? Really, it is. If you've got them amenities in there. (*R003*)

Similarly:

> In public toilets, the (sharps) facilities some of them have, I think, should be made more widespread ... but only on the basis that we can go to these places discretely, with discretion and without the fear of having that *bang, bang, bang*. "We're (police) outside waiting for you". (*R001*)

Nevertheless, the ambiguity and function of settings equipped with sharps bins is perhaps superfluous in the context of *street-based* injecting, especially when considered alongside associative issues such as drug dependency, homelessness, avoiding arrest and reducing withdrawal symptoms. Indeed, when situated within these particular experiences of injecting drug use, any environmental ambiguity associated with places of shelter is diminished in the pursuit of 'feeling well again'. For example:

> ... put it this way, if you're feeling that rough and you've got a bag (of heroin), you've got your works on you, you'll find a way of doing it and you *will* find a place to do it. And obviously if those toilets are there and they've got sharps facilities to be used then I think it's probably better for everyone concerned to (inject there) ... . but I don't think it's promoting you to do it there because (street-based injecting) is not everyone's cup of tea. (*R009*)

Similar sentiments to each of the aforementioned points are further articulated by R001. In this extract, this individual recognises the value attached to the safer design features within the relevant public toilets. However, the added inference regarding an absence of more specialised harm reduction provision for drug users ('us'), who may continue to inject within public conveniences adds poignancy to this particular observation.

> I'm assuming it's the council that have obviously put this all into process. But when the toilets were going to be built, (they must have said) "Right, well let's put this into the equation to make it better". I don't think it's better for *us* ((laughs)) but it is better for the general public. (*R001*, emphasis added)

Indeed, the limited harm reduction value afforded by toilet cubicles is further noted in the following comment. In this extract, the respondent articulates how the immediate and positive benefits afforded by 'place' may be forever reduced by the negative consequences of injecting drugs behind locked doors of public conveniences (whether they are equipped with sharps bins or not).

> ((*sighs*)) ... it's a good thing as in that you've got somewhere to go. But it's a bad thing because if you lock yourself in, and you go over (overdose), then you're *fucked* ... (*R013*, emphasis added)

Comparing Environments of Public Convenience

In the previous section, visual data were used in conjunction with a variety of verbal and written accounts to demonstrate the positive outcomes associated with public conveniences fitted with innovative mechanisms for disposing of drug related litter and other sharps. In short, the previous section concerned the impact of environments that had been deliberately modified to enable the reduction of potential harm in community settings (caused by discarded injecting equipment). As a means of further consolidating and concretising this position, it is an equally valid process to refer to comparative data that demonstrates how the absence of the relevant intervention within similar environments may perpetuate and/or preserve opportunities for harm production. In the following section, a summary of the views of frontline service personnel employed within public toilets *not* equipped with bespoke discarding facilities is presented. In providing contrasting and oppositional perspectives in this manner, the harm reduction value attached to the environmental and spatial design described above will be made more apparent.

The settings described in each of the following Fieldnotes may be regarded as 'traditional', high-street, public toilets that are each located in the central business district of the relevant urban centre. Furthermore, each of the public conveniences described below are characterised by regular, high-volume, public attendance. Furthermore, they are settings that are partially-supervised, as the relevant cleansing personnel rotate between numerous similar sites during the course of their daily routines. Each setting are also frequently attended by drug users for injecting purposes and throughout the period of fieldwork, emergency services were regularly noted attending to drug-related incidents (overdose, arrest) in the various venues concerned. Finally, none of the following settings of public convenience had installed facilities for discarding sharp items. However, in one location, signage pertaining to the collection of 'hypodermic needles' was recorded (Figure 7.18). This notice was particularly ambiguous given the public setting of the toilet facility, and it remained unclear throughout fieldwork to whom the message was targeted towards (whether non-drug users, toilet attendants, injecting drug users or all/none of the above). Nevertheless, despite the presence of this highly visible sign, the following fieldnote perhaps demonstrates its limited impact upon toilet patrons:

> (The public toilet) has a notice on the wall stating that discarded needles may be given to the attendant for disposal. Respondent stated that *drug users* occasionally observe this and may tap the window of the canteen to give it to the attendant for disposal in a sharps box. These were described as the 'conscientious druggies' as injecting paraphernalia is typically left in all kinds of 'hiding holes' within the cubicles. Examples of the latter included 'behind the S-bend of the toilet, in cracks behind the toilet, *in* the toilet, and sometimes pins (needles) are placed into the roll of toilet paper positioned on the side of the wall'. Another hiding place included 'on the top of door ledges so that they will fall onto the next person entering the toilet cubicle'. (Respondent believed all these discarding strategies are attempts by drug users meant to deliberately cause harm to attendants and members of the public). (*Fieldnotes, Public Convenience*)

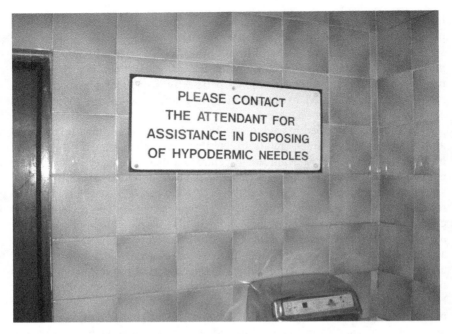

Figure 7.18   Ambiguous Signage

Similarly, at another location (without any signage regarding the collection of hypodermic needles):

> Respondent described the regular presence of drug related litter to include blood, tin foil, cans and the ever presence of needle caps. (Respondent) stated that if she found needle caps but no needles she became very cautious as she believed there would invariably be a needle somewhere else in the toilet cubicle/area. Needles and/or syringes are deposited and put in the toilet, behind toilet, on the door ridge, in plug holes, sanitary bins. (Respondent) was able to describe the different types of barrel and needle size, adding that she tends to find a lot of 'long needles' (suggesting more frequent episodes of groin injecting). (*Fieldnotes, Public Convenience*)

Figures 7.19 and 7.20 depict some of the 'hiding places' described in the above accounts. Indeed, a further observation of these environments (that may contain potentially hazardous items) was the subsequent impact drug related litter awareness had upon how toilets were actually cleansed by the relevant staff. For example:

> As a result of the frequency of discarded needles found in the toilet, (respondent) stated she has to remain alert and observant, especially since experiencing needlestick injury and will advise less-experienced staff on how to clean whilst

The Management of Drug Related Litter in UK Settings

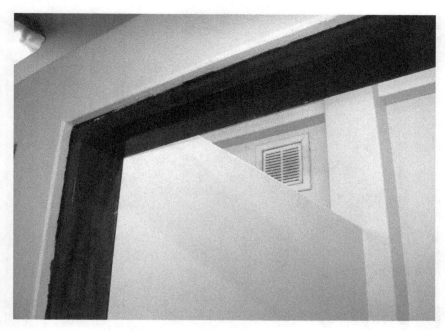

Figure 7.19 'Hiding Places' (1)

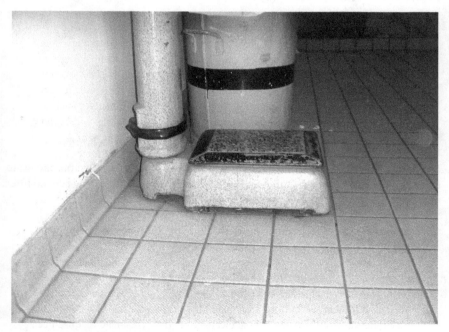

Figure 7.20 'Hiding Places' (2)

214   *An Applied Visual Sociology: Picturing Harm Reduction*

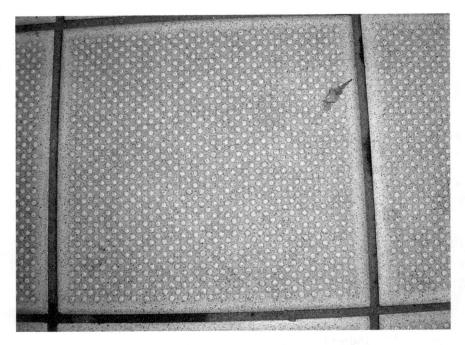

Figure 7.21 '**Hiding Places**' (3)

being observant of possible hazards. She showed me an example of how *not* to clean upper surfaces (partitions, ledges and shelves) that are above head height (i.e. without gloves) as these are places where needles and syringes are occasionally discarded. Furthermore, she demonstrated how the 'sweeping motion' of cleaning may cause the sharp item to 'fly-off' the shelf and, in effect, be transformed into a dart/missile flying across the toilet area. As such she always uses and advises the use of a wet mop so that any sharps will become 'clogged' into the fibres of this tool. (*Fieldnotes, Public Convenience*)

In addition to influencing the application of more safety-conscious approaches to cleaning surfaces within the toilet cubicles, the presence of some drug related litter made cleansing more arduous and time consuming. For example:

(Respondent) has received training in safe disposal of sharps and will put any used injecting equipment into 'haz-mat' (hazardous materials) bags using either tongs or gloves and will apply advisory procedures for removing blood spillage/splatter in toilet cubicles. (Respondent) stated that the floor surface within the toilet area consists of raised and bubbled tiles (see Figure 7.21) and added that this makes it more difficult to clean due to the uneven surface. Related to this is a further difficulty concerning the cleaning of white chocolate that has been trodden into the tiled surface of the floor. (Respondent) stated that cleaning this was 'like getting shit off a blanket'. White chocolate on the floor was another attendant observation that was regarded as a further 'tell-tale sign' that drug users were accessing the cubicles. This was because respondent believed drug users will buy the chocolate only for the tin foil wrapper so that they can smoke heroin in the cubicle. On other days respondent added there will be 'huge sheets of kitchen tin foil' on the floor. Other litter found on a daily basis includes 'half coke tins all burnt on the inside' (cookers) and 'plastic bottles with pipes coming out of them' (bongs/crack pipes). Respondent added that the large steel bin under sink basins is also used by drug users/toilet attendants to discard used equipment (as well as under the weighing machine in the 'ladies' room) (see Figures 6.13 and 7.20 respectively). (*Fieldnotes, Public Convenience*)

In addition to shared experiences regarding the presence of drug related litter in specific working environments, a further mutual response was noted within the same settings with regard to the presence of injecting drug users. Indeed, the following responses typify how frontline service personnel managed the presence of those who may be engaged in the consumption of illicit substances within their particular workplace.

When asked to describe his work, (respondent) stated he will 'turn a blind eye' to anybody that may be using drugs in toilets so long as they are not causing offence or disturbance to the public. If things do 'get out of control when they are off their heads' (shouting, swearing, becoming abusive) then respondent stated he will call for police assistance. However, once individuals have left the cubicle(s) respondent stated he will clean the toilet(s) they accessed, adding that blood splatter on walls was often the most difficult to clean. Any/all drug related litter is put into haz-mat bags for incineration. In short, his informal policy is to ignore drug users as they attend; not to intervene in order to avoid any personal danger and to clean-up after they leave to minimise any community contact with any discarded equipment. (*Fieldnotes, Public Convenience*)

The Common Ground of Drug Related Litter

This chapter has focused upon how drug related litter is formally *and informally* managed by frontline service personnel in settings that are affected by episodes of street-based injecting. These accounts have also been contrasted with similar views and opinions of injecting drug users. When compared as a single dataset, it is perhaps noteworthy that both respondent cohorts (injecting drug users and frontline service personnel) stand on some common ground. Namely, both cohorts expressed support for initiatives that sought to reduce opportunities for needlestick injury to occur within public places. Similarly, there was undisputed agreement amongst *all* respondents that the maintenance of public health and community safety are values to be supported. In addition, the various strategies of drug related litter management described throughout this chapter further demonstrate varying degrees of support for the practice and principles of harm reduction. More specifically, this support was often expressed overtly or inferred by actions, sentiments and various viewpoints that were noted during semi-structured interviews and/or ethnographic observation.

Nevertheless, each of the findings described throughout this chapter have been contextualised against the backdrop of an advisory document published by the Department for Environment, Food and Rural Affairs, (a section within the UK's Central Government). This document concerns good practice guidelines on how statutory bodies and community partnerships may play a more proactive role *Tackling Drug Related Litter* in municipal settings (Defra 2005). Whereas this document does not seek to make mandatory its various recommendations, it does provide a template for the appropriate management of public environments affected by drug related litter and/or street-based injecting. Accordingly, throughout this chapter, mixed qualitative data have been used to demonstrate the positive impact of various recommendations forwarded by Defra (2005). Similarly, these mixed data have also been used to highlight more negative outcome of procedures that may be regarded less favourably in the management of drug related litter and/or street-based injecting.

Furthermore, throughout the previous *three* chapters, visual images have been used to complement verbal and written testimony from a range of individuals in order to validate various lived experiences of injecting spaces located within public places. The application of visual methods, the analysis of visual data and presentation of the latter as empirically-generated data have served to demonstrate the categorical range of injecting environments in public places (and associated harms); the contentious nature of drug related litter (and how it is perceived an understood from oppositional perspectives) and have assisted in the depiction of benefits and outcomes of environments specifically modified to accommodate disposal facilities for injecting paraphernalia. In essence, these collated inter-related qualitative materials have been used as a mechanism for 'picturing harm reduction' and to demonstrate the value of solution-focused, applied-visual-sociological, research.

Whereas the latter view may be regarded as a form of subjective self-appraisal by the author (whose clarity may have been distorted by a research-focused 'tunnel vision'), the following chapter seeks to confirm the alleged and purported 'applied value' of visual data used throughout this sociological research.

PART III
An Applied Visual Sociology

Chapter 8
The Value of Applied Visual Data in 'Real World' Settings

In the concluding three chapters of this book, emphasis is now placed upon the applied and academic value of visual data that may be generated as part of sociological research. Whilst this discussion centres primarily upon the empirical research described during this book, it is important to note that the issues raised throughout Part III are equally valid, and as relevant, in studies that *do not* necessarily concern injecting drug use. As such, the following chapters may be regarded as an explanatory template and/or empirical framework for those who may wish to consider the use of visual data as part of applied/academic sociological inquiry.

In order to proceed however, it is perhaps helpful to provide a summary recap of this book's content thus far as an *aide-mémoire* to the final construction of an applied visual sociology.

Part I: Review

The initial chapters of this book provide a review of the literature pertaining to the central themes of this work. Namely, Chapter 1 provides an overview of visual research and a summary of how visual data may be considered within social scientific inquiries. Chapter 2 follows this format and presents a similar overview of the development and spread of harm reduction as a response to the hazards associated with injecting drug use (such as blood borne virus transmission, dependency etc.). This review of harm reduction demonstrates that the evolution of such intervention is essentially political at heart, as exemplified by its origins of grassroots activism, its current role in international drug policy and its concomitant status as a globally recognised intervention.

Part II: Empiricism

Part II however, (Chapters 3–7 inclusive), presents a summary of how visual methods may be incorporated into a specific research project alongside a range of other qualitative techniques. More specifically, these five chapters detail the use of visual methods (and analysis) employed in a series of studies concerning street-based injecting drug use. In addition, all photographs and images contained within Chapters 3–7 represent visual data generated as part of solution-focused, empirical, studies of drug-related harm in various locations throughout the south of England during 2006–2011.

Part III: An Applied Visual Sociology

In relation to the latter point, the empirical application of all visual research methods described throughout Part II occurred in a series of studies that were commissioned and/or funded by organisations outwith the academic institution in which they took place. For these reasons, Part II of this book may be subsequently regarded as an example of 'real world research' (Robson 2011) due to its focus upon 'live' issues pertaining to public health and community safety.

According to Robson (2011, 3–4) 'real world' research tends to prioritise policy-related issues, and especially those that involve problems that impact directly upon people's lives. Robson (ibid.) adds that research of this nature is often dedicated to developing responses and/or recommendations to address social problems; is concerned with affecting change and/or providing outcome to better inform the relevant stakeholder organisations who may intervene as necessary. However, Robson (ibid.) categorically states that real world research is typically less concerned with developing an academic discipline (such as sociology) and does not necessarily seek to advance 'contributions to knowledge' in the relevant fields of inquiry.

In the following three chapters, this author seeks to challenge Robson's (2011) latter definition of real world research. More specifically, in asserting and advocating the construct of an 'applied visual sociology', the author aims to demonstrate how applied and academic research may be synthesised to generate findings that provide both *disciplinary* and *applied* value. Furthermore, in adopting a stance that boldly proclaims itself to be an 'applied visual sociology', the author also seeks to advocate the metaphorical building of bridges between academic institutions ('the academy') and applied settings (for example: stakeholder organisations with a mutual interest in solution-focused responses to social issues) in an attempt to produce research output that is, ultimately, 'written to be seen' (rather than 'seen to be written').

This advocacy of an applied visual sociology is therefore consolidated in the following three chapters. By way of introduction, this chapter presents a summary of the applied value of the visual data (relating to drug using environments) included throughout this book. This account is based upon an informal impact evaluation conducted by the author at a series of events at which drug-related photographs were included as part of research dissemination. In addition, this chapter seeks to demonstrate how visual data may be received amongst audiences (and respondents) who are employed in non-academic, service-relevant, positions and who themselves are focused upon addressing the complexities of drug-centred lifestyles. In Chapter 9 however, the aforementioned assertion of a developmental synthesis of applied and academic research is made more explicit in a discussion that clarifies the value and worth this study has brought to each side of this sociological coin. Finally, Chapter 10 provides a series of exercises dedicated to the development of competency and proficiency amongst those who may be considering an applied visual sociology for their own research purposes.

The Applied Value of Visual Data

As perhaps noted throughout this book, visual methods are undoubtedly a dynamic means of facilitating data generation and producing knowledge on specific issues (Hurworth 2004, Pain 2011). As such, visually-focused inquiries may provide immediate value for those directly involved and/or affected by the relevant research. For example, a wide range of research has utilised visual methods and associated data to inform public health *intervention* (Barrett 2004, Frohmann 2005, Hurworth and Sweeney 1995, Young and Barrett 2001). Similarly, other research demonstrates the value of visual data in assisting health intervention in various arenas containing substance use (Fitzgerald 2002, Forsyth and Davidson 2010, Haines et al. 2009, Mihai et al. 2006, Ranard 2002, Rhodes et al. 2006, Schonberg and Bourgois 2002, Taylor et al. 2004, Treloar et al. 2008).

Nevertheless, although each of these studies are commendable exemplars of visual research, little information is actually available on how these data are actually *perceived and received* by professionals and practitioners working in health fields beyond academic settings or by those who may be connected to the 'research topic' by professional association/interest only (that is, those within *applied* settings). Similarly, relatively little is known on how much visual data may impact upon health practitioners' knowledge of particular issues or if such data may advance professional intervention in any way whatsoever. Due to this paucity in the literature, the remainder of this chapter aims to address this absence of evidence in considering the 'applied-value' of visual data when extended beyond an 'academic' audience and/or research agenda.

Evaluating the Impact of Visual Data

This chapter is based upon an evaluation of responses to drug-related visual data that were presented at three conferences in addition to those displayed during a month-long public exhibition of drug-related photography (Parkin 2012). All visual data evaluated were photographs of drug using environments and/or of drug related litter. All images were taken by the author and many of which feature throughout this book. The evaluation of all drug related photography sought to demonstrate (or refute) the efficacy and impact of applying visual methods (and visual data) in research focused upon policy and practice. Each component of this impact evaluation (that is, the conference paper and the public exhibition) is described in more detail below.

The Conference Papers

During 2009–2010 the author delivered a series of conference papers at three regional events in the south west of England. These conferences were attended mainly by practitioners and professionals who had regular contact with injecting drug use/rs as a direct result of their employment (for example, health and social care; criminal justice, probation and policing). Each event was dedicated to summarising current trends, work in progress and emerging findings in the shared fields of substance use and hepatology (including hepatitis C transmission and treatment). The author was invited to deliver a conference paper at each of these events in order to summarise regionally relevant research concerning the issue of street-based injecting drug use. This invitation therefore not only assisted with the dissemination of locally-funded research (Parkin 2009a), but also advanced local understandings of injecting drug use from a city located in the relevant region of the conference events (the south west of England). Accordingly, the paper presented to the various audiences not only had *thematic* value, but equally provided contemporary detail on specific injecting-related behaviours that had immediate (local and regional) relevance.

The papers presented (Parkin 2009b, 2010a, b) to the various practitioner-based audiences summarised qualitative research that described a range of over 70 environments affected by street-based injecting drug use and the amplification of drug related harm (Parkin 2009a). The conference presentation sought to highlight that the categorisation of street-based injecting environments may be organised within a harm reduction framework that prioritises the issues of 'safety' and 'danger' (in relation to injecting drug use). This model, concerns the 'continuum of descending safety' (Parkin 2009a, 2013) as described in full detail throughout Chapter 5. In addition, the conference papers attempted to generalise the interplay of various environmental and social constants that collectively contribute towards the harmful effect of *place* upon health in the context of injecting drug use.

Each conference paper verbally and visually described the three environmental categories described in this book as 'Controlled', 'Semi-Controlled' and 'Uncontrolled' injecting environments. In this framework, 'control' refers to the range and availability of amenities within the immediate injecting environment that may facilitate/impede safer injecting practice (from the perspective of harm reduction). Accordingly, those settings considered 'more controlled' provide greater opportunities to reduce drug-related harm (such as access to more hygienic locations, providing access to discarding facilities, running water and other sanitation). In contrast, 'lesser controlled' environments serve to produce (and *re*produce) existing and established hazards normally associated with injecting drug use (such as needlestick injury, paraphernalia sharing, overdose, violence and death). As such, those places categorised as Semi-Controlled and Uncontrolled within the typology were found to be the most harmful and most hazardous from the perspectives of injecting drug users (Parkin 2009a, 2013, Pearson, Parkin and Coomber 2011).

The Visual Data in the Conference Paper

In order to demonstrate the socio-spatial model of the 'continuum of descending safety' to the various practitioner audiences, 24 photographs of drug using environments were included in the presentation. This dataset visualised the aforementioned categorisation of drug using environments as well as the associated descent from environmental safety to physical danger. Similarly, the images displayed were selected on the basis that they each represented and typified the environmental settings of 'control' observed during the relevant period of fieldwork. Many of the photographs presented in Chapter 5 were amongst the 24 images used in the presentations.

Frontline: A Photo-ethnography of Drug Using Environments

In June 2012, the author was granted an award to stage a photography exhibition of drug using environments based upon a selection of approximately 100 images accrued throughout the period 2006–2011. This award was made available by the University of Huddersfield in an attempt to maximise the impact and reach of various research outputs produced by the author as part of a process aimed at 'public engagement' with academic research.

The exhibition was designed to address the issue of injecting drug use in a manner that was accessible and instructive for an audience possibly unfamiliar with issues such as harm reduction and related drug policy. In addition, the exposition sought to challenge audience perceptions about street-based injecting and to emphasise the environmental conditions in which drug related harm may occur on a regular, day to day, basis. To facilitate the overall design, the event was promoted as: '*Frontline: A 'Photo-Ethnography of Drug Using Environments*'. The term 'photo-ethnography was chosen to purposely avoid any preconceived notions associated with the term 'exhibition' (for example, relating to sensationalism and exploitation) and equally sought to distance the author from issues of power (such as subservience and dominance) connected to 'photographic expositions' (cf. Lidchi 2006). Accordingly, 'photo-ethnography' aimed to demonstrate the combined application of 'visual' and 'ethnographic' methods when conducting fieldwork, in which the author is 'participant-photographer' (Morton 2009, 252), as part of research with a policy and practice remit.

As such, as a public installation, the photo-ethnography of drug using environments had five key aims. These aims related explicitly to the issue of 'public engagement with research' and, more specifically, were:

- to increase the impact of various academic articles regarding street-based injecting and harm reduction published by the author (Parkin 2013, Parkin and Coomber 2010, 2011).
- to promote applied visual methods as valid and innovative research within

sociology and social science *per se.*
- to disseminate research findings to a wider audience (to include the general public and relevant practitioners).
- to emphasise the harms and hazards associated with street-based injecting drug use.
- to advocate the need for continued harm reduction intervention at a national level (especially in a policy era currently defined by 'recovery' from drug dependency).

With the above goals, the open-access, public event within the University of Huddersfield aimed to provide a visual and provocative insight into the environmental conditions that house the lives of some of society's most vulnerable members. The photo-ethnography did not aim to glorify or demonise injecting drug use/rs, but instead portray the harsh reality of the environmental settings that may be associated with drug dependency and homelessness. As explained in the promotional literature attached to the event (Parkin 2012), the photo-ethnography was a 'genuine attempt to raise awareness of the harms associated with street-based injecting drug use'. Similarly, it was anticipated that the exhibition would illustrate that public injecting drug use should not necessarily be associated with chaotic, anti-social behaviour and, instead, may be considered alongside aspects of dependency, poverty and socio-economic exclusion/deprivation.

The Content of the Photo-ethnography Exhibition

The photo-ethnography exhibition concerns the topic of drug use and, more specifically, the range of public environments affected by episodes of injecting substances such as heroin, crack-cocaine and amphetamine sulphate. This exhibition emerged from almost five years of ethnographic fieldwork conducted by the author as part of various studies of public injecting environments located throughout the UK (Parkin 2013). Collectively, these studies involved visits to over 400 public settings affected by injecting episodes and/or drug-related litter[1] and a combined dataset of over 1000 digital images. The exhibition consists of approximately 100 images taken during ethnographic data collection and are organised into three distinct themes. These themes are consistent with the concomitant chapters contained within this book relating to, 'place' (Chapter 5), 'litter' (Chapter 6) and 'spatial management' (Chapter 7).

---

1 It should also be noted that all visual material used in the photo-ethnography (as with this book) was presented with permission from the relevant research commissioners. This permission was obtained for the purposes of 'reproduction' – as the author was no longer a member of staff at the original academic institution where all data generation took place.

Place

This aspect of the photo-ethnography visually demonstrates the range of public places that may be temporarily appropriated for injecting purposes. When viewed as a collective work, this section of the display aims to depict the descent from environmental safety to physical danger from the perspectives of injecting drug users and from a viewpoint supportive of harm reduction. In this regard, the theme of 'place' presents an 'environmental triptych' that reflects the overall 'lived-experience' of street-based injecting drug use.

Litter

The second theme relates to the issue of discarded injecting paraphernalia and other drug-related litter. These images are included in the photo-ethnography in an attempt to provoke harm reduction responses by statutory bodies whilst simultaneously depict the harms and hazards that may be associated with discarded equipment.

Management

The final section of the photo-ethnography depicts the range of methods currently used by various authorities in managing drug related litter. From these images it may be noted that an entire industry has emerged dedicated to drug-related litter management in public places. This aspect of the exhibition aims to reveal this industry to a public largely unaware of the way in which, an otherwise 'invisible', community-focused harm reduction is applied in public settings by the relevant authorities.

Although all images were mounted on a range of display boards, no explanatory text accompanied any of the photographs, other than the exhibition brochure (Parkin 2012). This absence of text was designed to emphasise the qualities attached to visual methods and associated data in which the audience were invited to consider the image without any external influences. Similarly, the combined themes of the event were an attempt to raise awareness (by visual inference) of the environmental hazards associated with street-based injecting drug use. As such, each image on display was purposely selected in an attempt to promote the need for continued harm reduction intervention in community settings throughout the UK (and beyond).

Finally, the 'open-access' photo-ethnography event was funded by, and hosted within, the University of Huddersfield for a period of 26 consecutive days during September–October 2012.[2]

---

2 The 'Frontline' exhibition was subsequently held at the 23rd Harm Reduction International Conference in June 2013 (Vilnius, Lithuania). A third staging of the exhibition was held at the 17th World Congress of the International Union of Anthropological and

Evaluating Impact

At each of the events summarised above, conference delegates/university visitors were invited to complete an evaluation form that related to the content of visual material displayed at the relevant works. (A copy of the evaluation form can be found in Appendix II). At conference events, the evaluation form was circulated prior to the author's oral presentation and completed at a convenient time by delegates following the paper's conclusion. The same evaluation form was used in association with the exhibition of photo-ethnography, in which visitors to the gallery were able to complete the same form made available throughout the relevant venue.

The evaluation was not concerned with the subject matter of the presentation/photo-ethnography nor with the author's performance at any event. Instead, the evaluation aimed to consider the *applied* value and relevance, (within non-academic contexts), of the visual data used throughout each presentation/exposition. That is, the evaluation sought to determine whether (or not) such images were beneficial in assisting understanding of street-based injecting environments *from the perspective of the respondents' employment, profession or other vocation (academic or otherwise)*.

Accordingly, the survey instrument consisted of six questions that related to the effectiveness and value of visual data. Each question combined a Lickert-type scale with opportunities to respond to more open-ended questions. Whereas the former requested respondents to state how much they *professionally* agreed/disagreed with a particular statement relating to the relevance of the visual data to their employment/vocation (that is, photographs of drug-injecting environments), the latter provided opportunities for individuals to include more subjective, and more non-specific, qualitative responses.

Analysis

A total of 77 evaluation forms were completed and returned to the author. All returns and responses were subject to quantitative analysis using the Statistical Package for the Social Sciences (SPSS 18). Similarly, of a possible 462 potential 'qualitative' responses (obtained from six open-ended questions), a total of 279 remarks and comments were entered as 'string' data (Pallant 2005). These responses were collated as a single document and entered as a corresponding file for coding/analysis using NVivo8 (a software package used in qualitative data analysis). These qualitative comments pertaining to visual data were subsequently arranged into appropriate themes (or 'fields') that emerged from analysis and coding of the document's content. The findings obtained from these quantitative and qualitative processes are summarised below.

Ethnological Sciences Conference in August 2013 (University of Manchester, UK). The images were not evaluated at these two events however.

Evaluation Findings

Over half of all responses (n= 39/77, 51 per cent) were obtained from delegates attending a one-day conference held at Buckfastleigh, (Devon) (Parkin 2010a). A further 21 responses (27 per cent) were gathered from participants attending *Annual Hepatology Meetings* during 2009 and 2010 (Parkin 2009b 2010b). The remaining 17 (22 per cent) responses were obtained from visitors to the photo-ethnography exhibition held at the University of Huddersfield during September–October 2012 (Parkin 2012).

Employment

A wide range of individuals provided an evaluative response regarding the value of drug-related images in the context of their line of employment/vocation. These occupations are summarised below in Table 8.1 and it may be noted that 'nurse specialists' (including community practice nurses, blood borne virus nurses) provide the greatest representation of respondents involved in the impact evaluation. Other notable respondents include senior managers of health services (including commissioners), harm reduction practitioners (drug workers, needle and syringe managers, outreach staff), police officers, senior consultants (from hepatology, phlebotomy and representatives from the Coroner's Office) and social workers (from criminal justice and probation services). A further response was provided by

Table 8.1   Evaluation Respondents' Occupation/Profession

Occupation/Profession	Frequency	Percent
Nurse Specialist	22	26
Health Manager/Senior Officer	13	19
Harm Reduction Practitioner	8	10
Consultant (senior GP)	8	10
Police Officer	5	6
Criminal Justice Worker	4	5
Service User/Former Drug User	4	5
Social Worker	4	5
Student	3	4
Higher Education (Staff)	3	4
Youth Worker	1	1.3
Missing	2	2.6

four 'former injecting drug users' who described their current role as a 'service user representative' for various drug and alcohol services in relevant settings. Accordingly, the respondent sample reflects a wide range of experience and seniority within the health, medical and social care professions; each of which invariably encounter issues relating to injecting drug use on a regular (if not daily) basis. Other individuals who may not necessarily encounter injecting drug use/rs as regularly as their health-related counterparts also contributed to the evaluation of applied photography. These included students, those employed in higher education (researchers, lecturers and 'teachers'), social workers and youth workers.

'Helpfulness' of Photographs

Respondents expressed resounding support for the use of photographs as a mechanism for appreciating drug-injecting environments in street-based settings. More specifically, 91 per cent (70) of respondents stated that the images were either 'very helpful' or 'helpful' and provided employment-relevant data for all professions/occupations concerned. Only four individuals (two of which represented police constabularies) thought that the photographs were 'unhelpful'. However, the entire cohort of nurse specialists (all 22 respondents) found the images 'most helpful'; followed by health managers (9/13 respondents) and harm reduction practitioners (all 8 respondents).

Overall, when asked to elaborate upon 'why' the images were perceived 'helpful' or 'useful' (or not), a wide range of responses were provided by individuals. These open responses were subsequently organised and categorised into the appropriate 'field' that emerged from qualitative data analysis. Respondents believed that the visual images 'reflected the reality of public injecting practice' (27 per cent); emphasised the 'value of visual research methods' to assist comprehension of injecting drug use (17 per cent), 'assisted with recognising street-based injecting sites' *per se* (14 per cent), or 'provided an appreciation of the typology framework' (12 per cent). Furthermore, it was those respondents more aligned with health and medicine that appeared to express greater appreciation of visual images. Although 18 per cent (14) of the cohort did not provide any added opinion regarding the 'utility' of image, only two individuals believed that the method underlying the use of photographs to contextualise drug issues was 'not a new idea' (again, this less positive view was expressed only by police officers).

Nevertheless, the following qualitative comments demonstrate the overwhelming positive opinion expressed by respondents regarding the general 'usefulness' of visual data in the context of individual employment/occupation. For example, the following responses illustrate the 'realities of public injecting environments' as the photographs:

> Helped to establish context and dispel myths (Community Psychiatric Nurse: Substance Misuse)

> (Provided an) insight of what is going on 'out there' (Blood Borne Virus Nurse)
>
> Show(ed) reality of public injecting and makes it real (Harm Reduction Nurse)
>
> Gain(ed) an insight into the lives of injecting drug users (Gastroenterology: Trainee)

Similarly, the value of visual data may be noted in the following responses in which photographs of injecting sites are viewed as thus:

> Photographs provide a reference point for the levels of risk and bring the reality of public injecting sites into focus (Community Psychiatric Nurse)
>
> Photos provide a poignant example of the breadth of injecting practice (Advanced Nurse Practitioner: Hepatology)
>
> Photographs give a perspective and context to verbal reporting of service users (Service Manager)

For others, the photographs provided a wider understanding and appreciation of drug using environments located in street-based settings. This may be noted in the following responses.

> I've never really thought about the different types of injecting sites ('Education')
>
> I have thought little of public injecting previously and tend to think more of drug using in a house or on traveller sites (Advanced Nurse Practitioner: Hepatology)
>
> They highlighted the difficult public decisions on how to manage these sites (Employment Not Stated)
>
> The photos show the locations could be anywhere (Social Work)

Similarly, the impact of the 'continuum of descending safety' (Chapter 5) underlying the theme of place may be noted in the following responses:

> I thought the model of safety-danger was a great way of informing health professionals (Advanced Nurse Practitioner: Hepatology)
>
> We need to recognise that different environments influence the effect of risk to patients (Consultant)
>
> Visuals help me to understand the different types of site (Care Worker)

Provides insight into aspects of drug use and homelessness I wouldn't ordinarily come across (Podiatrist)

Informative Impact

When asked to consider if the photographs used in the presentation informed the respondents' work in any way, 53 per cent (n=41) said 'yes', 26 per cent (n=20) were 'not sure' and the remainder (17 per cent, n=13) said 'no'.

Similarly, the open question regarding *how* the images may have informed individual working practices provided 41 qualitative responses. These latter data were categorised into one of two fields concerned with 'training staff and/or clients' (19 per cent, n=15), and/or 'understanding injecting environments' (35 per cent, n=27). However, those that found the visual data most informative were once more typically situated within the health professions.

However, regardless of profession, the informative impact of images for training staff and/or clients may be noted in the following comments:

When giving advice, (I'll be) able to inform service users of the pros and cons of using (drugs) in certain areas (Needle Syringe Programme Worker)

(Photographs of sites) are an area to consider when discussing harm reduction with service users and helps with service development (Nurse Consultant: Hepatology)

(Images) made me think how we work with street wardens to address potential drug-related harm (Service Development Officer)

Perhaps most poignant in this regard however was the following statement:

I deal with the deceased and speak with families regularly. (The photographs would) help me explain some matters to the (grieving) family (of injecting drug users) (Coroner)

Similarly, as part of an informative process of 'understanding injecting environments', the following statements were proffered:

(Images) gave me a better understanding of environs when talking to clients (Blood Borne Virus Manager)

I am now more fully aware of the risks patients are prepared to go to when injecting drugs – i.e. reflecting their desperation (Consultant Hepatologist)

Seeing the lifestyle, making it real. Realising the increased risks and seeing it from a service user perspective (Criminal Justice: Service Manager)

A good way of showing problems about risks in public sites. As police we often don't think of the other side of the story, so good to think about it. (Police Sergeant)

Stimulus for reflection on lifestyle of patients and cannot assume 'the message' about litter, blood borne virus is known to or followed by all who inject (Director of Drug/Alcohol Service)

Revelatory Impact

The third evaluation question asked respondents to consider if the photographs revealed information about street based injecting environments of which they were not previously aware. Almost half of the cohort (49 per cent, n=38) agreed that the photographs did indeed assist awareness of this issue, in contrast to the seven respondents who were 'not sure' (9 per cent) or who disagreed (36 per cent). Nevertheless, it was mainly individuals located within the health professions (at all levels of experience and seniority) who typically agreed with this statement.

Thirty-six qualitative comments were provided in response to the relevant open question attached to the revelatory value of the photographs. These responses were subsequently arranged into one of two fields; namely 'improved awareness of injecting environments' (18 responses) and awareness brought about by a visual explanation of the 'continuum of descending safety' (17 responses). Examples of the former category may be noted in the following comments:

(Awareness of) safety issues that the user is facing daily and of differing dangers (Social Work)

Unaware of the importance of places like public toilets (Liver Transplant Assessment)

I was not aware of the use of blue lights in toilets and why they were used (Nurse Specialist: Hepatology)

I'm very new to post, so very good for me to see the realism of the variety of public areas and the safety issues involved (Viral Hepatitis Nurse)

Perhaps most significant was the comment that perhaps reflects the overall impact of visual data upon the whole cohort involved in the impact evaluation. Namely:

Someone not on the frontline is not able to picture different environments without this type of assistance (Senior Consultant)

Indeed, this particular response was so influential that it actually informed the main title of the open-access, public exhibition (as staged at the University of Huddersfield (Parkin 2012), the Harm Reduction International Conference in Lithuania (Parkin 2013b) and the International Union of Anthropological and Ethnological Sciences World Congress at the University of Manchester (2013)).

In addition, respondents also provided positive comments regarding the environmental diversity associated with street-based injecting settings and the concomitant *visually-oriented* typology of harmful and hazardous environments of injecting drug use. For example:

> The different categories is a helpful way of looking at risk (Blood Borne Virus Nurse)

> It had never occurred to me that 'location' had an impact on drug-related death (Drug and Alcohol Counsellor)

> The categorisation was useful rather than considering an overall 'clump' of public injecting sites (Service Manager: Drugs and Alcohol)

> Drug using environments are more varied than the general assumption (Social Work: Student)

Understanding Drug Using Environments

A fourth evaluation question asked respondents if the images provided a 'better' understanding of drug-using environments. This elicited the second most positive response (following 'helpfulness') from the evaluating cohort. Namely, 70 per cent (n=54) said 'yes'; 18 per cent (n=14) said 'no' and only five respondents (6 per cent) were 'not sure' of this issue. Those who felt that the images did not assist comprehension of drug-using environments were representatives from police constabularies and those involved in criminal justice. Similarly, those who expressed uncertainty were either nurse specialists or harm reduction practitioners; whereas those expressing agreement with the statement were predominantly health-based professionals.

When asked to elaborate upon this issue in the relevant open-ended question, 37 comments were provided that clarified of this comprehension from the perspective of each individual respondent. These comments were subsequently ordered to establish that the images predominantly 'visualised injecting conditions' (21 per cent, n=16) or 'visualised harm and hazard' (14 per cent, n=11). Other lesser categories included the depiction of the 'continuum of descending safety', 'unhygienic environments', and of 'injecting practice'.

The following comments typify those regarding 'injecting conditions' and 'harm and hazard'.

> Especially useful for people who have no knowledge of public injecting to see these pictures to help understand risk (Blood Borne Virus Nurse)
>
> They highlighted different environments used and a lot of nurses are not aware if not working with injecting drug users (Community Psychiatric Nurse)
>
> They made me more aware of the difficulties people who inject face and how closed-minded non injecting people are (Nurse Specialist: Hepatology)
>
> It provides info on where the user is in respect of how bad their usage is (Service User Representative)
>
> I am not overly familiar with the whole drug-taking fraternity and this has helped my understanding (Coroner)
>
> Not an area I have had much exposure to so useful to see. May help to underline strategic work ('Trainee')

It is perhaps also worthwhile to note that some respondents considered the visualisation of the continuum of descending safety as a useful model for understanding street-based of drug-using environments. For example:

> I was aware of 'controlled' and 'uncontrolled' environments but not so much about the areas injecting drug users use socially and of the risks involved in sharing H2O (water) (Viral Hepatology Nurse)
>
> I hadn't really thought about the variety and difference in harm which can come alive through the categorising of sites (Criminal Justice Worker)
>
> Categories made it easier to understand and easy to remember (Harm Reduction Nurse)

Blood Borne Virus Transmission

Due to the specific drug-related themes underlying each event (relating to harm reduction, hepatology, hepatitis, HIV and drug-related death), a fifth question sought to determine how relevant the images were in providing 'insights of the social and environmental situations concerning blood borne virus (BBV) transmission'. This was a question purposely included in the evaluation in an attempt to consider if visual data may be used to assist understanding of more complex behaviours associated with spatially situated injecting drug use.

Over half (58 per cent, n=45) of all respondents agreed that the images *did* provide an understanding of the social and environmental situations concerning viral (hepatitis/HIV) infection. A further 13 per cent (n=10) were 'not sure' about this issue; whereas only 14 (18 per cent) respondents 'disagreed' with the statement. Those who believed the images provided an understanding of these more epidemiological matters were typically specialist nurses, harm reduction practitioners, consultants and service users.

Over 30 additional comments complemented answers to this question, most of which were responses that considered the photographs in relation to the social aspects of blood borne virus transmission. For example:

> (The images) show the worst environments for increasing the risk of BBV transmission (Blood Borne Virus Manager)

> Showed lack of (sharps) bins in public places. Ideas on how to prevent BBV could now perhaps be put into practice (Harm Reduction Worker)

> (Photographs illustrate) how the vicious circle does not allow injecting drug users to think of BBV transmission, it's the least of their priorities. (Harm Reduction Nurse)

> I was aware of the risks about transmission – but am now aware what would help more; sharps bins in semi-controlled areas, safer injecting rooms etc. (Social Worker)

> There are more chances of BBVs spreading in semi-controlled and uncontrolled areas than controlled areas (Employment Not Stated)

> It suggests that more controlled environments have helped the prevention of BBV or can prevent drug related death (Community Psychiatric Nurse)

> (The photographs provide) the enhanced understanding of the impact of a shared environment (Service Development Officer)

Informing Responses to Drug-Related Harm

The final evaluation question was perhaps the most important of the survey (from a research perspective), in asking respondents if the images could inform professional responses to drug-related harm. For this question, a Likert-type scale was not provided and the response left open in anticipation of specific 'work-related' responses. This was a purposive design of the evaluation in an attempt to note the applied value of images that are epistemologically grounded in (and theoretically framed by) the philosophy of harm reduction.

A total of 36 (representing 46 per cent of respondents) qualitative comments were provided in response and were each coded as one of three fields that emerged from analysis. Namely, 'general harm reduction' (23 per cent, n=14), 'inform local/national drug policy' (22 per cent, n=13) and 'training aid' (15 per cent, n=9). The following comments typify the use of the images as a means of informing a 'general harm reduction' response to drug-related harm.

> Definitely an excellent tool for illustrating BBV transmission risks – with clients and workers (Blood Borne Virus Nurse)

> (Use with) awareness raising and understanding the implications of risk and harm (Blood Borne Virus Manager)

> I can advise clients on safer injecting sites – especially to relatively new injecting users (Housing Officer: Drug Intervention Programme)

> Can provide more information for clients upon release from prison and the dangers of different environments (Blood Borne Virus Manager)

> Useful in terms of drug-related death prevention and the harm reduction advice we can offer our service users (i.e. categorisation of sites) (Needle and Syringe Programme: Manager)

> (I would use these) images in treatment process with service users during safer injecting intervention/session (Chief Executive Officer: Drugs and Alcohol Service)

Similarly, the following comments reflect the potential value of photographs for informing local and national policy on matters relating to injecting drug use (particularly in relation to a call for state-sanctioned safer injecting facilities/drug consumption rooms):

> Can we influence local authority or police behaviours with this evidence? (Clinical Lead: Drug and Alcohol Services)

> It would help to inform public perception of the environments used. It might hasten developments in pilots for safer injecting facilities (Community Psychiatric Nurse)

> Supports the 'drug consumption room' argument and raises awareness for others (Employment Not Stated)

> Take your presentation to local councils! (Criminal Justice Worker)

> The realisation that a multi-agency response to closing down a public injecting site can, and does, force injecting drug users towards more dangerous environments is a concern (Police Officer)

Finally, the use of the photographs as a generic 'training aid' (or pedagogical device) for employees/students/service users is evident in the following:

> Really useful for staff teaching (Community Psychiatric Nurse)

> Would use these in my teaching sessions or assist in provision of education for patients (Consultant: Hepatology)

> For education purposes to disseminate to other groups (Primary Care Hepatitis Nurse)

> Would be very helpful to present to local authorities, needle exchanges and specialist drug agencies – so they know where to spend money and not ignore the problem (Community Psychiatric Nurse)

> (Useful) for educating junior doctors to help understand the environment in which drug users exist (Senior Consultant: Hepatology)

The Value of Applied Visual Data in Real World Settings

The findings outlined in this chapter have been obtained from a small-scale evaluation of drug-related visual data, in which responses were provided by a conference delegates and exhibition visitors located in the south west and north of England. For these reasons, there is perhaps a need to acknowledge the limited range of this study for evaluating visual data *per se*, as it does not necessarily reflect findings that may emerge from a more structured and focused survey of diverse geographic settings that encompasses a greater range of occupations.

Nevertheless, these limitations may actually be viewed positively due to the esoteric and 'specialised' nature of the photography under evaluation and because the images were collected to inform specific (equally esoteric) audiences with a particular interest in substance use issues. This is made yet more significant given that the original research methodology underlying the collection of visual data is one that prioritises the practice and principles of harm reduction and the logics of specific, drug-related, cultural 'practice'. This is perhaps made evident in the design and application of the 'continuum of descending safety' (Chapter 5) which seeks to advise, inform and educate those affected by street-based injecting issues in a manner that reflects the 'lived-experience' of drug use/rs.

Street-based injecting drug use and harm reduction are issues that directly and indirectly affect a multitude of workplaces across a wide spectrum of public sectors (health, social work, environment, policing, housing and criminal justice). Similarly, they are issues that are regularly encountered by street-based services (cleansing operatives, outreach workers, security officers, police officers, public attendants) and addressed by those within established institutions (hospitals, hostels, local government departments, drug and alcohol services and community-based facilities) and third sector organisations (addressing homelessness, outreach, poverty, sex-work). For these reasons, the specificity of the respondent cohort in this evaluation may actually add increased credibility to the findings summarised above due to its 'professional grounding' in drug related issues. In addition, the findings obtained in this evaluation would appear to suggest that the public health value of the photographs presented at conference and as part of an exhibition of photo-ethnography has positively enriched and enhanced understandings of street-based injecting drug use. More specifically, photographs of drug injecting environments are typically viewed favourably by practitioners and professionals involved in drug-related employment (whether harm reduction, treatment or prevention orientated). Indeed, such photographs are viewed as helpful and informative in regard to a particular applied knowledge of drug use/rs. Similarly, the images were found to be revelatory in providing social and environmental context concerning injecting episodes located in street-based settings. In addition, the latter finding noted that visual data assisted with an overall appreciation of street-based injecting environments and of the way in which *place* may have a subsequent impact on producing and reproducing established harm and hazard associated with injecting drug use.

These conclusions are encouraging results as they essentially reflect the methodological framework within which the field research (and data generation) took place. In short, the favourable responses expressed above appear to reflect the epistemological orientation of the study design in which ethnographically situated visual data seeks to generate applied value beyond academic interpretation. This is made perhaps more significant with the overriding support expressed by *health* professionals during the evaluation of visual data. Indeed, the less positive opinions expressed by those people not employed in health professions (such as those employed in criminal justice) further emphasises the methodological orientation of the visual data. In short, the public health 'ethnographicness' of images that reflect a particular disciplinary visuality (Chapter 1) have been noted in this evaluation to be most helpful within the intended target audience of an applied visual sociology (that is, harm reduction and health care professionals).

Accordingly, the collected findings summarised throughout this chapter indicate that theoretically and epistemologically informed photography *does* provide applied and pedagogic 'added-value' to qualitative research. Furthermore, images such as those contained within this book *can* assist practitioners working directly (or indirectly) with particularly 'sensitive' issues (such as harm reduction, injecting drug use, blood borne virus transmission and drug using environments), provided they are appropriately anchored within a robust methodological framework (that is, not generated for the purposes of illustration).

This conclusion subsequently raises a number of implications regarding the dynamic and innovative use of visual data generated during street-based, ethnographic research. More specifically, images that assist in the development of an applied visual sociology (with particular reference to the practice and principles of harm reduction) can have both applied and academic merit and provide meaningful contributions to debates regarding policy and practice. In the following chapter these implications are presented and discussed in further detail in an attempt to provide a 'positioning paper' concerning the author's claims of an applied visual sociology.

Chapter 9
Towards an Applied Visual Sociology

In this penultimate chapter attention re-turns to the central issue of 'applied visual sociology', in which this section clarifies the research concept that forms the main title of this book. Indeed, the term has been used regularly throughout this work with limited clarification of what the applied research model actually involves. As such, the reader has thus far possibly been forced to draw their own conclusions regarding the definition of the expression 'applied visual sociology'.

To some extent, this lack of clarification has been a deliberate 'writing strategy'. This is because the purpose of this chapter is to define and consider the concept as a model of research worthy of singular attention. In bringing together the main conclusions from the respective chapters in this book, this final section provides a 'position paper' on the topic of applied visual sociology. Accordingly, it would appear logical to situate this positioning in this concluding chapter in order to present a closing and definitive argument in support of the model.

As such, presented below is a descriptive and explanatory account of a model of qualitative research that has emerged from the process of 'serial triangulation' described in Chapter 3. Whereas 'picturing harm reduction' (Chapters 3–7) represents the empirical application of an applied visual sociology, the following pages provide a more general account regarding the evolution of the academic construct of an applied visual sociology, including the way in which it has informed academic output, provided relevance to harm reduction practitioners and local policies relating to street-based injecting. This 'position' chapter concludes with an assessment of the perceived strengths and benefits of conducting applied visual sociology as empirical research.

Applied Visual Sociology Defined

The inclusion of *visual* research within the methodological design of this qualitative and sociological study of street-based injecting drug use sought to synthesise two key functions of research *per se*. As Robson (2011) notes, social research may be characterised by an interest in positively changing 'real world' concerns, or conversely by developing knowledge only to advance the theoretical qualities of particular disciplines. These different aspects of social inquiry are generally referred to as 'applied' and 'academic' research respectively, and are procedures that may be further defined by either quantitative or qualitative frameworks. However, the distinction inferred by the term 'real world' in relation to 'applied' research perhaps inadvertently dismisses more 'academic' oriented studies as somehow disconnected from reality, as 'unreal research' and, by association, as less relevant, meaningful and/or significant. In short, such an assumption undervalues (and perhaps devalues) the 'disciplinary visuality' (Rose 2003) associated with any social science inquiry that may include visual methods.

A further inference made by the existence of two seemingly divergent research paradigms is that applied and academic studies cannot be bridged and that 'never the twain shall meet'. For these reasons, the author seeks to unite these functions of sociological research in devising a methodological framework that provides academic value in combination with applied output (with intervention and/or policy-related relevance). In building a metaphorical bridge consisting of visual methods between these two designs, it was envisaged that the respective research would inform the academy (with contributions to knowledge via a doctoral thesis/qualification, research outputs and publications), whilst simultaneously generate 'real world' findings to inform multi-agency intervention and social change at a local (and potentially, national) level.

The bridging and unifying qualities of visual methods attached to all research conducted during 2006–2011 may be noted in Table 9.1. For example, the conventional academically-focused requirements of sociology (as a discipline) may be noted in the key components attached to the theoretical and epistemological framework. Similarly, the rationale for conducting community-based studies with those affected by, and participant in, street-based injecting may be noted in the section termed 'applied sociology'. This tabular representation of the research also includes a summary of the way in which these academic and applied qualities of the study were synthesised via the employment of visual methods. Whether viewed collectively, or as individual items, it may be noted that each aspect of this 'bridge' has both *academic* value (for the researcher, the research and the 'researched') as well as *applied* value (for the research-stakeholders, research participants and research outcome). Indeed, the multi-faceted value of this particular sociological approach to injecting drug use may be further noted in the different goals attached to each aspect of the study (at the foot of Table 9.1).

In short, the goals associated with this model of applied visual sociology follow a disciplinary tradition within sociology regarding a drive towards social reform and challenging structural problems. As such, the core principles underpinning applied visual sociology may be succinctly stated *Knowledge-Action-Change*.

The Influence of Established Research Methods upon Applied Visual Sociology

It should be stressed that the author does not, in any way, claim to have devised a 'new' and unique form of sociological inquiry in advocating the notion of applied visual sociology. Indeed, the model of applied visual sociology defined

Table 9.1 Visual Methods as 'the Bridge' between Applied and Academic Sociology

Academic Sociology: Theoretical and Epistemological Framework

To consider the role of structure and agency in the topic of public injecting drug use

To conduct an empirical assessment of Pierre Bourdieu's 'habitus' construct

To generate phenomenological accounts of street-based injecting from divergent perspectives (drug users and frontline service personnel)

To prioritise the practice and principles of harm reduction during data generation/ analysis

To identify the relationship between drug related harm and drug using environments

(synthesis) Visual Methods as 'The Bridge' (synthesis)

To provide opportunities to 'relive' ethnographic experiences

To provide 'documentation' of injecting environments (not 'documentary')

To provide polysemic representations of injecting environments

To provide visual material that complements more traditional forms of (text-based) qualitative data

To provide material with pedagogic value for drug users and frontline service personnel

Applied Sociology: Informing Harm Reduction Intervention

To foster collaboration between drug users, frontline service personnel and drug services in environments (street-based settings) affected by injecting drug use

To document *emic* (not *etic*) accounts of injecting environments from multiple perspectives to increase understanding of associated issues and concerns

To inform strategic and service intervention (with a harm reduction remit) in regard to public health/community safety in local settings

The Goals

Academic: To provide a valid contributions to knowledge in the fields of injecting drug use, harm reduction and public health sociology (relating to methodology, theory, structure and agency)

Applied: To develop harm-reduction responses to drug related harm that is informed, structured and guided by methodological innovation (i.e. theoretical, epistemological and ontological framing and all associated qualitative methods of data generation/ analysis). Responses to benefit wider community and not only individuals.

above actually draws upon, and has been directly influenced by, a variety of established modes of inquiry that characterise social science research. These influences include 'action research'; 'community based research' and 'applied visual anthropology'. A summary of each of these influences is presented below in order to further contextualise the development and evolution of the applied visual sociology concept.

Action Research

According to McKernan (1991, 3), action research is a form of inquiry that aims to 'render the problematic social world understandable' and intends to improve the quality of life in those settings. For these reasons, it may be regarded as 'unconventional' research due to its designated focus upon seeking resolutions to the difficulties experienced by (mainly non-academic) practitioners in the context of daily, employment-related, schedules. These practices may be situated within fields such as public health; education, social work, business, industry, transport, crime prevention and/or community safety. Similarly, an earlier definition by Rapoport (1970) emphasises that the applied nature of action research also contributes to a *social science* agenda as a result of collaborative partnerships between the academy and practitioners. In addressing social problems as part of a formalised, cooperative enterprise, the action researcher therefore aims to identify satisfactory responses to the relevant issues in order to inform the efficacy and performance of the relevant practice/practitioner. Or more succinctly:

> action research is the systematic collection of information that is designed to bring about social change. (Bogdan and Biklen 1982, 215)

In addition, action research further differs from traditional, academic inquiry as the former does not necessarily prioritise reports and other written outputs as a primary concern (McKernan 1991, 4). Indeed, this view resonates with that of Karl Lewin,[1] who stated:

> research that produces nothing but books will not suffice. (Lewin 1948, 203)

Lewin's (1948) proposed outline of action research consists of a linear and progressive process that is punctuated by cyclical phases of reflection, analysis, explanation and redefinition (of problem and action). Periods of reflection are purposely incorporated into a longitudinal research process in order to facilitate any necessary modification to the over-all design and delivery of emerging responses to the problem under scrutiny. Similarly, this cyclical process further enables on-going analysis to occur, as and when an action research project is underway. In practice, Lewin's model appears to permit a continuous process of reflexive analysis, coupled with modified proactive and reactive responses to social issues, in which the process is only concluded when a satisfactory outcome (to the problem) has been achieved.

---

1 Often cited as the original architect of action research.

Community Based Research

A further category of social investigation, which is closely aligned to that described above, is known as 'community based research'. This form of inquiry may also be referred to as 'community based participatory research' or 'participatory action research' 'co-production' and/or 'co-inquiry' (Durham Community Research Team (DCRT) 2011). However, regardless of the term chosen, when located in the field of public health, all terminology typically describes research that addresses social and structural inequality through active involvement by community members, stakeholder organisations and professional researchers (Israel et al. 1998). Furthermore, each participatory sector contributes their own area of expertise to the problem in hand and all are united in providing the optimal outcome for the relevant community (ibid.).

At first glance, this model of collaborative partnerships between professional researchers and institutional bodies appears almost identical to that described above and defined as 'action research'. DCRT (2011) however, attempts to clarify the two approaches in a 'discussion paper' regarding ethical challenges involved with establishing such partnerships. Namely, DCRT contends that both approaches to solution-focused research may be placed on a continuum of 'community participation', in which 'action research' perhaps more accurately provides a more conventional 'top-down' approach to methods of data collection/analysis. This translates as research that is generally controlled and led by professional researchers with greater or lesser degrees of community participation attached to the study. In such projects, the professional researcher may seek guidance from a community based 'working/steering group'; may be assisted by community members who provide specific data for the study by participatory methods (such as taking photographs) and/or may receive support in data collection/analysis from community-trained researchers (DCRT 2011, 6). At the opposite side of this spectrum of participation are those projects that are designed as 'bottom-up' approaches to research, in which there is *no* involvement from professional researchers and *all* work is controlled, managed, designed and delivered *by* community members *for* community members. DCRT further note that in-between these two extremes are collaborations that are controlled by community organisations in which professional researchers are managed by community members. In addition, other collaborative partnerships may be organised as equitable enterprises in which there is joint ownership of projects, production and output. All four models within this 'bottom-up' (or 'top-down') hierarchy may be regarded as models community based participatory research. However, those that incorporate a greater amount of participation by *community* members (that is, 'bottom-up') perhaps represent a greater degree of grassroots activism and project ownership at a *community* level.

Applied Visual Anthropology

Finally, in addition to the above, Sarah Pink (2007a) has been prominent in advancing a theoretical framework that seeks to compartmentalise distinctions between visual data collected for *academic* and *non*-academic purposes. These advances have been made in anthropological research in which Pink describes a difference between 'academic visual anthropology' and 'applied visual anthropology' in which the latter is described as:

> ... using visual anthropological theory, methodology and practice to achieve non-academic ends ... entailing problem solving and engaging in cultural brokerage. (Pink 2007a, 6)

As such, Pink's construct of applied visual anthropology aims to address social problems in collaboration with research respondents as part of an attempt to initiate some form of social change (via intervention). Such objectives therefore differ from 'academic visual anthropology' that possibly only informs the relevant disciplinary discourse and does not necessarily seek to improve the lives of those affected by the issues recorded (Pink 2007). It is due to the added-value potential of 'applied visual anthropology' that Pink considers this to be a useful term to highlight the positive enterprise generated from researchers engaging with organisations beyond academic settings. However, Pink also emphasises that academic and applied visual anthropology should not be viewed as mutually exclusive endeavours. Instead she argues that each may complement the other and 'simultaneously integrate and develop academic and applied agendas (and) be productive of both social interventions and academic contributions' (Pink 2007a, 14). As evidence of a possible disciplinary amalgamation within her field of anthropology, Pink's (2007c) *Visual Interventions* collates numerous ethnographic studies that have each utilised visual methods as part of an interventionist agenda.

Towards an Applied Visual Sociology

In the absence of any equivalent resource similar to *Visual Interventions* (Pink 2007c) within the field of sociology, the application of visual methods within this body of research (concerning street-based injecting drug use) sought to develop the synthesis of academic and applied visual sociology outlined in Table 9.1 (above). Furthermore due to the non-existent model of sociological practice noted in any previous endeavour, the author drew upon previous experiences of conducting applied research for inspiration in this venture. As such, at the onset of this project (in 2006) the author sought to develop methodological innovation regarding the use of visual methods for sociological purposes, relating to the shared issues of harm reduction and substance use. Similarly, the pioneering spirit attached to developing an applied visual sociology was, and continues to be, concerned with academic endeavour (towards a qualification and making valid on-going contributions to knowledge) and applied outcome (informing harm reduction as part of solution-focused, public health intervention). In the following section, the evolution of this development is summarised in an attempt to illustrate how previous experience in established research methods facilitated the author's re-*vision*ing of the above formats of qualitative inquiry for both applied and academic purposes.

Applied Visual Sociology: Re-visioning Established Research Methods

During the period 1995–2006 the author conducted (and assisted with) a number of health-related studies that incorporated an action research design. This body of research typically consisted of collaborative partnerships between academy institutions and various stakeholder groups within regional and local authorities. Amongst the many issues addressed in this body of action research were problems such as methadone leakage, HIV/AIDS awareness amongst sex worker populations, community responses to local health facilities, in addition to problematic and 'recreational' drug use.

The same period of research was also characterised by the author's involvement in various projects that adopted more community-focused approaches to drug-related issues. Notable research here includes an ethnographic study of community responses to local drug problems, in which the research was a collaborative venture with a quasi-autonomous, non-governmental organisation (or 'quango') dedicated to reducing social and economic exclusion via increased community inclusion (McKeganey, Neale, Parkin and Mills 2001). During this study, the author assisted with the formation and delivery of a 'breakfast club' for disadvantaged schoolchildren.[2] This community-based initiative was organised as a part of a public health initiative to launch the collaborative research project in the relevant community. This project also provided a means of validating the author's ethnographic research presence in a setting where both the researcher and community residents were unfamiliar with each other. Throughout this study the author also collected visual data relating to sectarian/gang-related graffiti as a means of complementing ethnographic data regarding these issues in which the relevant images were used as 'documentary' evidence of tensions underlying the affected setting. Similarly, assisting Alasdair Forsyth's community-based, observational study of bar-room violence in Scotland (Forsyth and Cloonan 2008, Forsyth 2012) provided further preparation for the author in assessing the effect of environments upon health and social behaviour.

The only written documents to emerge from those studies that contained an action research agenda were the final confidential and unpublished reports made available to the various commissioners, stakeholders and associated steering

---

2   Under the direction and supervision of Professor Joanne Neale (now of King's College, London)

groups (for example, Parkin 1996, Parkin and Kaner 1996, Parkin and McKenna 1997, Barnard and Parkin 1999). This absence of published material should therefore be regarded as representative of the fundaments (rationale and design) of action research projects, as the aim of such work is to influence positive change with structural and community assistance. Similarly, those studies that adopted a more community-based approach to the relevant issues provided both confidential and *published* material (such as Parkin and McKeganey 2000, McKeganey, Neale, Parkin and Mills 2001), in which the former provided advisory recommendations to the relevant collaborating partnerships, whereas the latter considered the same research findings from more theoretical perspectives attached to various academic disciplines.

These experiences of applied and academic research partnerships therefore had a significant influence (perhaps consciously *and* unconsciously) upon the methodological design and delivery of the work documented throughout this book. In addition, the foundational concepts underlying the model of an applied visual sociology do not necessarily represent any radical departure from established and orthodox research methods that typify the social sciences. However, the model does aim to re-*vision* methodological and applied innovation in a process that advances qualitative methods. This re-*visioning* strives towards establishing a package of *complementary* and *complementing* techniques of inquiry that equally inform academic and applied inquiry of *social problems*. Indeed, it is these guiding principles – originally developed during the author's doctoral research (and subsequently applied as solution-focused, harm reduction research as part of Plymouth University's Public Injecting Rapid Appraisal Service (Parkin, Coomber and Wallace 2010))that continue to inspire and drive the notion of applied visual sociology.

The Rationales of Applied Visual Sociology

In the following section, an account of the perceived and actual benefits brought to the research by the use of visual methods is presented and discussed. This account commences with a critical review of the benefits established by visual methods designed to inform the *academic* framework of the study. This review is then repeated in the context of *applied* research and demonstrates how 'harm reduction' intervention has benefitted from the same visual methods employed throughout the study. Collectively, these perceptions of visual methods are used as the bases for developing and advocating the framework of applied visual sociology.

The Rationale of Academic Visual Methods

The rationale for including visual methods to increase academic understandings of street-based injecting aimed to provide meaningful and original contributions to the literature in regard to methodological and theoretical developments in the discipline of sociology. This rationale therefore directly relates to the well-versed mantra in which original contributions to knowledge are a prerequisite and defining feature of academic-oriented research (Oliver 2004). The predominant contribution of visual methods in this respect therefore relates to the generation of alternative perspectives regarding the social organisation of drug using environments physically situated in public settings. More accurately, these varied perspectives of injecting drug use were visually and verbally obtained from individual, collective and multiple experiences and from various cohorts that were directly affected by street-based injecting (such as frontline service personnel and drug users). As such, analysis and interpretation of these verbal and visual experiences assisted in making the desired contributions to knowledge and the associated sociological discourse pertaining to illicit drug use (see Parkin 2009a, Parkin 2013).

Learning-by-Doing

The application of visual methods also enhanced and enriched the wider research process. More specifically, visual data generated from field-based interviews typically included a wide-range of emotional, sensory and situational factors that are embedded within street-based drug use and are experiences that may not necessarily have been made obvious by conventional academic inquiry (that is, asking questions). The application of visual methods within several hundred drug using environments therefore provided voluminous qualitative insights of activity *affecting*, and *affected* by, injecting episodes within the 'naturalistic' settings of such events. For example, the application of participant observation in these street-based locations provided a baseline appreciation of the environmental and spatial qualities of 'hidden places' in public settings. However the actual *process* of collecting and recording *visual* data (using various cameras) required 'observant participation' methods that developed a 'situated knowing-how-to' within the same environments (Wacquant 2005, 466). More simply, the inclusion of visual methods established sensory cognisance and spatial appreciation of injecting environments through a process of 'learning-by-doing'. Accordingly, all physical actions connected to the conduct of visual methods further increased awareness of drug using environments as the author was required to access/attend/exit particular places in a manner that emulated the relevant participant groups. As an illustration, during observant-participation sessions with drug users within injecting environments, participants verbally and physically articulated movement and motion, experience and knowledge of injecting episodes that was recorded on- and off- camera (fieldnotes, audio-visual recording equipment). Similarly, in conducting observant participation fieldwork, the research was influenced and informed by the 'skilled vision' (Grasseni 2004) of those with direct experience of street-based injecting issues. Cumulatively, these experiences of visual data collection *allegorically* transmitted injecting experience from participants to researcher via a process of 'total pedagogy (that) tacitly guides social agents in their familiar universe' (Wacquant 2005, 465). Through this research focused activity, a spatial and corporeal appreciation of injecting spaces was obtained through the (researcher's) reproduction of (participant) practice that subsequently assisted in developing more academic appreciations of these *embodied* and *harmful* experiences (see Parkin (2013) for a full account of the embodiment of harm noted here).

Methodological Orientation

Furthermore, the inclusion of visual methods assisted in circumventing any preconceived constructions of drug using environments held by the author. More significantly, the use of visual methods avoided considering street-based injecting episodes in an analytical (and perhaps clichéd) framework that prioritised 'risk' and/or 'risk-taking'. Instead, *all* data generation focused upon the relational interplay between health, place and lived experience – *as described by respondents* – in an attempt to identify *actual* (and not perceived or potential) harm and hazard that is associated with street-based, drug using environments (Parkin 2013). As a consequence of prioritising this particular *methodological* paradigm, more phenomenological accounts of injecting drug use emerged. For example, by purposely avoiding subjective and positivist constructions of 'risk' associated with *individual* behaviour, the employment of visually-focused methods in *social* settings of drug use assisted in recording the *shared* and symbolic meanings attached to injecting drug use within street-situated environments. As such, a more *constructivist* interpretation, characterised by *critical* appraisals of 'place' (relating to structure and agency), emerged from data analysis that totalised the lived experiences of those directly involved in (or affected by) such issues.

The *methodological* rationale underlying visual methods in this work was therefore to obtain multiple representations of street-based injecting and provide academic explanations of the way in which drug related harm is made manifest on a day-to-day level by those concerned. In accordance with this logic of practice, image-based data serves to 'visualise verbal accounts' of street-based injecting episodes, whereas language-based responses seek to 'verbalise visual representations' of street-based injecting environments. In this way, mixed qualitative datasets may be collapsed towards more complementary and symbiotic associations that, in turn, concretise the various theoretical, epistemological and empirical frameworks underpinning the entire research design.

Consolidation by Visual Means

The visual methods described in this work not only accompany more conventional qualitative techniques (such as interviews, observations), but also assist in the validation and confirmation of findings obtained from the four different geographic areas of the multi-site study. This is made possible by the process of *serial triangulation*, (described in Chapter 3), in which the longitudinal repetition of methods creates a naturally-occurring template for achieving 'completeness' of understanding (Quine and Taylor 1998). Furthermore, due to the *ethnographic* design of the project, all visual methods became a form of social inquiry 'embedded in real time situations that (sought) to capture collective constructions' (Auyero and Swistun 2009, 140) of spatially-mediated injecting drug use. Therefore, the academic visual sociology underlying this work *methodically* and *methodologically* attempts to explicate the varied social, political and cultural contexts attached to street-based injecting episodes; identify drug-related harm associated with this behaviour and provide a valid critique of the contained relationships that are constructed by structure and agency in particular 'places' (that is, drug using environments).

Structure and Agency Visualised

A more *theoretically* focused rationale for employing visual methods was also attached to this study. As noted throughout, the visual images contained within this book were generated from a longitudinal qualitative study of drug-using environments that incorporated photography and video as part of ethnographic fieldwork (Parkin 2009a, 2013). However, from the perspective of *structure and agency* (perhaps *the* most central tenet of all sociological inquiry), each of the respective studies conducted during 2006–2011 were also empirical assessments of Pierre Bourdieu's *habitus* construct. Namely, each individual study aimed to describe socially/culturally constructed performances situated within specific environments that characterise Bourdieu's theories of habitus, capital and practice. Whereas this book has focused almost exclusively upon the applied value of this collected research, the more theoretical inclinations of the same work have been presented in *Habitus and Drug Using Environments: Health, Place and Lived Experience* (Parkin 2013).

Visualising the Habitus of Drug Using Environments

In an attempt to summarise the thesis contained within the latter text, it is perhaps necessary to emphasise that Bourdieu used the following formula to summarise the logic of social *practice* within particular social arenas (*fields*):

[(habitus) (capital)] + field = practice (Bourdieu 1984, 101)

Bourdieu's formulaic approach for explaining social action was subsequently adopted by the author (Parkin 2009a, 2013) within the context, settings and practice of injecting drug use/rs, in which an interpretivist epistemology of harm reduction framed all data collection and analysis. Furthermore, the absence/presence of harm reduction techniques by drug users within environments of street-based injecting was considered in order to note the constructed nature of injecting environments (social and physical characteristics), in addition to the presence (or not) of amenities to facilitate 'un/safer' injecting episodes. This constructivist interpretation of injecting environments influenced the creation of a similarly Bourdieusian framework (by the author) that attempts to provide a theoretical explanation of harm production and/or reduction in street-based settings. More accurately, the following formula provides a theoretically-informed device to determine the nature of *how* drug related harm may be made manifest within drug using environments *per se*. Namely:

Harm Pro-/Re-duction = [(Social Environment) + (Physical Setting) + (Opportunities for Hygiene) + (Concealment) + (Marginality)] (Parkin 2009a, 156)

When these two formulas for social action are combined they establish theoretical and epistemological convergence that explains a drug-centred *habitus* and locates (street-based injecting) *practice* within a 'continuum of descending safety' (Parkin 2009a 156). This theoretically-driven and visually-informed formula was, in-part, generated by visual data that were directly informed by the aforementioned 'skilled visions' (Grasseni 2004) of all research participants and the author's own embodied experiences of 'learning by doing' whilst situated in street-based settings.

Further conclusions attached to this theoretical framework note that the relationship between structural forces and social agency within drug affected environments shape action towards the amplification of harmful practice and hazardous outcome (including death). In essence, the lived-experience of these drug related hazards was not regarded as 'risk behaviour' by the cohort of injecting drug users. Instead, these experiences of drug-related harm in public settings were generally perceived as everyday inconveniences to be avoided and simultaneously emphasised the *illusio*[3] construct associated with a 'public injecting habitus' (Parkin 2013).[4] Consequently, injecting drug user responses typically acknowledged the

---

3   Bourdieu uses the term '*illusio*' to describe individual dedication to a particular form of social action or shared practice. The *illusio* emerges from a commitment to the belief that these practices produce various benefits and validate a desired outcome (see Parkin (2013) for a detailed account of the *illusio* construct attached to street-based injecting drug use).

4   It is also necessary to emphasise that the drug-related harms associated with street-based settings are not necessarily exclusive to public injecting practice. Indeed, it is probable that similar experiences of injecting drug use will be encountered throughout any population of injecting drug users regardless of injecting environment. However, it is equally important to reiterate that these findings relate to *environmental* influences upon injecting episodes and how *place* shapes harm within the habitus of public injecting.

harm-producing qualities that may result from injecting episodes within street-based environments and equally accepted drug-related harm as an everyday occurrence in the lived-experience of public injecting drug use.

In addition to the above academic contributions to knowledge generated by the inclusion of visual methods, image-based material obtained from this research also provides significant import to a variety of practitioners holding 'real world' positions. This includes those individuals with a professional (or personal) interest in public health, harm reduction, community safety, spatial management and all related policy. Accordingly, in order to validate this claim, the following section details the outcome attached to the *applied* visual methods connected to this study.

The Rationale of Applied Visual Methods

As noted in Table 9.1, the use of visual methods in this research aims to develop a meaningful synthesis of academic and applied sociology, similar to that which is emergent in other social science disciplines (Pink 2007a). As such, in the context of applied research, this visual approach to sociological inquiry of injecting drug use sought to generate pedagogic and instructional material that prioritises the practice and principles of harm reduction. Indeed, from the onset of all research, it was envisaged that visual data would, in the very least, provide pragmatic data for multi-agency *intervention* at a local level (and potentially, extend reach towards national and international settings given the universality of injecting drug use). In formulating this particular strategic outcome of the study, the various logics underlying 'action research' and 'community based research' are perhaps made evident in the *applied* design of this study. Namely, the application of visual methods in this work are to be regarded as hypothetical bricks and mortar that assist the construction of the metaphorical bridge between methodology and intervention; as symbolic masonry that connects academic and applied research as part of a robust and rigorous unit of inquiry.

In order to construct this bridge however, it was also necessary to become involved in a procedure termed 'cultural brokerage' (Chalfen and Rich 2007, Pink 2007a). This process requires the collation of views of one group (for example, injecting drug users) and *re-*presenting these opinions/experiences to a distinctly different group (for example, harm reduction practitioners, research commissioners and funders). Implicit within this process is the transformation of the researcher towards an 'agent of change' (Ropoport 1970, 499), as the expectation of any knowledge transfer obtained from cultural brokerage is that it should influence positive intervention. Pink (2007a) emphasises that it is this 'applied' aspect of visual research that differentiates it from more 'academic' orientations, as the former is more likely to contribute to social change as a result of participatory, collaborative research with participants from a given field. Indeed, the various applied outcomes of this collected research perhaps confirm Pink's contention in this regard.

Visually Informed Service Outcome

To illustrate the above claim, during the course of this 56-month (2006–2011) study of street-based injecting, a series of annual, unpublished and confidential reports were produced for the various funders and commissioners of research. Whilst the specific content of these commissioned documents cannot be made public in this text (for reasons relating to 'confidentiality'), it is possible to include a more generic summary of outcome achieved from this collective body of ethnographic research. As such, listed below are the key outcomes to emerge from research and fieldwork carried out in four different geographic areas of southern England. Furthermore, the processes of applying visual methods, in conjunction with analysis of visual data, were influential in advocating the relevant recommendations pertaining to the various issues outlined below.

This applied, visual and *sociological* studies of street-based injecting throughout the UK described in this book have contributed towards the following *service developments* in harm reduction intervention[5]:

1. the provision of bespoke recommendations relevant to local settings regarding local responses to the management of public injecting drug use
2. the enabling of service commissioners to better target intervention and training for service providers and service users
3. advancing local policies aimed at mitigating (rather than increasing) drug related harm
4. the development of partnerships designed to reduce fatalities associated with street-based injecting
5. a *strategic* review of the way in which homeless/roofless individuals may access injecting paraphernalia
6. a *strategic* review of various policies within hostels regarding the possession of injecting paraphernalia
7. an internal review of the way in which public injecting environments may be policed
8. an internal review of the public health value attached to 'blue lights' (as a measure to prevent injecting drug use in some public settings) and the physical removal of blue lights from some public locations
9. the scaling-up of needle and syringe distribution in certain locations
10. an internal review of how mobile needle and syringe programmes may extend reach
11. an internal review and/or introduction of methods to improve the monitoring and surveillance of public injecting sites and/or drug related litter
12. an internal review of how assertive outreach services may become more focused towards settings of street-based injecting drug use

---

5 These are presented as non-site specific and generalise the overall success of all research conducted during 2006–2011

13. the implementation of pilot research to consider more innovative measures of delivering harm reduction intervention in environments affected by injecting drug use
14. the identification of populations who may benefit from hepatitis (A and B) vaccinations
15. a review of the implementation and management of drug related litter bins located in public places – including systems to improve visibility and management (location, collection procedures, advertising)
16. a review of training programmes for individuals in workplaces affected by injecting drug use
17. consideration of outreach intervention in residential areas affected by street-based injecting
18. a review of the way in which public toilets are policed and accessed by outreach services
19. notification to central government's Department for Food and Rural Affairs, Department for Health and the National Treatment Agency (now Public Health England) of the harmful associations attached to blue light installations within public conveniences
20. invitations to the author to provide harm reduction training and/or workshop sessions (UK-wide) regarding environmental influences upon drug-related harm to various practitioner audiences (including health consultants, nurse specialists, drug and alcohol workers, statutory bodies and third sector organisations)

Visually Informed Pedagogy

The 20-point list of outcome presented above confirms absolutely the applied value of visually-assisted research dedicated to issues surrounding street-based injecting drug use. However, in addition to these various developments of harm reduction in local settings is the *pedagogic* legacy of this particular *applied visual sociology*. More specifically, a number of language and image based publications[6] have been generated from this combined study that lasted almost five years in total. Collectively, these outputs have been used regularly to demonstrate the physical and environmental conditions that perpetuate drug related harm; explain a metaphorical environmental descent from 'safety and hygiene' towards 'dirt and danger', provide useful contributions to harm reduction intervention and make recommendations in the relevant areas of social policy (such as public health, community safety, spatial management and design).

---

6 Parkin 2009a, 2011, 2012, 2013, Parkin and Coomber 2009 a,b, 2010, 2011, Parkin, Coomber and Wallace 2010, Pearson, Parkin and Coomber 2011

The Continuum of Descending Safety Made Visual

The pedagogic and instructive value of these documents has been complemented by relevant image-based data that qualifies the various claims made in relation to the environmental influences upon drug-related harm. For example, perhaps the most significant, service-relevant, finding to emerge from this study is the development of a framework for classifying street-based injecting environments from a harm reduction perspective. This model, the topic of Chapter 5, is termed the 'continuum of descending safety' also provides a template for predicting (and responding to) drug related harm in those settings described as 'controlled', 'semi-controlled' and 'uncontrolled' injecting environments (Parkin 2011).

Furthermore, as a consequence of the serial triangulation attached to the study, this environmental framework (and template of harm) has been developed and empirically tested on numerous occasions in a variety of urban settings throughout the south of England. Perhaps more accurately, the 'continuum of descending safety' emphasises the harmful relationship between environmental setting and injecting practice, in which the former may *produce* and *reproduce* established injecting-related harms in an *amplified* manner. As such, this visual representation of a particular health-place nexus serves to highlight a challenge faced by harm reduction practitioners in disseminating advice and information relating to assumptions of what is considered 'clean', 'sterile' 'safe' and 'sanitary' in the *lived experience* of street-based injecting. For these reasons, the model portrayed and described in Chapter 5 represents a credible and legitimate tool that may be used for instructive, pedagogic and/or educational purposes by all those with a vested interest (whether personally or professionally) in drug-related issues. For example, this framework may be easily adapted and applied within settings such as Needle and Syringe Programs (NSP) whereby service providers can initiate discussions with service users regarding the effect of 'place' on drug related harm during the relevant provision of injecting paraphernalia. Similarly, as noted elsewhere in this book (Chapters 2 and 3), drug user requests for specific types of paraphernalia provide an indication of *where* individuals inject; both bodily and environmentally. As such, requests for certain equipment could provide an *entrée* to a service relevant discussion regarding settings of injecting episodes and the harms associated with the 'continuum of descending safety'

Practitioner Evaluation

The applied harm reduction value attached to the visually-oriented representation of injecting environments (known as the continuum of descending safety) may be noted throughout Chapter 8. More specifically, the pedagogic, service-relevant value of this model is widely supported and commended by the various testimonies provided by the 77[7] individuals (from a wide range of professions) that participated in the evaluation of visual material relating to street-based injecting environments.

Almost all of the positive responses and supportive testimony obtained from this evaluation (and documented throughout Chapter 8) confirm that methodologically-informed visual images generated from studies of harm reduction provide *pedagogic, political and instructive* value to the intended target populations of the applied research agenda (that is, *health* professions). According to the practitioner evaluation responses, ethnographically-contextualised images, such as those used throughout this book, provide opportunities for enriched communication and understanding when used to sensitively portray the everyday settings of injecting episodes. This was particularly apparent in the relevant remarks pertaining to the *polysemic* visual material to assist interaction and intervention between service-providers and service-users *within harm reduction settings*.

Similarly, as noted in Chapters 6 and 7, theoretically-informed visual data analysis may also be used to advocate the secure and discrete installation of street-based sharps bins in areas most affected by public injecting (in order to collect, and make safe, used and unused injecting paraphernalia). Likewise, as stated above, visual datasets of drug-using environments may be adapted to provide instructive material for use amongst the relevant local municipal authorities responsible for town planning, local services and the management of public space. Perhaps more controversially is the suggestion noted in Chapter 8 that drug-related photography may also be a useful mechanism for advocating the introduction of safer injecting facilities (or drug consumption rooms) in UK settings. Such facilities are currently not available in the UK. However, according to responses from the 'Practitioner Evaluation' (Chapter 8), coupled with the environmental settings of drug related harm, drug related litter and their management (Chapters 5–7 respectively) the visual data such as those within this book provides evidence to validate current harm reduction lobbying for such service provision, (if only on a pilot/trial basis). Nevertheless, in the absence of any similar legally-sanctioned facility in UK settings, the (empirically-tested) visual research described throughout this book offers practitioners a range of legitimate responses and interventions that may be discussed, developed and adapted in local, regional and/or national settings as less controversial responses to street-based injecting drug use.

Structural Challenge and Deconstruction via Applied Visual Sociology

Chapter 6 of this book focused upon the emotive issue of drug related litter in community settings. More specifically, it attempted to provide new perspectives of this issue that aimed to facilitate harm reduction and prevent the undermining of

---

7   These respondents are *in addition* to the 240 qualitative/interview responses gathered during the five year research project (that is, a cumulative total of 317 individuals contributed to the study)

valid intervention (needle and exchange provision) by structural forces (within the media). This chapter also seeks to challenge the demonisation of drug use/rs and circumvent health-related hysteria regarding discarded injecting paraphernalia. Throughout Chapter 6, visual data played a significant part in formulating these alternative perspectives that openly confront structural misrepresentations of drug use/rs and discarded injecting paraphernalia (further assisted by the provision of a relevant (reproducible) resource contained within Appendix I). Accordingly, the central aim of Chapter 6 is to 'deconstruct' more dominant representations of drug related litter that prove to be less helpful in generating pragmatic, harm reduction responses to a politically sensitive, public health issues.

A further structural challenge offered by sustained visual analysis may also be noted throughout Chapter 6. More specifically, this challenge relates to the author's claims that suggest drug-related images may be used as a *forensic* resource in developing and advocating applied harm reduction intervention. The value inherent in this contention may not be immediately apparent, but has significant connotations that connect to the discussion above regarding the public consumption of drug-related images, especially when obtained from street-based settings.

To elaborate upon this issue, one should consider how all images of drug related litter re-presented throughout this book may be interpreted by, for example, journalists, police officers, nurses, school teachers or refuse collectors and in a manner without any accompanying analysis or commentary. One may anticipate that each of these individuals would provide their own *subjective* analysis that would typically concur with a negative portrayal of street-based injecting drug use. Indeed, it is entirely probable that such images would justify demands for sanctions and reprisals against those considered 'responsible' for injecting drug use and/or those agencies that legitimately distribute injecting paraphernalia. Accordingly, such subjectivity would perhaps inadvertently overlook attempts by drug users to employ 'informal' (street-based) harm reduction practices that seek to minimise the various harms associated with used, discarded needles in drug using environments (see Chapter 6).

Indeed, some may argue that the multi-layered meaning and polysemic content of photographic images demonstrates the unreliability of visual methods as a valid research process. However, as Henley (1996) suggests, such varied interpretations of images may actually enrich ethnographic description. Henley further suggests that visual data typically indicate a 'quality of thick *in*scription' (Henley 1996, 12, original emphasis) and become a source of 're-analysis and re-interpretation' (ibid.) that can contribute to the resituating of initial visual readings. Indeed, this became evident in the present study, in which images of drug related litter were initially viewed by the author as collections of randomly discarded syringes. Subsequent re-analysis, following drug user accounts of their experiences of street-based injecting episodes, provided far richer (and perhaps more provocative) interpretations of the images concerned. Namely, the author's re-analysis of the seemingly random distribution of used injecting paraphernalia appeared to confirm respondent accounts of discarding practices that partially neutralised the harmful effects of exposed sharps. That is, a forensically-oriented re-analysis of images was adopted to substantiate particular injecting experiences in specific locations. Indeed, this focused analysis appears to confirm that injecting drug users do (on occasion) apply indigenous strategies reported during interviews that are dedicated to reducing harms associated with used injecting equipment.

The Applied Politics of Drug Related Litter

The challenge presented to structural understandings of drug related litter continued in Chapter 7 in which an account of the formal *and informal* management strategies employed by frontline service personnel provides further significant (and previously understated) accounts of street-based injecting drug use. When these experiences of frontline service personnel are compared to those of injecting drug users, one may recognise certain areas of common ground shared by both cohorts. For example, the respective work routines and lifestyles of the two groups share characteristics such as 'movement and motion' across wide geographic areas within city environs; both involve a degree of transience and operating independently to complete necessary 'chores' and, most importantly, both parties aim to perform their respective 'tasks' (cleaning/injecting) in a manner that is rapid in order to 'save time' and be most efficient in their respective practice.

Whereas these similarities clearly relate to opposing roles that may be defined as licit (employment) and illicit (drug use), the commonalities of mobility, transience and rapidity serve to facilitate competent performance (completing jobs *vs.* administering drugs), in a manner that avoids interference from authority (line managers/supervisors *vs.* police/public); in which all of the above need to occur within a specific time-frame (that is, as quickly as possible). Moreover, as noted in Chapter 5, environments characterised by rushed and rapid injecting practice contribute towards injecting-related harm amongst drug users.

Accordingly, it is perhaps of little coincidence that rushed, rapid and informal cleansing procedures conducted by frontline service personnel within similar environments may also produce 'drug related harm' in the form of needlestick injury. As a result of this applied visual sociology, it has become apparent that those frontline service personnel whose work routines emulate the transient nature of public injecting drug use; whose cleansing routines adopt a 'common sense' approach to drug related litter management (despite having received training in drug issues and viral infection) and whose working practices are most characterised by rushed and rapid performance are those possibly most *susceptible* to drug related harm (needlestick injury). From an applied perspective these findings raise a number of significant issues for consideration by employers who provide health and safety training/awareness sessions for their employees. For example, work-based training issues may attempt to promote genuine awareness of the HIV and hepatitis viruses (all strains of the latter), the routes of infection and transmission, the longevity of each virus outside organisms and to provide accurate information regarding the probability of infection from needlestick injury.

Chapter 7 also provides applied value in presenting an informal evaluation of a government report published by the Department of Environment, Food, and Rural Affairs (Defra 2005) concerning ways in which local authorities may more effectively tackle drug related litter in community settings. Contained within Chapter 7 is confirmation that spatial management designs that indirectly incorporate harm reduction and community safety strategies can reduce harm and hazard associated with street-based injecting drug use. In essence, the empirical research that informs this chapter also endorses and supports (for the first time)[8] various recommendations by made by Central Government regarding suitable methods of intervention. More specifically:

1. Plans for managing drug related litter should include close liaison with those responsible for the design, maintenance and management of public toilets
2. Due to the increased risks to users and lack of evidence as to its efficiency, blue lighting should not be used in public toilets to deter drug use
3. Partnerships should fully explore the potential for sharps bins, liaising closely with drug users and services to ensure the siting and promotion of bins is as effective as possible (Defra 2005, 48)

The applied value of recommendations such as those above is that they seek to provide 'enabling environments' (Duff 2010) in which harm reduction may occur as a result of positive spatial design and manufacture.

Visualising the 'Frontline' of Street-based Injecting

A further image-based project to emerge from the visual dataset attached to this research is a public exhibition of 100 photographs generated during the multi-site study of street-based injecting drug use. This exposition (Parkin 2012) is named *Frontline: A Photo-Ethnography of Drug Using Environments* and has been included in various national and international events/settings (see Chapter 8). As part of the advertising surrounding the exhibition, photo-ethnography is described as the combined use of visual and ethnographic materials in an attempt to represent other social worlds in a sensitive and accessible manner. Similarly, the exhibition brochure (Parkin 2013, 1–2) states that the montage 'does not aim to glorify or demonise drug use or users. Instead it seeks to portray the environmental settings affected by drug dependency and homelessness' (ibid.). The brochure later notes that the exhibition aims to promote further understandings of environments

---

8   In addition to the author's previously published material on these topics (see Parkin and Coomber 2010, 2011).

associated with injecting episodes and 'reflect the physical conditions in which drug-related harm can and does occur' (ibid.). Finally, a more harm reduction polemic is perhaps inferred in the final aim of the exhibition in which images 'are presented explicitly to stimulate political debate, public engagement and encourage an appropriate response to this public health issue' (ibid.). Indeed, as a result of the UK's 2010 National Drug Strategy – that places increased emphasis upon a 'recovery' based policy agenda – this latter goal purposely sets about invigorating harm reduction intervention and placing street-based injecting on local radars and public health-related agendas. To emphasise this particular issue, a further declaration within the exhibition brochure states that 'each image ... is an attempt to promote the need for continued harm reduction intervention in community' settings throughout the UK and beyond' (ibid.).

In order to justify the above declaration of intent, the *Frontline Exhibition* is arranged into the three identical themes that are contained within this book. Namely, one section focuses upon the range of street-based environments appropriated for injecting purposes and provides a visual representation of the continuum of descending safety (cf. Chapter 5). A second section portrays the issue of discarded injecting paraphernalia (cf. Chapter 6) with a third section depicts the way in which drug related litter is managed in community settings (cf. Chapter 7). When these sections are viewed individually and collectively within the gallery space, the exhibition actually presents a photographic triptych that attempts to re-present the collective 'lived-experiences' of street-based injecting drug use (from the perspectives of injecting drug users and frontline service personnel). The arrangement of images in this format essentially guides the viewer through three distinct and divergent facets of injecting drug use, all of which are situated within a range of public environments. For these reasons the visual installation is regarded as an exercise in photo-ethnography, in which the viewer temporarily observes and visits the various accounts and settings of a particular, street-focused, lived-experience.

In June 2013, the *Frontline* exhibition was re-presented at the Harm Reduction International (HRI) annual conference in Vilnius, Lithuania. As noted on the HRI website,[9] the theme of the 2013 event 'calls on the urgent need to provide sufficient political and financial support to address the HIV epidemic driven by injecting drug use in many parts of the world, as well as the ethical basis of the harm reduction philosophy'. Whereas the initial outing of the *Frontline* exhibition at the University of Huddersfield intended to advance public interest in social science research (methods, analysis and content) and an engagement with harm reduction as a political/public health issue, the second staging in Vilnius was dedicated entirely to reproducing the themes contained within the title of the HRI event; namely *the value(s) of harm reduction*. Indeed, 'the value(s) of harm reduction' is made evident in all of the exhibition images as they are each dedicated to promoting the continued need for related intervention on a local, regional, national and global scale.

---

9   http://www.ihra.net/about-the-event-2 (accessed: 25 March 2013).

Informing Instructive Intervention – including Interaction

Other interest in the applied value of visual data gathered during this study has led to the development of a collaborative project between the author and the Irish Needle Exchange Forum (Parkin et al. 2013). This project aims to collate *video* material generated during fieldwork (described in Chapter 3) to develop a practitioner-focused film-production that details the environmental, social and spatial concerns surrounding street-based injecting. This short film (in the form of a DVD package and/or online, open-access presentation) will be available to international practitioners of harm reduction as well as be presented to people who inject drugs (or are affected by those who inject drugs in public places) in relevant settings.

This collaborative video production therefore aims to further maximise the pedagogic and instructive content associated with the continuum of descending safety and further demonstrates the applied visual sociology advocated and summarised throughout this book. For example, any online presence of this film production will increase public access to material designed to provide pragmatic value and be further representative of the proactive qualities attached to 'action research'.

A Proactive Pedagogy

The combined pedagogic and political value of all data contained within this book would therefore suggest that health promotion and public health intervention may be significantly assisted with relatively cost-effective research methods specifically designed to provide beneficial health outcome. Similarly, the findings from the evaluation summarised in Chapter 8 also provide optimism for the continued construction of an applied visual sociology and holds promise for the continued proliferation of visual methods throughout the applied social sciences. For example, in this study, visual data has been empirically-tested in numerous settings and have been found to provide meaningful contributions to harm reduction intervention when expertly considered by professional and practitioner audiences. Similarly, the same visual data were noted as enabling improved understanding of injecting episodes and environments and assisted in the invocation of applied professional responses and appropriate reflection. In short and more simply stated, these particular conclusions confirm the value of visual media for 'educational' and 'applied' purposes in the field of health promotion and intervention (Hurworth 2004, Killion 2001, Rhodes and Fitzgerald 2006).

The Caution of Social Scientists

However, as previously noted by Schonberg and Bourgois (2002), as much as photographs may paint a thousand words so they may equally articulate a thousand lies! For example, as indicated earlier, images of drug-injecting environments lacking appropriate theoretical and epistemological grounding may be appropriated by others with an interest in sensationalising drug use in media reports; furthering the demonisation/stigmatisation of drug users or influence the intensification of street-based enforcement procedures. For these reasons there is a great need for social scientists and visual researchers (especially those engaged in studies of 'sensitive' issues) to adopt a methodological responsibility that seeks to advance an appreciation of the issues contained within (and around) an image *in a manner that is actively constructed rather than passively received* (Schwartz 1989). Failure to recognise this methodological principle is likely to produce images that are misrepresented and exploited in non-academic settings by those with less altruistic/academic interests. Images that fail to be consistent with *any* disciplinary visuality will ultimately generate superfluous, illustrative material. If there is an expectation to avoid this during more conventionial (word-based) social science research, then there has to be an equal and identical expectation to maintain such precedents when engaging with visual media during research endeavours.

Towards Applied Visual Sociology: The Final Words

In contrast to the above cautionary note, the visual methods designed for application throughout this study have provided a number of benefits that fundamentally strengthen the epistemological positioning and political orientation (see Chapter 3) of this research. These benefits have been of *academic* value (Parkin 2013) but also include the development of local harm-reduction drug services and *applied* intervention (this chapter).

In summary, the applied visual sociology contended throughout this book appears to have successfully contributed towards a range of research outcomes via innovative inquiry and generated the relevant evidence required to initiate change in particular policy agendas with a drug-focused remit. Furthermore, when each of the above applied and academic principles are considered, the 'literal representation' of images, purely for illustrative purposes (as exemplified in this book's *Introduction*), would appear to have been successfully avoided throughout this entire study of street based injecting. In this regard, the use of visual methods towards applied and academic outcome would appear to have been commensurate with established protocols underlying the central tenets of social science scholarship. Namely:

> (t)he research problem or issue should be described clearly, and contextualised within the relevant literature of that subject. There would also usually be an explanation and justification of the research design and of the data collection and analysis methods. As part of this one might also expect an explanation of the way in which the study is located within a specific theoretical tradition or perspective. Finally, there would be a careful analysis of the data and a summary

of the conclusions drawn (Oliver 2004, 6: describing the content and organisation of a doctoral thesis)

In conclusion, the visual data attached to this book appears to comply with established academic traditions within the social sciences. Furthermore, visual data used specifically to *picture harm reduction* as part of an *applied visual sociology* equally demonstrates an 'allegorical expression of a thesis' (Bourdieu 1965, 93) due to the complementary dialogical synthesis of syntax and images towards initiating social change and/or intervention.

Additionally, whilst Sarah Pink (2011) correctly notes her anthropological influence upon this author's work in applied social science, she also *incorrectly* associates it with her vision of an 'applied visual anthropology'. Although this is no great criticism in itself, it is however, fundamentally, *an inaccurate comparison*. This is because this work (and all associated publications attached to the study) is steadfastly and resolutely anchored within a sociological research paradigm. Furthermore, the relevant methodological framework purposely deconstructs structure and agency as part of solution-focused research towards public health intervention and harm reduction advocacy in real world settings. For these reasons, this author's vision of an *applied visual sociology* should not be directly associated with an applied visual anthropology due to an emphasis that is purposely placed upon structural challenge and intended reform (of the relevant health intervention).

And Finally ...

Based on the conclusions summarised throughout this chapter, further and future developments *towards an applied visual sociology* appear entirely positive and plausible. Perhaps more significantly, the combined outcomes described throughout this book clearly demonstrate Lewin's (1948) conviction that social science research with an activist agenda *can* produce more than books alone.

Chapter 10
Practical Exercises in Applied Visual Sociology

This final chapter provides a series of exercises that have been designed for the readership to practise the principles of the applied visual sociology advocated throughout this book (and especially during Chapter 9). Each exercise aims to develop competency and proficiency with fundamental methodological issues underlying applied visual sociology. Presented below are a number of 'assignments' that reflect a hierarchical model of progression (from 'Beginner' to 'Advanced') and may be completed by researchers at any stage of their academic career. Similarly, all exercises below are suitable for individual contemplation as part of self-study; or as part of extracurricular activity relating to structured coursework within academic and/or non-academic settings in which focus is upon visual methods and the social sciences (especially sociology). Similarly, these assignments are equally transferable to a wide range of pedagogic activities relating to visual research methods and/ or active learning (such as organised pair-work, group-work, discussion groups, debating societies, workshops and seminar groups).

Each assignment below requires a consideration of situations that have been informed by actual events and reflect research tasks previously completed by the author. Similarly, each task involves individual/shared reflection upon various *methodological* processes (including epistemological orientation, theoretical framing, critical thinking, analytical awareness, ethical considerations and ethnographic observation) attached to visual research and how these issues may assist/hinder visual *methods* and data collection. In addition, each assignment requires a need to consider visual research, methods and data from both applied and academic perspectives and how any emergent dilemmas may be appropriately reconciled. All of the tasks below are essentially exercises in 'practical theory' and 'theoretical practice'. Each exercise provides *foundational* templates for developing proficiency (and sensitivity) in conducting applied visual sociology as independent research.

As a means of further assisting research development, this chapter concludes with a checklist for consideration during any visually-informed study in the social sciences. Reflection upon the issues presented in this checklist aims to provide a more coherent rationale and explanation for including any visual approach to sociological inquiry. Similarly, in considering the questions posed, it is anticipated that the researcher will avoid gratuitous and illustrative representations of visual data such as that outlined in the opening vignette of this book (see *Introduction*).

'Learning by Doing'

The underlying rationale for including these exercises as a form of 'cloze' within this book is purely pedagogical. 'Cloze' may traditionally be regarded as a method of examination, in which respondents typically complete 'missing text' with appropriate responses. However, in this chapter the 'clozing' tasks are intended to provide a light-hearted, informative and instructive conclusion to a tome that has addressed solemn issues surrounding street-based injecting drug use. In addition, a further *raison d'être* of this 'clozing' chapter is to validate the concept of an applied visual sociology (described in the previous chapter) in a process that emulates aspects of 'observant-participation', or 'learning by doing' (see Chapter 3).

Accordingly, whilst genuine academic and applied endeavour is attached to this chapter, it is also necessary to state that the tasks below are designed to draw this book to a more informal, yet *practical*, conclusion. As such, a personal message to all/any who may consider attempting the following tasks would be to *regard each exercise as an informal and instructive project to be completed at an appropriate pace in an entertaining and enjoyable manner*. Furthermore, it is important to reiterate that there are no correct/incorrect responses to any of the tasks below. Indeed, all items presented are left open for discussion, subject to debate and audience interpretation. However, all responses (whether positive, negative or indifferent) need to be defended so that they are commensurate with academic and applied purposes, in which a coherent argument is presented, explained and justified so that the various rationales appear logical, relevant and valid. Finally, all tasks below should not be regarded as a test of what has gone before; but more as preparation for what might yet come!

Visual Methods: Beginner Level ('Undergraduate')

The first assignment ('Family Album') involves the practical management of a visual dataset that contains several hundred (possibly thousands of) photographs that span several generations. This exercise aims to develop/introduce skills relating to analyses of image-based data. Issues to consider in this task will relate to many of those discussed in Chapter 4 concerning analysis and data coding.

The second task ('Haphazard Street Pictures?') is a practical exercise that consists of arbitrary image-taking followed by a period of focused analysis. The arbitrary image-taking emulates the often 'haphazard' nature of visual data collection that may occur during ethnographic/observational research. In attempting this 'practical' exercise in generating visual data, one may become more familiar with the actual processes attached to such fieldwork. Similarly, in practising this process with the topic suggested below, the novice visual researcher may learn to recognise (and respond to) the difficulties associated with the method. Equally, the pleasure and creativity associated with conducting visually-based research will also be experienced. The secondary task of focused data analysis introduces the researcher to content analysis and thematic interpretation. In addition, this task also provides opportunities to describe visual data with succinct text-based explanations that aim to generalise the entire dataset (and emulate processes that typify qualitative research).

1. Family Album

The Brief

- Imagine you are a sociologist visiting your own family/relatives/friends for an extended period of fieldwork. Your family/relatives/friends have lived in a former industrial centre in the North of England for several generations.
- You have been presented with the entire collection of your family's/relatives'/friends' photograph albums that span several generations (and include paper [monochrome] and digital [colour] photographs).
- The collection contains at least 100,000 images.
- Although you are known to your family/relatives/friends, you should view this collection of images as if you were a sociologist conducting fieldwork in the hometown of your family/relatives/friends. The fieldwork you are conducting relates to a study of gender roles in a de-industrialised town/city.

The Task

- What difficulties would you envisage in doing this exercise?
- How would you address these difficulties?
- When engaged in this task, is it possible to view the images as an 'objective researcher'? Why/not?
- How would you organise and arrange individual photographs contained within the photograph albums/digital dataset?
- What categories would you devise, create or formulate for arranging and analysing these images?
- Why would you select these categories and how would they help you in your fieldwork or in understanding the 'society' which you are studying?

Reflexive Issues

- Would you use any of the images in your written work?
- What decisions would you make regarding the inclusion/exclusion of images in any text you produce?
- How does this exercise help your understanding of *applied* visual research (including methods, data, analysis and interpretation)?
- Does this exercise assist you in understanding sociological constructs of 'power' in any way? (If yes, how and why?)

2. Haphazard Street Pictures?

The Brief

- In a city of your choice, take approximately 100 haphazard snapshots of street locations. However, in each photograph you *must not* include the *facial* image of any person. All photographs must be taken in a single day within a three hour time period. Do not begin this exercise with any preconceived ideas or plans about the type of scene you wish to photograph.

The Task

- When complete, collate the 100 snapshots into visual themes (or categories) you identify within the collection.
- Identify the most recurring theme.
- Select five images from the most recurring theme.
- Use these images to write a 1500 word report on the theme identified and its relevance to the city concerned (that is, what do the five images tell you about the location?)
- (TIP 1: the five images selected should best reflect the theme you have identified. The task in hand is to explain *why* they best reflect this theme).
- (TIP 2: Allocate approximately 200 words per image for your report)

Reflexive Issues

- How does this exercise help your understanding of *applied* visual research (including methods, data, analysis and interpretation)?
- Does this exercise assist you in understanding sociological constructs of 'power' in any way? (If yes, how and why?)

Visual Methods: Intermediate Level ('Postgraduate')

The following two exercises introduce the researcher to elements of ethnographic research that incorporate visual data generation. In 'Watching Tourists' the researcher is required to complete a period of ethnographic observation and subsequently produce a reflexive account of other people taking photographs of objects/subjects. The central concern of this task is 'interpretation'; of image, of image-takers and image-makers. The rationale for this task is to initiate reflexive accounts, based upon the observations of others, on how a fieldworker may subsequently manage their own performance (comportment, image-making) whilst gathering visual data in public settings.

The second intermediate assignment, 'Ethics of Photography', provides further opportunities to consider visual data generation whilst conducting observational and ethnographic fieldwork. In this exercise, more emphasis is placed upon sensitivity and awareness of others whilst taking pictures and the implications of capturing images of other people *without* their consent.

3. Watching Tourists

The Brief

- Visit a popular tourist destination of your own choice. The destination should be popular with overseas visitors and is preferably a setting that is picturesque and popular with photographers (amateur or professional). Examples here may include popular landmarks, historic buildings or living history museums.
- (TIP: a pen and notepad will be invaluable in this exercise!)

The Task

- Find a comfortable position and spend at least two hours observing tourists and visitors taking photographs.
- Notice the people and objects that are the subject of their photography.
- What commonalities do you notice in how photographs are taken?
- What similarities do you notice regarding the framing of the tourists' images?
- How do people react in front of the camera?
- What can you say about 'pose'? Does this affect the image taken in any way?
- What similarities do you notice in the performance of all the photographers you observe?
- Do you notice any form of '*etiquette*'? What does this involve?
- How do people not involved with the photograph/er respond to the presence of a camera?

Reflexive Issues

- As an ethnographer, how would you interpret the photographs that you imagine have been taken?
- Write a 2000 word report that summarises your observations.
- Include an account of the positive and negative aspects of taking photographs in public places that is based upon your observations.
- How does this exercise help your understanding of *applied* visual research (including methods, data, analysis and interpretation)?
- Does this exercise assist you in understanding sociological constructs of 'power' in any way? (If yes, how and why?)

1. Ethics of Photography

The Brief

- As you walk around an urban setting on a daily basis, make a mental note of where, when and whom you see taking photographs in public settings. This can include people taking photographs or making videos with mobile devices (telephones, tablets, cameras); whether they are amateur or professional photographers, alone, in couples (pairs) or organised groups.
- As part of your mental observations, notice how people not directly connected to the video/photograph respond to the presence of another person's camera/ or to the presence of a photographer (if relevant).

Task 1

- At a convenient time/place, make a written note of each observation. This should essentially be a personnel reflection on what you thought about the 'photographic event' (and whether you viewed it as positive, negative, critical or commendable). Create a field journal that documents these observations.
- After a period of one week (or one month) of collecting reflexive fieldnotes, conduct a thematic and focused analysis of your reflections. What conclusions do you draw from this analysis?

Task 2

- You should now consider your analytical conclusions as if you are a member of a Research Ethics Panel.
- You have been presented with a research application that involves a team of professional academics taking pictures of public places for no purpose other than 'illustration'. Your contribution to the Panel requires a decision to comment upon this visual component of the project.
- Based upon your earlier observations, what elements of this photography-based research proposal would you approve/disapprove as formal, applied research?
- What advice, (if any), would you suggest to the researchers applying for ethical approval of their project?

Reflexive Issues

- How does this exercise help your understanding of *applied* visual research (including methods, data, analysis and interpretation)?
- Does this exercise assist you in understanding sociological constructs of 'power' in any way? (If yes, how and why?)

Visual Methods: Advanced Level ('Applied Research')

The final two exercises ('Which Bin?' and 'Colliding Interventions?') are concerned with more 'real world' issues, in which the applied visual data analysis and applied decision-making of the reader will inform the (hypothetical) policy and practice of a (hypothetical) organisation.

These two assignments are exercises in considering 'wider' issues attached to interpretations of visual data, in which the researcher needs to be mindful of how their work (research, data and outcomes) may affect *entire* communities (rather than specific populations within it). Similarly, both tasks require the researcher to consider any (overt and covert) specific policy-related dilemmas – in conjunction with the lived experiences of injecting drug users and frontline service personnel – as documented throughout Chapters 5–7.

3. Which bin?

Figures 7.4–7.8 show an assortment of dedicated sharps bins that the author has noted in numerous settings throughout the UK. This range of drug related litter bins vary in design, installation and environmental setting. Furthermore, each image is of a sharps box that is an example of real world intervention. Each image therefore portrays receptacles that are currently used for collecting/disposing injecting paraphernalia in public settings.

In addition to this drug-related visual dataset is a further image below (Figure 10.1). This photograph is of an entirely different receptacle and depicts an intervention designed to reduce the discarding of cigarette butts and chewing gum in public locations. Readers may note that this container is cylindrical in shape and features a 'birdhouse' design to assist in discarding items in a more considered way.

The Brief

- Become familiar with the Department for Environment, Food and Rural Affairs (Defra 2005) recommendations regarding drug related litter bins in public places (Chapter 7).

The Task

- All of the following questions relate to Figures 7.4–7.8 and Figure 10.1
- Is the range of bins consistent in design, location and environmental setting?
- Are any of the bins better/worse than others in terms of design and installation? (Which? Why?)
- Are there any bins in Figures 7.4–7.8 you would remove/change? (If yes, which one(s) and why?)
- Would you endorse/support any of the bins? (If yes, which one(s), and why?)
- Are there any bins that concern (or trouble) you in any way? (Which? Why?)

270 *An Applied Visual Sociology: Picturing Harm Reduction*

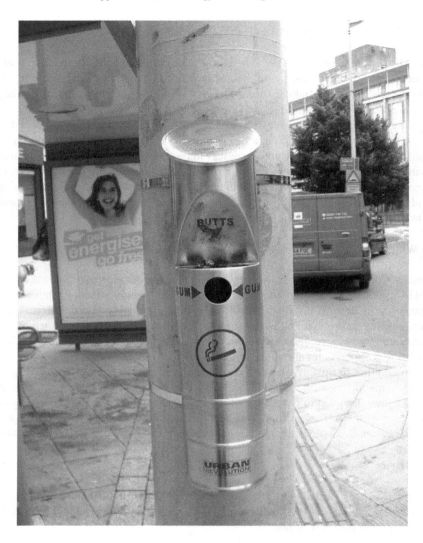

Figure 10.1   Gum and Butt Bin

- Are there any inconsistencies with Defra's (2005) recommendations regarding *Tackling Drug Related Litter*? (If yes, what are they and what challenges do they pose?)
- What are the advantages/disadvantages of each particular bin?
- Which of these bins would you recommend for installation in your local high street? (Why?) Where would you recommend they are installed and who would finance the project?
- Could the bin in Figure 10.1 be used for collecting drug related litter and/

or needles/syringes? (If yes, why? If no, why not?)
- Is the design of the bin in Figure 10.1 consistent with any of the recommendations by Defra?
- Do your answers to the two previous questions conflict in any way? Do they conflict in any way with your answers to all previous questions in this task?

Reflexive Issues

- What are your personal conclusions regarding drug related litter bins?
- What are your policy-related conclusions regarding this particular exercise in analysis of specific visual data?
- How does this exercise help your understanding of *applied* visual research (including methods, data, analysis and interpretation)?
- Does this exercise assist you in understanding sociological constructs of 'power' in any way? (If yes, how and why?)

4. Colliding Interventions?

This final exercise is concerned with using visual data to understand social issues, community problems and how images may be used to initiate debate on matters such as drug related policy and practice.

The aim of this exercise is to assist the reader in conducting critical analyses of drug-related, community-based dilemmas in order to provide pragmatic recommendations for relevant policy and practice. Similarly, this exercise aims to demonstrate the flexibility of visual data and how images may initiate and inform critical debate surrounding sensitive issues.

The Brief

- Refer to Figure 10.2 and consider the various drug related intervention that have been labelled upon this image. These labels reflect 'real world' intervention in an area associated with, and affected by, street-based injecting drug use. The reader should assume that all interventions labelled on the image are active and currently operational at the time of viewing the image.
- However, the decision to introduce 'blue lights' into the toilet cubicles (that currently contain sharps bins) will depend upon the reader's conclusions and recommendations. (Blue lights are typically installed in public places with the specific intent of preventing injecting drug use in the relevant settings. This is because the blue lighting effect makes injecting more arduous and difficult to complete).

272   An Applied Visual Sociology: Picturing Harm Reduction

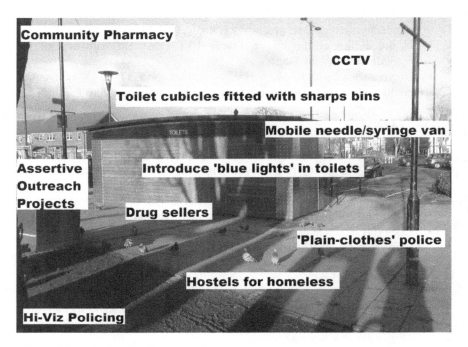

Figure 10.2   Colliding Interventions

The Task

- Establish two lists of intervention based upon the labels presented in this image. List 1 should contain those interventions that facilitate harm reduction. List 2 should be those that problematise harm reduction.
- After completing these lists, what conclusions may be drawn about current drug related intervention in this setting? Evidence your conclusions with reference to the image.
- What conclusions relating specifically to current 'harm reduction intervention' in this setting may be drawn from the two lists? Evidence your conclusions with reference to the image.
- What recommendations would you make regarding the overall management of drug related intervention in this setting? Evidence your suggestions with reference to the photograph.
- Would you recommend that a single organisation/institution co-ordinates and manages all drug related intervention in this setting? Or would you recommend a partnership approach? Evidence your suggestions with reference to the photograph.
- If you recommend a partnership approach, which agencies and organisations would you suggest? And why? Evidence your suggestions with reference to

the photograph.
- What are your recommendations regarding the existing drug related litter bins in the public toilets? Do you recommend scaling-up further installations (throughout the city) – or would you suggest the opposite? Evidence your suggestions with reference to the photograph.
- Finally, you have the final decision on whether 'blue lights' should be installed in the relevant public toilets? What is your decision? What is this decision premised upon? Evidence your suggestions with reference to the photograph.

Reflexive Issues

- What are your conclusions regarding this particular exercise in visual data analysis?
- How does this exercise help your understanding of *applied* visual research (including methods, data, analysis and interpretation)?
- Does this exercise assist you in understanding sociological constructs of 'power' in any way? (If yes, how and why?)

A Checklist for Conducting Visual Research

An appropriate point of closure for this book, concerned with an applied visual sociology, is to provide a checklist for use with any proposed/planned study that aims to include visual methods and/or visual data.

The following checklist has been influenced and informed by O'Toole et al.'s (2003) *Table for Proposed Process for Describing Community-based Participatory Research Findings*. As with the latter, this checklist has been designed to provide a more coherent rationale and explanation regarding the use of particular methods attached to social science research. In this book, the concern is with visual methods and the following checklist is dedicated to how the latter may be incorporated most effectively within qualitative, sociological studies. In adopting the methodological rigour that this checklist provides, visual research output will typically avoid gratuitous and illustrative representations of image-based data.

A Checklist for Rationalising the Use of Visual Methods as Part of an Applied Visual Sociology (inspired by O'Toole et al. 2003)

The Research Topic

1. What is the issue under investigation? What is the policy relevance of the research?
2. Are there population groups more affected than others?

3. Does the proposed research aim to access so-called 'hidden populations'? If yes, why? If yes, what are the implications (positive and negative) for using visual methods with these people as research respondents?
4. What are the limitations posed by traditional qualitative inquiry that would validate the use of visual methods in the research (regardless of population)? What would visual methods/data add to the study?
5. Would visual methods in this study provide any new contributions to knowledge of the topic under investigation? Why/not?
6. What are the advantages and disadvantages of using visual methods in this research? How do you explain the latter?
7. State the intended outcome of applying visual methods. State the intended use of visual data. Explain how both will be managed and conducted during and after fieldwork.
8. How would visual data meaningfully inform the policy surrounding the research topic? (see Question 1 above)
9. Is the research population a particular 'community'? How will the research access this community? How does this community reflect the policy concerns of the study?

Methodology and Methods

1. Which visual methods are to be employed? Why those in particular?
2. What ethical challenges are presented by the use of visual methods in the research? How have they been addressed?
3. How do the visual methods reflect the relevant methodological framework (in terms of ontology, epistemology and theory)?
4. Will the visual study involve community participation in applying/assisting with methods chosen? Why/not?
5. Will any respondents gather/own the visual research data? Why?
6. How will the research design address inclusion, participation, ownership and dissemination of visual research?
7. Who will interpret all visual data? Why?
8. What analytical frameworks have been chosen? Why? How does this reflect methodology?
9. What ethical and practical safeguards have been included to ensure methodological rigor and implementation of all visual research?
10. Does the visual representation generated by the researcher/population actually inform the relevant policy questions asked?
11. What difficulties are anticipated whilst in the field and how are they to be addressed?
12. What methodological decisions have influenced answers to each of the above questions?

Findings

1. How has confidentiality and anonymity been addressed?
2. How has respect, dignity and esteem of community/participants been addressed?
3. How did you obtain consent to reuse images/film? What are the implications of this consent?
4. What do the visual data add to the study that language-based data does not provide?
5. Do the visual data make new contributions to the policy and academic discourse on the relevant topic?
6. How will the findings impact upon the community? Research participants? Who has benefitted from visual research? (Why/not?)
7. What academic and applied developments are expected follow these findings?
8. What decisions have been made in regard to publication? Is the research written for academic or applied audiences? What differences exist? What protocols have been established in regard to ownership of text/image, manuscript contribution, authorship and design of research output?
9. What are the implications of publishing material from this research? Would a confidential (unpublished) document be more appropriate? Validate answers to these responses.

Post-Fieldwork Reflexivity

1. What challenges were encountered during data generation? How were these resolved?
2. What were unexpected outcomes of visual research methods? How did these unexpected events usefully inform the study? How are these events relevant to the policy concerned? Are they relevant to the academic discipline with which the research is aligned?
3. How are the results of the study to be disseminated at a policy level? Academic level? And community level? What differences exist? Why do these differences exist?
4. Does the inclusion of visual data make the study any more/less generalizable than if they had not been included? How does the researcher validate responses to this question?
5. What limitations are attached to the visual data gathered during fieldwork?
6. Do the visual data provide bases for further academic/applied visual research?
7. What *methodological* issues have emerged from this research?
8. Does the research provide any further insight on issues of power-domination between researcher and researched? What are the academic and applied implications of the answer to this question? How has the research findings addressed these implications?

References

ACMD, 1988. *AIDS and Drug Misuse. Part 1* (Report by Advisory Council on the Misuse of Drugs). London: HMSO.
Auyero, J. and Swistun, D.A., 2009. *Flammable: Environmental Suffering in an Argentine Shantytown*. Oxford: Oxford University Press.
Ball, M.S. and Smith, G.W.H., 1992. *Analyzing Visual Data*. London: Sage.
Banks, M., 2007. *Using Visual Data in Qualitative Research*. London: Sage.
Barnard, M., 2006. *Drug Addiction and Families*. London: Jessica Kingsley Publishers.
Barnard, M. and Parkin, S., 1999. *Young People's Routes into Drug Misuse in Shetland*. Centre for Drug Misuse Research, University of Glasgow, Glasgow.
Barrett, D., 2004. *Photo-documenting the Needle Exchange: Methods and Ethics. Visual Studies* 19, 145–9.
Barrett, D., Cook, C., Lines, R., Stimson, G. and Bridge, J., 2009. *Harm Reduction and Human Rights. The Global Response to Drug-Related HIV Epidemics*. International Harm Reduction Association, London.
Bateson, G. and Mead, M., 1942. *Balinese Character: A Photographic Analysis*. New York: New York Academy.
Bazeley, P., 2007. *Qualitative Data Analysis with NVivo*, Second ed. London: Sage.
Beck, U., 1992. *Risk Society: Towards a New Modernity*. London: Sage.
Becker, H.S., 1967. Whose side are we on? *Social Problems* 14, 239–48.
Becker, H.S., 1974. Photography and Sociology. *Studies in the Anthropology of Visual Communication* 1, 1–26.
Becker, H.S., 1978. Do photographs tell the truth? *Afterimage*, 9–13.
Becker, H.S., 1996. The epistemology of qualitative research, in *Ethnography and Human Development: Context and Meaning in Social Inquiry*, edited by R. Jessor, A. Colby and R.A. Shweder. Chicago, IL: University of Chicago Press, pp. 53–71.
Becker, S. and Bryman, A., 2004. *Understanding Research for Social Policy and Practice: Themes, Methods and Approaches*. Bristol: Policy Press.
Berg, B.L., 1998. *Qualitative Research Methods for the Social Sciences*. Boston, MA: Allyn & Bacon.
Berridge, V., 1994. AIDS and British Drug Policy: History repeats itself … ?, in *Drugs and Drug Use in Society. A Critical Reader*, edited by R. Coomber. London: Greenwich University Press, pp. 154–70.
Best, S. and Kellner, D., 1997. *The Postmodern Turn*. New York: Guilford Press.

Beynon, C.M., Taylor, A., Allen, E. and Bellis, M.A., 2010. Visual versus written cues: a comparison of drug injectors' responses. Have surveys using the written word underestimated risk behaviors for Hepatitis C? *Substance Use and Misuse* 45, 1491–508.
Bhaskar, R., 1978. *A Realist Theory of Science*. Hemel Hempstead: Harvester Wheatsheaf.
Bhaskar, R., 1989. *Reclaiming Reality: A Critical Introduction to Contemporary Philosophy*. London: Verso.
Blacklock, S., 2010. *Guidance for Operatives Involved in the Removal of Drug Related Litter*. www.hiwecanhelp.com.
Blenkharn, J.I., 2008. Clinical wastes in the community: Local authority management of discarded drug litter. *Public Health* 122, 725–28.
Bloor, M., 1997. Addressing social problems through qualitative research, in *Qualitative Research: Theory, Method and Practice*, Second ed., edited by D. Silverman. London: Sage.
Blume, A.W., Anderson, B.K., Fader, J.S. and Marlatt, G.A., 2001. Harm Reduction Programs: Progress rather than Perfection, in *Addiction Recovery Tools: A Practical Handbook*, edited by R.H. Coombs. London: Sage, pp. 367–82.
Bogdan, R.C. and Biklen, S.K., 1982. *Qualitative Research for Education: An Introduction to Theory and Methods*. Boston, MA: Allyn & Bacon.
Bourdieu, P., 1965/1990. *Photography: A Middle-brow Art*. Cambridge: Policy Press.
Bourdieu, P., 1977. *Outline of a Theory of Practice*. Cambridge Cambridge: University Press.
Bourdieu, P., 1984. *Distinction: A Social Critique of the Judgement of Taste*. London: Routledge and Kegan Paul.
Bourgois, P., 2000. Disciplining addictions: The bio-politics of methadone and heroin in the United States. *Culture, Medicine and Psychiatry* 24, 165–95.
Bourgois, P., Lettiere, M. and Quesada, J., 1997. Social Misery and the Sanctions of Substance Abuse: Confronting HIV Risk Amongst Homeless Heroin Addicts in San Francisco. *Social Problems* 44, 155–73.
Bourgois, P. and Schonberg, J., 2009. *Righteous Dopefiend*. Berkeley, CA: University of California Press..
Briggs, D., 2011. *Crack Cocaine Users: High Society and Low Life in South London*. London: Routledge.
Bukowski, K. and Buetow, S., 2011. Making the invisible visible: A photovoice exploration of homeless women's health and lives in central Auckland. *Social Science and Medicine* 72, 739–46.
Buning, E.C., van Brussel, G. and van Santen, G., 1992. The impact of harm reduction drug policy on AIDS prevention in Amsterdam, in *The Reduction of Drug Related Harm*, edited by P.A. O'Hare, R. Newcombe, A. Matthews, E.C. Buning and E. Drucker. London: Routledge, pp. 30–38.

Carlson, R.G., 2000. Shooting Galleries, Dope Houses and Injection Doctors: Examining the Social Ecology of Risk Behaviors among Drug Injectors in Dayton, Ohio. *Human Organisation* 59, 325–33.

Casswell, S., Mortimer, D. and Gilroy, C., 1982. The minimal effects and methodological problems in the evaluation of a harm reduction drug education program in a high school setting. *Journal of Drug Education* 12, 345–52.

Chalfen, R. and Rich, M., 2007. Combining the Applied, the Visual and the Medical: Patients Teaching Physicians with Visual Narratives., *Visual Interventions: Applied Visual Anthropology*, edited by S. Pink. New York: Berghahn Books, pp. 53–70.

Chen, J., 2011. Beyond human rights and public health: Citizenship issues in harm reduction. *International Journal of Drug Policy* 22, 184–88.

Clark, D., 2006F. The Drug Experience: Heroin, part 9., *Drink and Drug News*, p. 15.

Cohen, J., 2009 Not Enough Graves: The War on Drugs, HIV/AIDS, and Violations of Human Rights Human Rights Watch, NYC, pp. http://www.hrw.org/reports/2004/2007/2007/not-enough-graves.

Coleman, A.D., 1987. Private lives, public places: street photography ethics. *Journal of Mass Media Ethics* 2, 60–66.

Collier, J. and Collier, M., 1986. *Visual Anthropology: Photography as a Research Method*. Alberquerque, NM: University of New Mexico Press.

Coomber, R., 2002. 'Signing your life away?' Why Research Ethics Committees (REC) shouldn't always require written confirmation that participants in research have been informed of the aims of a study and their rights – the case of criminal populations. (Commentary)', Sociological Research Online.

Coombs, R.H., *2001. Addiction Recovery Tools: A Practical Handbook*. London: Sage.

Coomes, P., 2012. Picture power: Living dead of the drug war News in Pictures @ BBC.

Cresswell, J.W., 2003. *Research Design: Qualitative, Quantitative and Mixed Methods Approaches*, Second ed. London: Sage.

Crofts, N., 2012. Foreword, in *Harm Reduction in Substance Use and High-risk Behaviour: International Policy and Practice*, edited by R. Pates and D. Riley. Oxford: Blackwell, pp. ix–x.

Crossley, N., 2007. Researching embodiment by way of 'body techniques'. *The Sociological Review* 55, 80–94.

Csete, J. and Cohen, J., 2003. Abusing the User: Police Misconduct, Harm Reduction and HIV/AIDS in Vancouver Human Rights Watch, New York.

DCRT, 2011. Community-based Participatory Research: Ethical Challenges. Centre for Social Justice and Community Action, Durham University, Durham.

DEFRA, 2005. Tackling Drug Related Litter: Guidance and Good Practice. Department for Environment, Food and Rural Affairs, London.

Derricott, J., Preston, A. and Hunt, N., 1999. *The Safer Injecting Briefing: An Easy to Use Comprehensive Reference Guide to Promoting Safer Injecting.* Liverpool: HIT.

Des Jarlais, D.C., Paone, D., Milliken, J., YTurner, C.F., Miller, H., Gribble, J., Shi, Q., Hagan, H. and Friedman, S.R., 1999. Audio-computer interviewing to measure risk behaviour for HIV among injecting drug users: A quasi-randomised trial. *The Lancet* 353, 1657–61.

Douglas, M., 1966. *Purity and Danger: An Analysis of Concepts of Pollution and Taboo.* London: Routledge.

Dowdall, G.W. and Golden, J., 1989. Photographs as data: An analysis of images from a mental institution. *Qualitative Sociology* 12, 183–207.

Duff, C., 2010. Enabling places and enabling resources: new directions for harm reduction research and practice. *Drug and Alcohol Review* 29, 337–44.

Emerson, R.M., Fretz, R.I. and Shaw, L.L., 1995. *Writing Ethnographic Fieldnotes.* Chicago, IL: University of Chicago Press.

ENCAMS, 2005. Drugs-Related Litter Survey – 2005. Environmental Campaigns (ENCAMS), Wigan.

Engelsman, E.L., 1989 Dutch policy on the management of drug-related problems *British Journal of Addiction* 84, 211–18.

Erickson, P.G., 1995. Harm reduction: What it is and is not. *Drug and Alcohol Review* 14, 283–5.

Fitzgerald, J.L., 1996. Hidden populations and the gaze of power. *Journal of Drug Issues* 26, 5–21.

Fitzgerald, J.L., 2002. Drug photography and harm reduction: reading John Ranard. *International Journal of Drug Policy* 13, 369–85.

Flick, U., 2007. Introduction, in *Using Visual Data in Qualitative Research*, edited by M. Banks. London: Sage, pp. ix-xiii.

Foddy, W., 1993. *Constructing Questions for Interviews and Questionnaires: Theory and Practice in Social Research.* Cambridge: Cambridge University Press.

Forsyth, A.J.M., 2013. Barroom Approaches to Prevention, in *Alcohol-Related Violence: Prevention and Treatment*, edited by M. McMurran. London: John Wiley & Sons.

Forsyth, A.J.M. and Davidson, N., 2010. The nature and extent of illegal drug and alcohol-related litter in Scottish social housing community: A photographic investigation. *Addiction Research & Theory* 18, 71–83.

Fraser, S. and Moore, D., 2011. *The Drug Effect: Health, Crime and Society.* Cambridge: Cambridge University Press.

Fraser, S. and Seear, K., 2011. *Making Disease, Making Citizens: The Politics of Hepatitis C.* Farnham: Ashgate.

Friedman, S.R., De Jong, W., Rossi, D., Touze, G., Rockwell, R., Des Jarlais, D.C. and Elovich, R., 2007. Harm reduction theory: Users' culture, micro-social indigenous harm reduction, and the self-organization and outside-organizing of users' groups. *International Journal of Drug Policy* 18, 107–17.

Friedman, S.R., de Jong, W.M. and Des Jarlais, D.C., 1988. Problems and dynamics of organizing intravenous drug users for AIDS prevention. *Health Education Research: Theory and Practice* 3, 49–57.

Frohmann, L., 2005. The Framing Safety Project: Photographs and Narrative by Battered Women. *Violence Against Women* 11, 1396–419.

Fry, C. and Dwyer, R., 2001. For love or money? An exploratory study of why injecting drug users participate in research. *Addiction* 96, 1319–325.

Geertz, C., 1973. *The Interpretation of Culture*. London: Hutchinson.

Giddens, A., 1990. *The Consequences of Modernity*. Polity Press, Cambridge

Giddens, A., 1991. M*odernity and Self Identity: Self and Society in the Late Modern Age*. Cambridge: Policy Press.

Gomez, J.C., Rodriguez, F.R., Navarro, G.M. and CGonzalez, S.M.I., 1998. Accidental contact with syringes used by intravenous drug users (IDU): a decade of study. An Esp Pediatr (*Anales españoles de pediatría*) 49, 375–80.

Grasseni, C., 2004. Video and ethnographic knowledge: Skilled vision in the practice of breeding, in *Working Images: Visual Research and Representation in Ethnography*, edited by S. Pink, L. Kurti and A.I. Afonso. London: Routledge, pp. 15–30.

Green, J. and Thorogood, N., 2004. *Qualitative Methods for Health Research*. London: Sage.

Grund, J.P., 1993. *Drug Use as a Social Ritual. Functionality, Symbolism and Determinants of Self-regulation*. Rotterdam: Instituut voor Verslavingsonderzoek, .

Guba, E.G. and Lincoln, Y.S., 2004. Competing paradigms in qualitative research: theories and issues, in *Approaches to Qualitative Research: A Reader on Theory and Practice*, edited by S.N. Hesse-Biber and P. Leavy. Oxford: Oxford University Press, pp. 17–38.

Haines, R.J., Poland, B.D. and Johnson, J.L., 2009. Becoming a "real" smoker: cultural capital in young women's accounts of smoking and other substance use. *Sociology of Health and Illness* 31, 66–80.

Hammersley, M., 1992. *What's Wrong with Ethnography?* London: Routledge.

Hammersley, M., 1995. *The Politics of Social Research*. London: Sage.

Hammersley, M. and Atkinson, P., 1995. *Ethnography: Principles in Practice*, Second Edition ed. London: Routledge.

Harper, D., 1988. *Visual Sociology: Expanding the Sociological Vision*. The American Sociologist Spring, 54–70.

Hathaway, A., 2006. Harm Reduction, *Drugs and Society*: Volume 2, edited by Anon, Marshall Cavendish, New York, pp. 433–35.

Henley, P., 1998. Film-making and Ethnographic Research, in *Image-based Research*, edited by J. Prosser. London: Falmer Press.

Hertz, R., 1997. *Reflexivity and Voice*. London: Sage.

Hockings, P., 1995. *Principles of Visual Anthropology*, Second ed. Berlin and New York: Mouton de Gruyter, .

HPA, 2012. Shooting Up: Infections among people who inject drugs in the United Kingdom 2011. Health Protection Agency, Health Protection Scotland, Public Health Wales, and Public Health Agency Northern Ireland, London.

Hughes, E.C., 1971 (1989). *The Sociological Eye*. New Brunswick, NJ: Transaction.

Hunt, N., Albert, E. and Sánchez, V.M., 2010. User involvement and user organising in harm reduction, in *Harm Reduction: Evidence, Impacts and Challenges. European Monitoring Centre for Drugs and Drug Addiction*, edited by T., Rhodes and D. Hedrich. Lisbon, pp. 333–56.

Hurworth, R., 2004. The Use of the Visual Medium for Program Evaluation, in *Seeing is Believing? Approaches to Visual Research*, edited by C.J. Pole. Elsevier, Oxford, pp. 163–81.

Hurworth, R. and Sweeney, M., 1995. The use of the visual image in a variety of Australian evaluations. *Evaluation Practice* 16, 153–64.

IFRC, 2003. *Spreading the Light of Science: Guidelines on Harm Reduction Related to Injecting Drug Use*. International Federation of Red Cross and Red Crescent Societies, Geneva.

IHRA, 2010. What is Harm Reduction? A position statement from the International Harm Reduction Association. London: International Harm Reduction Association.

IHRA, 2013. *Global Overview*. London: Harm Reduction International.

Killion, C.M., 2001. Understanding Cultural Aspects of Health Through Photography. *Nursing Outlook* 49, 50–54.

Kincheloe, J.L. and McLaren, P.L., 1994. Rethinking critical theory and qualitative research, in *Handbook of Qualitative Research*, edited by N.K. Denzin and Y.S. Lincoln. London: Sage, pp. 138–57.

Latkin, C.A., Vlahov, D. and Athony, J.C., 1993. Socially desirable responding and self-reported HIV infection risk behaviours among intravenous drug users. *Addiction* 88, 517–26.

Letherby, G., 2003. *Feminist Research in Theory and Practice*. Milton Keynes: Open University Press.

Lewin, K., 1948. *Resolving Social Conflicts*. New York: Harper.

Lidchi, H., 2006. Culture and constraints: further thoughts on ethnography and exhibiting. *International Journal of Heritage Studies* 12, 93–114.

LiPuma, E., 1993. Culture and the Concept of Culture in a Theory of Practice, in *Bourdieu: Critical Perspectives*, edited by C. Calhoun, E. LiPuma and M. Postone. Cambridge: Polity Press, pp. 14–34.

Lloyd, G.E.R., 1996. *Adversaries and Authorities: Investigations into Ancient Greek and Chinese Science*. Cambridge: Cambridge University Press.

Lupton, D. and Tulloch, J., 1999. Theorizing fear of crime: Beyond the rational/irrational opposition. *British Journal of Sociology* 50, 507–23.

MacDonald, D. and Patterson, V., 1991 *A Handbook of Drug Training: Learning about Drugs and Working with Drug Users*. London: Routledge.

Maher, L., 1997. *Sexed Work: Gender, Race, and Resistance in a Brooklyn Drug Market*. Oxford: Oxford University Press.

Malinowski, B., 1932 (1922). Argonauts of the Western Pacific: An Account of Native Enterprise and Adventure in the Archipelagoes of Melanesian New Guinea Second Edition ed. London: Routledge.

Marks, D.F., Murray, M., Evans, B., Willig, C., Woodall, C. and Sykes, C.M., 2005. Health Psychology: *Theory, Research & Practice*, Second Edition. London: Sage.

Mason, J., 2002. *Qualitative Researching*, Second Edition. London: Sage.

May, T., 1997. *Social Research: Issues, Methods and Process*, Second ed. Milton Keynes: Open University Press.

McCann, E.J., 2008. Expertise, truth, and urban policy mobilities: global circuits of knowledge in the development of Vancouver, Canada's 'four pillar' drug strategy. *Environment and Planning A* 40, 885–904.

McDermott, P., 2005. The great Mersey experiment: The birth of harm reduction, in *Heroin Addiction and the British System*: Volume 1, edited by J. Strang and M. Gossop. Abingdon: Routledge, pp. 139–56.

McKeganey, N., 2000. Rapid assessment: Really useful knowledge or an argument for bad science? *International Journal of Drug Policy* 11, 13–18.

McKeganey, N., 2001. To pay or not to pay: Respondents' motivation for participating in research. *Addiction* 96, 1237–8.

McKeganey, N., 2011. *Controversies in Drugs Policy and Practice*. Basingstoke: Palgrave Macmillan.

McKeganey, N. and Barnard, M., 1992. *AIDS, Drugs and Sexual Risk: Lives in the Balance*. Milton Keynes: Open University Press.

McKeganey, N.P., Neale, J., Parkin, S. and Mills, C., 2004. Communities and Drugs: Beyond the Rhetoric of Community Action. *Probation Journal* 51, 343–61.

McKernan, J., 1991. Curriculum Action Research: A Handbook of Methods and Resources for the Reflective Practitioner, Second ed. London: Kogan Page Limited.

Mead, M., 1995. Visual anthropology in a discipline of words, in *Principles of Visual Anthropology*, edited by P. Hockings. Berlin and New York: Mouton de Gruyter, pp. 3–12.

Mihai, A., Damsa, C., Allen, M., Baleydier, B., Lazignac, C. and Heinz, A., 2006. Viewing videotape of themselves while experiencing delirium tremens could reduce the relapse rate in alcohol-dependent patients. *Addiction* 102, 226–31.

Millar, T., 2009. From underground peer needle exchange to professional partnerships – the drug user group experience, National Conference on Injecting Drug Use, Glasgow.

Mills, C.W., 1959/2000. *The Sociological Imagination* (40th Anniversary Edition). Oxford: Oxford University Press.

Moon, R., 2000. *The Language of Photography: The Etymology of Photographic Words*. Source, Belfast.

Morton, C., 2009. Fieldwork and the participant photographer: E.E. Evans-Pritchard and the Neur rite of gorot. *Visual Anthropology* 22, 252–74.

Murray, S.A., Tapson, J., Turnbull, L., McCallum, J. and Little, A., 1994. Listening to local voices: adapting rapid appraisal to assess health and social needs in general practice. *British Medical Journal* 308, 698–700.

Newcombe, R., 1992. The reduction of drug-related harm: A conceptual framework for theory, practice and research, in *The Reduction of Drug Related Harm*, edited by P.A. O'Hare, R. Newcombe, A. Matthews, E.C. Buning and E. Drucker. London: Routledge, pp. 1–14.

Nourse, C.B., Charles, C.A., McKay, M., Keenan, P. and Butler, K.M., 1997. Childhood needlestick injuries in the Dublin metropolitan area. *Irish Medical Journal* 90, 66–9.

Nyiri, P., Leung, T. and Zuckerman, M.A., 2004. Sharps discarded in inner-city parks and playgrounds: Risk of blood borne virus. *Communicable Disease and Public Health* 7, 287–8.

O'Hare, P., 2007. Merseyside, the first harm reduction conferences, and the early history of harm reduction *International Journal of Drug Policy* 18, 141–4.

O'Hare, P.A., 1992. Preface: A note on the concept of harm reduction, in *The Reduction of Drug Related Harm*, edited by P.A. O'Hare, R. Newcombe, A. Matthews, E.C. Buning and E. Drucker. London: Routledge, xiii-xvii.

O'Hare, P.A., Newcombe, R., Matthews, A., Buning, E.C. and Drucker, E., 1992. *The Reduction of Drug-Related Harm*. London: Routledge.

O'Shea, R.S., 2010. Hepatitis C, in *Current Clinical Medicine*, edited by W.M. Carey, Second ed. Philadelphia, PA: Saunders Elsevier, pp. 545–8.

O'Toole, T.P., Aaron, F.D., Chin, M.H., Horowitz, C. and Tyson, F., 2003. Community-based Participatory Research: Opportunities, challenges and the need for a common language. *Journal of General Intern Medicine* 18, 592–4.

Oldrup, H.H. and Carstensen, T.A., 2012. Producing geographic knowledge through visual methods. Geografiska Annaler: Series B, *Human Geography* 94, 223–37.

Oliver, P., 2004. *Writing Your Thesis*. London: Sage.

Ong, B.N., Humphris, G., Annett, H. and Rifkin, S., 1991. Rapid appraisal in an urban setting: an example from the developed world. *Social Science and Medicine* 32, 909–15.

Pain, H., 2011. Visual methods in practice and research: A review of empirical support. *International Journal of Therapy and Rehabilitation* 18, 343–49.

Pain, H., 2012. A literature review to evaluate the choice and use of visual methods. *International Journal of Qualitative Methods* 11.

Parker, H., Bakx, K. and Newcombe, R., 1988. *Living with Heroin*. Milton Keynes: Open University Press.

Parkin, S., 1996. The Bede Centre: White Elephant or Phoenix Rising? Department of Primary Health Care, University of Newcastle, Newcastle.

Parkin, S., 2008. Visual Methods within the Addictions: The Pulp-Fictionalisation of Reality TV?, in *Proceedings of the Plymouth Post-Graduate Symposium*

2007, edited by A. Barton, J. Lean, M. Williams, and M. Wright. University of Plymouth, Plymouth, pp. 139–47 ISBN 1753–7053 (Print).

Parkin, S., 2009a. *The Effects of Place on Health Risk: A Qualitative Study of Micro-injecting Environments* (Unpublished PhD Thesis), Faculty of Health. University of Plymouth, Plymouth.

Parkin, S., 2009b. Places of Risk, Places of Harm: Visualising Public Injecting Drug Use in Plymouth, South West Hepatology Nurses' Group Meeting, Exeter, Buckerell Lodge.

Parkin, S., 2009c. Public Injecting Drug Use and Applied Visual Research: Design, Collaborative-Implementation and Outcome, First International Conference on Visual Methods, University of Leeds.

Parkin, S., 2009d. Visual Research Methods and Public Injecting Drug Use: Making the Invisible Visible, 20th International Harm Reduction Association Annual Conference, Queen's Park Hotel, Bangkok, Thailand.

Parkin, S., 2010a. The Effects of Place on Health (and Drug Related Death) Risk: Findings from a Qualitative Study of Public Injecting Drug Use in Plymouth, South West Drug Related Death Conference, Buckfast Abbey, Buckfastleigh, Devon.

Parkin, S., 2010b. Risk, Harm and Opportunities for Blood Borne Virus Transmission in Public Settings: Findings from a Qualitative Study of Injecting Drug Use in Plymouth (UK), British Association for the Study of the Liver: Nurses Forum, Royal College of Physicians, Edinburgh.

Parkin, S., 2011. Identifying and Predicting Drug-Related Harm with Applied Qualitative Research, in *Adult Lives: A Life Course Perspective*, edited by J. Katz and S. Peace. Bristol: Policy Press.

Parkin, S., 2012. *Frontline: A Photo-ethnography of Drug Using Environments* (Exhibition Brochure). University of Huddersfield, Huddersfield.

Parkin, S., 2013 *Habitus and Drug Using Environments: Health, Place and Lived-Experience*. Farnham: Ashgate Publishing.

Parkin, S., 2013b. Frontline: A photo-ethnography of drug using environments, Harm Reduction International, Vilnius, Lithuania.

Parkin, S., Bingham, T. and Bingham, A., 2013. 7x7 (7 Hits, 7 Days a Week). A short film about street-based injecting. (Collaborative Video Production by Parkin, S. (University of Huddersfield) and Bingham, T. (Irish Needle Exchange Forum, Republic of Ireland).

Parkin, S. and Coomber, R., 2009a. Public Injecting and Symbolic Violence. *Addiction Research and Theory* 17, 390–405.

Parkin, S. and Coomber, R., 2009b. Value in the Visual: On Public Injecting, Visual Methods and their Potential for Informing Policy (and Change). *Methodological Innovation Online* 4, 21–36.

Parkin, S. and Coomber, R., 2010. Fluorescent Blue Lights, Injecting Drug Use and Related Health Risk: Findings from a Qualitative Study of Micro-Injecting Environments. *Health and Place* 16, 629–37.

Parkin, S. and Coomber, R., 2011. Public Injecting Drug Use and the Social Production of Harmful Practice in High-Rise Tower Blocks (London, UK): A Lefebvrian Analysis. *Health and Place* 17, 717–26.

Parkin, S., Coomber, R. and Wallace, G., 2010. *Going Public, Drink and Drug News*. London, pp. 14–15.

Parkin, S. and Kaner, E., 1996. Substance Misuse in Blyth: Agency Interventions and Client Aspirations. Department of Primary Health Care, University of Newcastle, Newcastle.

Parkin, S. and McKeganey, N., 2000. The Rise and Rise of Peer Education Approaches. *Drugs: Education, Prevention and Policy* 7, 293–310.

Parkin, S. and McKenna, C., 1997. The Sex Industry in Lanarkshire and Related Needs of Female Sex Workers. Centre for Drug Misuse Research, University of Glasgow, Glasgow.

Pates, R., McBride, A. and Arnold, K., 2005. *Injecting Illicit Drugs*. Oxford: Blackwell Publishing (Addiction Press).

Pates, R. and Riley, D., 2012. *Harm Reduction in Substance Use and High-risk Behaviour: International Policy and Practice*. Oxford: Blackwell.

Pearson, G., 1987. *The New Heroin Users*. Oxford: Blackwell.

Pearson, G., 1992. Drugs and criminal justice: A harm reduction perspective, in *The Reduction of Drug Related Harm*, edited by P.A. O'Hare, R. Newcombe, A. Matthews, E.C. Buning and E. Drucker. London: Routledge, pp. 15–29.

Pearson, G., 2009. The researcher as hooligan: Where 'participant' observation means breaking the law. *International Journal of Social Research Methodology* 12, 243–55.

Pearson, M., Parkin, S. and Coomber, R., 2011. Generalizing applied qualitative research on harm reduction: the example of a public injecting typology. *Contemporary Drug Problems* 38, 61–91.

Philipp, R., 1993. Community needlestick accident data and trends in environmental quality. *Public Health* 107, 363–9.

Pike, K.L., 1954. Language in relation to a unified theory of the structure of human behavior. Summer Institute of Linguistics, Glendale, CA.

Pink, S., 2004a. *Home Truths. Gender, Domestic Objects and Everyday Life*. Berg, Oxford.

Pink, S., 2004b. Performance, Self-Representation and Narrative: Interviewing with Video., in *Seeing is Believing? Approaches to Visual Research*, edited by C.J. Pole. Elsevier, Oxford, pp. 61–78.

Pink, S., 2007a. Applied Visual Anthropology: Social Intervention and Visual Methodologies, *Visual Interventions: Applied Visual Anthropology*, edited by S. Pink. New York: Berghahn Books, pp. 3–28.

Pink, S., 2007b. Doing Visual Ethnography, Second Edition ed. London: Sage.

Pink, S., 2007c. *Visual Interventions: Applied Visual Anthropology*. New York: Berghahn Books.

Pink, S., 2007d. Walking with Video. *Visual Studies* 22, 240–52.

Pink, S., 2008. *Mobilising Visual Ethnography: Making Routes, Making Place and Making Images.* Forum Qualitative Sozialforschung/Forum: *Qualitative Social Research* 9.
Pink, S., 2009. *Doing Sensory Ethnography.* London: Sage.
Pink, S., 2011. Images, Senses and Applications: Engaging Visual Anthropology. *Visual Anthropology* 24, 437–54.
Pole, C.J., 2004. Visual Research: Potential and Overview, in *Seeing is Believing? Approaches to Visual Research*, edited by C.J. Pole. Oxford: Elsevier, pp. 1–8.
Prosser, J., 1998. *Image-based Research: A Sourcebook for Qualitative Researchers.* Abingdon: Routledge.
Prosser, J. and Loxley, A., 2008. *Introducing Visual Methods.* Economic and Social Research Council (National Centre for Research Methods).
Prosser, J. and Schwartz, D., 2004. Photographs within the sociological research process, in *Approaches to Qualitative Research: A Reader on Theory and Practice*, edited by S.N. Hesse-Biber and P. Leavy. Oxford: Oxford University Press, pp. 334–49.
Quine, S. and Taylor, R., 1998. Methodological Strategies, in *Handbook of Public Health Methods*, edited by C., Kerr, R. Taylor and G. Heard. Sydney: McGraw-Hill, pp. 17–23.
Ranard, J., 2002. A little less shock and more therapy. *International Journal of Drug Policy* 13, 355–67.
Rapoport, R.N., 1970. Three dilemmas in action research. *Human Relations* 23, 499–513.
RCP, 2000. Drugs: Dilemmas and Choices. Royal College of Physicians Gaskell, London.
Reavey, P., 2011. *Visual Methods in Psychology: Using and Interpreting Images in Qualitative Research.* Abingdon: Routledge.
Rhodes, T., Briggs, D., Holloway, G., Jones, S. and Kimber, J., 2006. Visual Assessments of Injecting Drug Use: A Pilot Study. National Treatment Agency for Substance Misuse, Centre for Research on Drugs and Health Behaviour Imperial College London.
Rhodes, T., Fitch, C., Stimson, G.V. and Kumar, M.S., 2000. Rapid assessment in the drugs field. *International Journal of Drug Policy* 11, 1–11.
Rhodes, T. and Fitzgerald, J., 2006. Visual data in addictions research: Seeing comes before words? *Addiction Research and Theory* 14, 349–63.
Rhodes, T. and Hedrich, D., 2010. *Harm Reduction: Evidence, Impacts and Challenges.* European Monitoring Centre for Drugs and Drug Addiction, Lisbon.
Rhodes, T. and Treloar, C., 2008. The social production of hepatitis C risk among injecting drug users: a qualitative synthesis. *Addiction* 103, 1593–603.
Rhodes, T., Watts, L., Davies, S., Martin, A., Smith, J., Clark, D., Craine, N. and Lyons, M., 2007. Risk, shame and the public injector: a qualitative study of drug injecting in South Wales. *Social Science and Medicine* 65, 572–85.

Rhodes, T., Zikic, B., Prodanovic, A., Kuneski, E. and Bernays, S., 2008. Hygiene and uncertainty in qualitative accounts of hepatitis C transmission among drug injectors in Serbia. *Social Science and Medicine* 66, 1437–47.

Riley, D., Pates, R., Monaghan, G. and O'Hare, P.A., 2012. A brief history of harm reduction, *Harm Reduction in Substance Use and High-risk Behaviour: International Policy and Practice*, edited by R. Pates and D. Riley. Oxford: Blackwell.

Ritchie, J. and Lewis, J., 2003. *Qualitative Research Practice: A Guide for Social Science Students and Researchers*. London: Sage.

Roberts, M., 2013. *The Public Health Reforms: What they mean for Drug and Alcohol Services*. London: Drugscope.

Robertson, R., 1990. The Edinburgh Epidemic: A Case Study, in *AIDS and Drug Misuse: The Challenge for Policy and Practice in the 1990s*, edited by J. Strang and G.V. Stimson. London: Routledge, pp. 95–107.

Robinson, D.E., 1976. Fashions in shaving and trimming of the beard: the men of the Illustrated London News 1842–1972. *American Journal of Sociology* 81, 1133–41.

Robson, P., 2011. *Real World Research*, Third ed. Chichester: John Wiley & Sons.

Rodman, M.C., 2003. Empowering Place: Multilocality and Multivocality, in *The Anthropology of Space and Place: Locating Culture*, edited by S.M. Low, D. Lawrence-Zuniga. Oxford: Blackwell, pp. 204–23.

Rose, G., 2001. *Visual Methodologies. An Introduction to the Interpretation of Visual Materials*. London: Sage.

Rose, G., 2003. On the need to ask how, exactly, is geography 'visual'? *Antipode* 35, 212–21.

Russell, F.M. and Nash, M.C., 2002. A prospective study of children with community-acquired needlestick injuries in Melbourne. *Journal of Paediatric Child Health* 38, 321–23.

Saldana, J., 2009. *The Coding Manual for Qualitative Researchers*. Sage: London.

Sayer, A., 2000. *Realism and Social Science*. London: Sage.

Schatz, E. and Nougier, M., 2012. *Drug Consumption Rooms: Evidence and Practice*. International Drug Policy Consortium.

Schembri, S. and Boyle, M.V., 2013. Visual ethnography: achieving rigorous and authentic interpretations. *Journal of Business Research* 66(9), 1251–4.

Scheper-Hughes, N., 1995. The primacy of the ethical: propositions for a militant anthropology. *Current Anthropology* 36, 409–40.

Scherer, J.C., 1995. Ethnographic photography in anthropological research, *Principles of Visual Anthropology*, edited by P. Hockings. Berlin-New York: Mouton de Gruyter, pp. 201–16.

Schonberg, J. and Bourgois, P., 2002. The politics of photographic aesthetics: critically documenting the HIV epidemic among heroin injectors in Russia and the United States. International *Journal of Drug Policy* 13, 387–92.

Schostak, J. and Schostak, J., 2008. *Radical Research: Designing, Developing and Writing Research to Make a Difference*. Abingdon: Routledge.

Schwandt, T.A., 1994. Constructivist, Interpretivist Approaches to Human Inquiry, in *Handbook of Qualitative Research*, edited by N.K. Denzin and Y.S. Lincoln. London: Sage, pp. 118–37.
Schwartz, D., 1989. Visual Ethnography: Using Photography in Qualitative Research. *Qualitative Sociology* 12, 119–54.
Schwartz, D., 1997. *Contesting the Superbowl*. London: Routledge.
Scott, J., 2005. Pharmaceutical aspects of injecting, in *Injecting Illicit Drugs*, edited by R. Partes, A. McBride and K. Arnold. Oxford: Blackwell Publishing (Addiction Press), pp. 33–46.
Seddon, T., 2005. Paying drug users to take part in research: Justice, human rights and business perspectives on the use of incentive payments. *Addiction Research and Theory* 13, 101–9.
Sheridan, J., 2005. Needle Exchange in Britain, in *Heroin Addiction and the British System*: Volume 2. London: Routledge, pp. 145–55.
Silverman, D., 2006. *Interpreting Qualitative Data: Methods for Analyzing Talk, Text and Interaction*. London: Sage.
Simmonds, L. and Comber, R., 2009. Injecting drug users: A stigmatised and stigmatising population. *International Journal of Drug Policy* 20, 121–30.
Singer, S., Simmons, J., Duke, M. and Broomhall, L., 2001. The challenges of street research on drug use, violence and AIDS risk. *Addiction Research and Theory* 9, 365–402.
Single, E., 1995. Defining harm reduction. *Drug and Alcohol Review* 14, 287–90.
Smith, C.B.R., 2012. Harm reduction as anarchist practice: A user's guide to capitalism and addiction in North America. *Critical Public Health* 22, 209–21.
Sohn, J.W., Kim, B.G., Kim, S.H. and Han, C., 2006. Mental health of healthcare workers who experience needlestick and sharps injuries. *Journal of Occupational Health* 48, 474–9.
Southall, M., 2009. Deploying peer-based needle exchange as an integral part of harm reduction services: a drug service manager's view, National Conference on Injecting Drug Use, Glasgow.
Stanley, L. and Wise, S., 1993. *Breaking Out Again Feminist Ontology and Epistemology*. London: Routledge.
Stimson, G.V., 1992. Public health and health behaviour in the prevention of HIV infection, in *The Reduction of Drug Related Harm*, edited by P.A. O'Hare, R. Newcombe, A. Matthews, E.C. Buning and E. Drucker.. London: Routledge, pp. 39–48.
Stimson, G.V., 2007. Harm reduction – coming of age: A local movement with global impact. *International Journal of Drug Policy* 18, 67–9.
Stimson, G.V., Alldritt, L., Dolan, K. and Donoghoe, M., 1988. Syringe exchange schemes for drug users in England and Scotland. *British Medical Journal* 296 1717–19.
Stimson, G.V., Fitch, C. and Rhodes, T., 1998. The Rapid Assessment and Response Guide on Injecting Drug Use, World Health Organization – Programme on

Substance Abuse. The Centre for Research on Drugs and Health Behaviour, London.
Strang, J. and Gossop, M., 2005a. The 'British System' of drug policy: Extraordinary individual freedom, but to what end?, in *Heroin Addiction and the British System: Volume 2: Treatment and Policy Responses*, edited by J. Strang and M.. Gossop. Abingdon: Routledge, pp. 206–19.
Strang, J. and Gossop, M., 2005b. *Heroin Addiction and the British System: Volume 2: Treatment and Policy Responses*. Abingdon: Routledge.
Strang, J., Griffiths, P. and Gossop, M., 2005. Different types of heroin in the UK: what significance and what relationship to different routes of administration, *Heroin Addiction and the British System: Volume 1 Origins and Evolution*, edited by J. Strang and M. Gossop. Abingdon: Routledge, pp. 157–69.
Suchar, C.S., 1997. Grounding Visual Sociology Research in Shooting Scripts. *Qualitative Sociology* 20, 33–55.
Sutton, R.M. and Farrall, S., 2005. Gender, Socially Desirable Responding and the Fear of Crime. *British Journal of Criminology* 45, 212–24.
Swartz, D., 1997. *Culture and Power: The Sociology of Pierre Bourdieu*. Chicago, IL: University of Chicago Press.
Taylor, A., 1993. *Women Drug Users: An Ethnography of a Female Injecting Community*. Oxford: Clarendon Press.
Taylor, A., Fleming, A., Rutherford, J., Goldberg, D., 2004. *Examining the Injecting Practices of Injecting Drug Users in Scotland*. Effective Interventions Unit, Scottish Office, Edinburgh.
Tempalski, B., Flom, P.L., Friedman, S.R., Des Jarlais, D., Friedman, J.J., McKnight, C. and Friedman, R., 2007. Social and Political Factors Predicting the Presence of Syringe Exchange Programs in 96 US Metropolitan Areas. *American Journal of Public Health* 97, 437–47.
Thompson, S.C., Boughton, C.R. and Dore, G.J., 2003. Blood-borne viruses and their survival in the environment: is public concern about community needlestick exposures justified? *Australian and New Zealand Journal of Public Health* 27, 602–7.
Treloar, C., Laybutt, B., Jauncey, M., van Beek, I., Lodge, M., Malpas, G. and Carruthers, S., 2008. Broadening discussions of 'safe' in hepatitis C prevention: a close-up of swabbing in an analysis of video recordings of injecting practice. *International Journal of Drug Policy* 19, 59–65.
VSSG-BSA, 2006. Statement of Ethical Practice for the British Sociological Association – Visual Sociology Group. British Sociological Association BSA – Visual Sociology Statement of Ethical Practice – October 2006.
Wacquant, L., 2004. *Body and Soul: Notebooks of an Apprentice Boxer*. Oxford: Oxford University Press.
Wacquant, L., 2005. Carnal Connections: On embodiment, Apprenticeship and Membership. *Qualitative Sociology* 28, 445–74.
Wacquant, L., 2008. Pierre Bourdieu, in *Key Sociological Thinkers*, Second ed., edited by R. Stones. Basingstoke: Palgrave Macmillan, pp. 261–77.

Wagner, J., 2001. Does Image-based Fieldwork Have More to Gain from Extending or Rejecting Scientific Realism?. *Visual Sociology* 16, 7–21.

Waldorf, D. and Reinarman, C., 1975. Addicts – Everything but Human Beings. *Journal of Contemporary Ethnography* 4, 30–53.

Walker, J., Thompson, C., Wilson, G., Laing, K., Coombes, M. and Raybould, S., 2011. *Family Group Conferencing in Youth Inclusion and Support Panels: Empowering Families and Preventing Crime and Antisocial Behaviour*? Youth Justice Board, London.

Wang, C.C., 1999. Photovoice: A Participatory Action Research Strategy Applied to Women's Health. *Journal of Women's Health* 8, 185–92.

Watson, J.D., 1999. *The Double Helix: A Personal Account of the Discovery of the Structure of DNA*. 2nd Revised ed. London: Penguin.

Webb, J., Schirato, T., Danaher, G., 2002. *Understanding Bourdieu*. London: Sage.

WHO, 2005. *Status Paper on Prisons, Drugs and Harm Reduction*. Copenhagen: World Health Organisation.

Williams, H. and Norman, M., 2005. Safer injecting: individual harm reduction advice, in *Injecting Illicit Drugs*, edited by R. Partes, A. McBride and K. Arnold. Oxford: Blackwell Publishing (Addiction Press), pp. 135–59.

Williams, T., Dunlap, E., Johnson, B. and Ansley, H., 1992. Personal safety in dangerous places. *Journal of Contemporary Ethnography* 21, 343–74.

Willig, C., 2011. Foreward, in *Visual Methods in Psychology: Using and Interpreting Images in Qualitative Research*, edited by P. Reavey. Abingdon: Routledge, xxv-xxvi.

Winn, P., 2009. Thailand's front page horror show. http://www.globalpost.com/dispatch/thailand/090511/thailands-front-page-horror-show.

Wodak, A. and McLeod, L., 2008. The role of harm reduction in controlling HIV among injecting drug users. AIDS. *Supplement* 2, S81–92.

Wyatt, J.P., Robertson, C.E. and Scobie, W.G., 1994. Out of hospital needlestick injuries. *Archives of Disease in Childhood* 70, 245–6.

Young, L. and Barrett, H., 2001. Adapting visual methods: Action research with Kampala street children. *Area* 33, 141–52.

Zinberg, N.E., 1984. *Drug, Set and Setting. The Basis for Controlled Intoxicant Use*. London: Yale University Press.

Appendix I
A Harm Reduction Response to Media Reports of Needlestick Injury/Drug Related Litter

In March 2013, Laurence Alvis of UnitingCare ReGen, (the lead alcohol and other drug treatment and education agency of UnitingCare Victoria & Tasmania), wrote an open letter to members of a local community following an account of needlestick injury (involving a young child) that had been reported in a local newspaper (*The Sunbury Leader*, 26th March 2013). The letter was written in order to avoid hysterical, 'kneejerk' and stigmatising responses by local authorities and officials in matters relating to street-based injecting.

The following 'harm reduction response' has been inspired by UnitingCare ReGen's proactive response to negative media reports of needles/syringes in community settings. The following 'letter' provides *a template* for similar action by relevant bodies based in the UK (harm reduction agencies, drug and alcohol workers, drug users).

Where the letter has (brackets), individuals/correspondents using the template should insert the details relevant to their particular geographical location.

The author advises and recommends using this letter as a template (adapt as required) to respond to press reports that seek to diminish and devalue the role of harm reduction in community settings and/or seek to over-sensationalise accounts of discarded paraphernalia in community spaces.

Dear (Journalist/Editor/Newspaper)

I am writing to you in connection with the recent story in your newspaper (online/print) regarding the incidence of (drug related litter/needlestick injury) in (name of town/area).

Although it is entirely natural for people to fear the consequences of needlestick injury (particularly in public spaces in community settings), the actual risk of *serious* harm to public/individual health from these types of injuries is relatively low. It is also important to emphasise that the epidemiological risk of contracting hepatitis C or HIV from these injuries is also very low (and no known incidence of serious blood borne infection from this form of injury exists in the research literature). Although I am not stating that there is completely 'no risk' of viral infection, you (as a broadcaster of information for public consumption) should be aware that research from the UK defined this 'low risk' as:

'the odds of sero-conversion following community acquired needlestick injury 'where the source is unknown but assumed to be an IDU [injecting drug user], is 12–31 per cent for HBV, 1.62 per cent for HCV and 0.003–0.05% for HIV' (Blenkharn 2008, 727). As such, there is perhaps only limited rationality in fear associated with virally contaminated needle/syringes in community settings' (Parkin and Coomber 2011, 1219)

All injuries involving sharp objects should be taken seriously (including blades, glass, razors and needles)and receive appropriate medical treatment. Injuries caused by needles however should not be a cause for panic or as a reason to mobilise discriminatory responses against people who inject drugs. The research shows that the chances of contracting a blood-borne virus like HIV or Hepatitis B or C from a used needle discarded inappropriately in community settings are minimal, as these viruses can only survive for a short time outside of the body. (That is why they are termed 'blood borne viruses'; because they need 'blood contact' to stay alive). As with any puncture wound there would also be a low level risk of tetanus, but this can be remedied by arranging a booster shot at a local Emergency Room or community GP.

Needles and syringes are distributed each year to members of the public through the UK's network of Needle and Syringe Programs (NSP), including the program run by (name of centralised agency) in (name of town/city/region/local authority) in your news story. NSP are regarded as an important part of public health policy in the UK and have been influential in reducing drug (and sex) related harms since their introduction to the UK in the mid-1980s. These programs are a key part of assisting people with drug problems and assisting them towards recovery from drug dependency.

People who discard <u>any form of litter</u> are acting irresponsibly, especially when there is a social expectation that people will manage their 'rubbish' in a responsible manner. This is especially so when littering involves cigarette butts, chewing gum, glass, sharp items, dog faeces and needles attached to syringes. While the story contained within your newspaper involved sharp items discarded by (one/two) individual(s), the specific actions of (this/these) individual(s) should not be regarded as sufficient evidence to support the moral outrage aimed at injecting drug users (inferred/noted) in your news story.

The stigmatisation and discrimination of people who inject drugs in our community is not a helpful response to difficult and challenging problems surrounding their drug dependency. Newspaper articles such as yours (date/title) may only influence negative responses towards people who may be vulnerable and in need of assistance. Accounts such as that in your paper may only push these people further away from seeking help with drug dependency and exacerbate their related health and social problems.

If you do have to report on such issues, a better approach may be to write an article that emphasises the need for parents/teachers/children to provide some form of awareness and training on the harms attached to handling sharp items, dog faeces, broken glass, barbed wire etc. For communities to respond positively to community issues, there is perhaps an equal moral responsibility for broadcasters such as yourself to provide the appropriate awareness needed for more positive action (and not promote fear and loathing that is directed towards already vulnerable people).

I look forward to your response,

Yours
(Name)

Reference

Blenkharn, J.I., 2008. Clinical wastes in the community: local authority management of discarded drug litter. *Public Health* 122, 725–28.

Parkin S, and Coomber R. 2011. Injecting drug user views (and experiences) of drug-related litter bins in public places: A comparative study of qualitative research findings obtained from UK settings. *Health & Place,* 17, 1218–27.

LETTER ENDS

Appendix II
Frontline: A Photo-Ethnography of Drug-Using Environments

Evaluation of Exhibition Photographs

Stephen Parkin (University of Huddersfield) is conducting an evaluation of the effectiveness and value of the drug-related photography used in the *Frontline* exhibition.

This evaluation aims to consider the relevance such images may (or may not) have in raising awareness of drug-related issues amongst professional and non-professional audiences. In short, the evaluation seeks to determine if such photographs are helpful or unhelpful in providing understandings of public health issues.

Presented below are a series of questions relating to the images used in the exhibition. Please consider each theme below and answer in terms of <u>*relevance*</u> to your line of employment/studies.

Your Job Title: _____

1. Overall, I found the *Frontline* exhibition photographs: (please circle)

    Useful   No Opinion   Useless

    Why?

2. Overall, I found the *Frontline* exhibition photographs: (please circle)

    Meaningful   No Opinion   Meaningless

    Why?

3. Do the photographs inform your profession/practice/ studies in any way? (please circle)

    Yes   Not Sure   No

    If Yes: how do they inform your work?

4. Do the photographs reveal anything about drug-using environments of which you were not already aware? (please circle)

   Yes   Not Sure   No

   If Yes: what do they reveal?

5. Do the images provide a better *understanding* of drug-using environments? (please circle)
   Yes   Not Sure   No

   Why (or why not)?

6. From the perspective of *your* profession (or studies), could these images inform responses to drug-related harm?
   Yes   Not Sure   No

   Why (or why not)?

7. Do the photographs provide a better *understanding* of social/environmental situations concerning blood-borne virus transmission? (please circle)

   Yes   Not Sure   No

   Why (or why not)?

Thank you for completing this evaluation.

Further details of any aspect of the *Frontline* Exhibition and this evaluation can be obtained from:

Dr. Stephen Parkin
Human and Health Research Building
School of Health and Human Sciences
University of Huddersfield
HD1 3DH

Index

A priori nodes 97, 103
'Academic community' 31
Academic paradigm 32
Academic research 7, 33, 133, 239
Academic sociology 60, 244
Academic visual anthropology 243
Academic visual methods 246
Action research 240–43, 260
'Activist science' 69
Advisory Council on the Misuse of Drugs 35–6
Analysis 93
Anonymity 29
Anthropology 21
Applied research 7, 20, 33, 69, 239
Applied sociology 60, 239, 244
Applied value 93, 217, 226
Applied visual anthropology 240–43
Applied visual data 219, 221
Applied visual methods 41
　rationale 251
Applied visual research 20, 60
Applied visual sociology 8, 29, 31–3, 93, 134, 173, 192, 217, 219–2, 237, 245
　defined 239–40
　outcomes 252–3
　rationale 246
ATLAS 96
Axial coding 99, 103

Balinese Character 22
Baseline analytics 94
Beards 18
'Blue lights' 113, 120
Bourdieu, P. 8, 13, 30, 33, 70, 95, 97, 100, 104, 249
'British System' 37

'Cambridge model' 199
Cash for questions 89
China 26
Codes 97
Coding frame 96
Coding Manual for Qualitative Researchers 99
Comfort letter 90
Community based research 240–43
Concealment 110
Conference papers 221
Confidentiality 29–30
Confucian philosophy 27
Confucianism 27
Consent 29, 31
Constructivism 10
Content analysis 18
Continuum of descending safety 101, 104–5, 110, 133, 182, 222, 249, 253, 258
　visualised 120
　control 111
　defined 111
Controlled environments 111–13, 118, 222, 253
　harm 115
Converging epistemology 69
Covert researcher 30
Covert visual methods 30
'Crack house' 76
'Critical distance' 16
Critical research 68
Critical theory 10
'Cultural brokerage' 251
Cultural relativism 26–7
　of suffering 27
　perspective 26

Data coding 96
Department for Food and Rural Affairs (DEFRA) 175–8, 190–91, 197, 199, 216, 257

recommendations 176, 191–2
Disciplinary visuality 9, 20, 23, 32, 240
'Discipline of words' 21
Drug related litter 54, 78, 80, 108, 173, 225
    ambiguous signage 212
    Blood borne virus 141–2
    clearance 177
    colliding perspectives 162
    community settings 140
    conflict 137
    content analysis 137
    continuum of descending safety 142
    controlled environments 186
    'dangerous bodies' 135
    epidemiological perspectives 142
    equipment 180
    facilitative space 162
    fear 135
    formal responses 180
    harm reduction 139, 206
    harmful 143, 147
    harmless 143
    hepatitis 141–2
    hidden harm 143, 154
    HIV 141–2
    indigenous discarding 158
    informal responses 180, 184
    malicious discarding 154, 162
    management 175, 178, 227
    massed harm 143, 151–2
    media reportage 137
    personal protective equipment (PPE) 177, 180, 185, 187
    politics of 139, 256
    'reflexive modernity' 138
    'risk society' 138
    Semi Controlled Environments 138, 147, 151–2, 161, 182, 186
    semi formal responses 182
    shaping space 168
    'snapping and dropping' 159–61
    social desirability responses 158
    'social threat' 135
    sociological perspectives 142
    symbolic associations 140
    training 180
    uncontrolled environments 138, 147, 186

Drug related litter bins 190–206
    politics of 190
Drug related relapse 91

Embodiment 247
Emic perspective 16, 20, 87, 104, 258
'Enabling environments' 258
Encampments 15
ENCAMS 190–91
EndNote 96
'Environmental liminality' 120
Environmental visual assessment (EVA) 74–9, 85–6, 91, 110
Epistemological orientation 237
Epistemological quantification 19
Epistemological stance 66
'Epistemological vigilance' 70
Epistemology 11, 66
Ethical approval 91
Ethical code of conduct 88
Ethnographic
    access 24
    method 24
    methodology 24
    observation 75, 84
    photographs 24
    research 14
Ethnography 71
Etic perspective 16, 20, 79, 104
Evaluation findings 226
Evaluation of visual data 225–37, 254
'Expository discourse' 25

Facial hair 18–19
Facilitative space 162
Family group conferences 17
Fear 175–6
Field-related concerns 88
First cycle analysis 97, 103–4
Focused coding 102
Forensic resource 255
Free node 97
Frontline: A Photo-ethnography of Drug Using Environments 8, 49, 223, 258–9

Generalisations 10
'Generative mechanisms' 63

Geography 21
Grassroots activism 38, 40, 243
Grassroots radicalism 40
Grounded theory 104

Habitus 249–50
Habitus and Drug Using Environments 8, 49, 60, 62, 91, 93–4, 249
Handbook of Drug Training 46
Harm reduction 7
  advocacy 68
  antithesis of 133
  control 111
  defined 34
  descending safety 121
  drug related litter 225
  global scale 47
  homelessness 224
  human rights 43
  humanism 44
  intervention 45
  origins 37
  outcomes 253–4
  practice 44
  pragmatism 44
  principles 42
  in UK 39
  visualising 7
Hepatitis 141–2, 222
HIV/AIDS 141–2, 245

'Ideological renegades' 39
'Illusio' 249
Illustrated London News 18
In vivo nodes 97
Incentives 89
INEF 259
Injecting environments 107
  environmental features 107
  typology 107
Injecting Illicit Drugs 50
Injecting paraphernalia 51, 143, 172
International Journal of Drug Policy 41
Interpretation 24, 28
Interpretivism 10
Interview procedure 83
Irish Needle Exchange Forum 259

Junkie Union 38
JunkieBonden 38–9

Knowledge-Action-Change 240

'Learning-by-doing' 87, 247, 249

Marginality 110
'Mental institution' 19
Mersey Drugs Journal 40
Merseyside 39
Methadone leakage 245
Method 75
Methodological orientation 248
Methodology 60, 63
Methods 60, 65, 133
Motivations 114, 116, 118
Moustache 18

'Naming and shaming' ritual 26
National Drug Strategy 77, 176, 258
Needle and syringe identification 53
Needle syringe exchange 39–40
Needle syringe programme (NSP) 40, 45, 47, 53, 80–81, 84
Negotiating access 76
Nodes 97
Numeric quotes 14
Nvivo 94, 96–7

Observant-participation 15, 87, 247
Ontology 11
  perspective 11
  positioning 63
Opioid substitution therapy (OST) 37, 45
Opportunistic contact 81
Overt visual methods 30

Participant-observation 15
Pattern coding 99, 101
Photo-elicitation 16
Photographs
  blood borne virus transmission 233–4
  helpfulness 230–31
  impact 229–31
  informative 229–30
  informing responses to harm 234–5
  revelatory impact 231

understanding drug using environments 230–33
lexicon 89
Photovoice 17
Placed-based cravings 91
Polysemic image 13, 24, 27–8, 32, 255
Positivism 10
'Postmodern turn' 20
Proactive pedagogy 260
Psychology 21
Public injecting habitus 66, 249
Purpose statement 62, 68

'Qualitative autopsy' 100
Qualitative Data Analysis with Nvivo 93
Qualitative research 10, 70
Question threat 81–2

Rapid appraisal 73
Real world research 219–20, 236, 239, 249
Realism 63
Realist ontology 64
Recovery 45, 47, 91, 258
Recreational drug use 245
Recreations of injecting episodes 86
Reflexivity 70
Relapse 91
Research design 32, 70
Research Ethics Committees 29, 43, 76, 91
Research paradigms 10
Researcher generated visual data 13
Respondent generated visual data 16
Righteous Dopefiend 15, 22, 27–8
Rolleston Report 37
Rotterdam JunkieBonden (RJB) 38

Safer injecting drug use 49
Safer toilet design 199
Secondary cycle analysis 99, 104
Semi controlled environments 112, 113, 115–16, 118, 207, 222, 253
harm 119
Semi referral 81
Semi structured interview 75, 80–81, 87
Serial triangulation 71, 72, 74, 248
Sex work 25, 29, 46, 80, 89, 106, 147, 236
Sex workers 25–6, 85, 106, 245

Shaping space 168
'Shooting gallery' 76, 151
'Shooting scripts' 79
'Site of production' 25
'Skilled vision' 87, 247, 249
Socially desirable responses 84
'Sociological sight' 79
Sociology 22–3, 28, 32, 68, 239, 244
Socratic philosophy 27
Stigma 26, 28, 82
Structure/Agency 10, 19, 249
Surveillance 30

Tackling Drug Related Litter 175–8, 197, 216, 257
The Reduction of Drug Related Harm 46
The Safer Injecting Briefing 50, 95, 111
Theoretical coding 99, 103
'Theorised subjectivity' 70
'Thick description' 70
'Thicker description' 85, 105
'Transformative intellectual' 69
Tree node 97
Tripartite research 78

Uncontrolled environments 112, 117–19, 207, 222, 253

Values of Harm Reduction 41
Verbal informed consent 83
Verbatim quotes 14
Visual analysis 18
    secondary sources 18
Visual data 66, 85, 105, 216
    academic 221
    as forensic resource 173
Visual ethnography 14, 89
Visual impact 225
Visual Interventions 244
Visual Methodologies 22
Visual methodology 12
    function 12
    purpose 12
    rationale 12
    realism 64
Visual methods 7, 60, 71, 90, 93, 221, 244, 247
    as 'bridge' 241

synthesis 244
Visual quotes 14
Visual research 7, 21, 60, 85, 88, 91
   ethics 28, 32
Visual Sociology 23
Visual sociology 22, 28, 79

Visual Studies 23
Visually informed pedagogy 253
'Voyeuristic pornography' 22

Written informed consent 83